No Place for Dy

No Place for Dying

Hospitals and the Ideology of Rescue

Helen Stanton Chapple

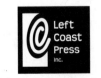

Walnut Creek, California

Left Coast Press is committed to preserving ancient forests and natural resources. We elected to print this title on 30% post consumer recycled paper, processed chlorine free. As a result, for this printing, we have saved:

4 Trees (40' tall and 6-8" diameter)
1 Million BTUs of Total Energy
370 Pounds of Greenhouse Gases
1,781 Gallons of Wastewater
108 Pounds of Solid Waste

Left Coast Press made this paper choice because our printer, Thomson-Shore, Inc., is a member of Green Press Initiative, a nonprofit program dedicated to supporting authors, publishers, and suppliers in their efforts to reduce their use of fiber obtained from endangered forests.

For more information, visit www.greenpressinitiative.org

Environmental impact estimates were made using the Environmental Defense Paper Calculator. For more information visit: www.papercalculator.org.

Left Coast Press, Inc.
1630 North Main Street, #400
Walnut Creek, California 94596
http://www.LCoastPress.com

Hardback ISBN 978-1-59874-402-6
Paperback ISBN 978-1-59874-403-3
eISBN 978-1-59874-703-4

Library of Congress Cataloging-in-Publication Data

Chapple, Helen Stanton.
 No place for dying : American hospitals and the ideology of rescue / Helen Stanton Chapple.
    p. cm.
 Includes bibliographical references.
 ISBN 978-1-59874-402-6 (hardcover : alk. paper) -- ISBN 978-1-59874-403-3 (pbk. : alk. paper)
 1. Palliative treatment. 2. Death. I. Title.
 R726.8.C4677 2010
 616'.029--dc22
                                    2009052717

Printed in the United States of America

∞™ The paper used in this publication meets the minimum requirements of American National Standard for Information Sciences—Permanence of Paper for Printed Library Materials, ANSI/NISO Z39.48—1992.

Cover design by Andrew Brozyna

Contents

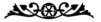

Introduction

As a hospice volunteer more than two decades ago, I enjoyed sitting with dying patients. Family members could rest or run errands, leaving us alone together. Sometimes I did needlework at the bedside. Sometimes I fetched things or helped the patient to the bathroom. It was peaceful. The closer the patient was to death, the more I liked to be there. When I needed a new career, nursing seemed like a logical choice to extend my hospice interest.

Neither my early years as a stockbroker nor that volunteer experience prepared me for the shock of nursing itself. After nursing school, as I cared for cancer patients undergoing clinical trials, suffering with complications, or dying in the hospital, I wondered why so many people with terminal illnesses never went to hospice. Meanwhile, on the weekends that I spent as a hospice home care nurse, I was nostalgic for the old volunteering days. Now I was too busy advising family members and adjusting medications to sit quietly with patients.

Over the years, my question about hospice persisted and became more complex. To my surprise, hospital colleagues linked hospice to giving up, even to hastening death. One nurse distrusted hospice because she connected it with Jack Kevorkian—how prevalent was that misperception, I wondered? Clinicians projected themselves into the dying situations of their patients and expressed their own preferences for a quick death, not wanting to imagine family members surrounding *their* deathbeds. Physicians avoided predicting death as a prognostic outcome so that patients who died in the hospital were not recognized or treated as dying before death occurred. Hospice care at home was distant, hidden away, out of the mainstream of health-care delivery, so how could its elaborate benefits be real to clinicians who never worked outside the hospital? Some patients with terminal cancer preferred to enter Phase 1 clinical trials that offered no personal benefit, hoping that the data from their experience would help others, but their consent processes did not include a description of hospice as an alternative path.

I began a study of bioethics, thinking that the answers I sought lay in the process of decision-making around the end of life. To get closer to the dilemmas of choice, I steered my nursing career into critical care. Meanwhile, bioethics studies left many questions unanswered. They did not probe deeply enough into the profound struggles I witnessed between clinicians and families who sought the "right" way to treat patients, even as they focused on every aspect of the all-important (it seemed) decision to forgo treatment. Bioethics discourses were not riveted by the troubling situation of the dying patient in the hospital without hospice, as I was. Outside of the controversy about administering pain medication according to the Rule of Double Effect (Sulmasy and Pellegrino 1999), the care of patients who were actually dying in the hospital did not seem to disturb the world of bioethics. What were the situations of these patients, unacknowledged by the system that held them? What was happening to them as they were dying? How had they become so lost, to hospice and to everyone else?

It was an anthropologist's criticism of the limitations of bioethics' cognitive approach that introduced me to a new set of questions. Exploring anthropology allowed me to see that being "in the field" was an appropriate description of my stance in hospital nursing, one of almost continuous questioning. Here was a discipline that explored how groups make meaning out of the world around them and transmit that meaning to one another. While asking "How did *this* come to be, right now, in exactly this way and no other?" anthropology turns over the rocks in the path to discover what is hidden underneath. The medical side of anthropology uses these questions and techniques to explore healing practices and their implications for the groups who engage in them. This lens enabled me to explore how dying occurs in the U.S. hospital, paying particular attention to the experiences and actions of clinicians. I have found that they practice according to a cultural expectation of rescue that has particular implications for the persons who happen to be dying among them. This book explores hospital practices around dying and how they came to be.

Rescue and the Hospice Ghetto

The hospice patients I had enjoyed sitting with as a volunteer had already been placed in the dying category. There was little question about this, even from the patients themselves. Open awareness reigned, ensuring that the patients' lack of a future exempted them from public concern (Glaser and

Strauss 1965). The line had been drawn. To be in hospice was and is to be bracketed out of public participation and public awareness. At the same time, to be in hospice (or in a hospital's palliative care unit) is to be refuged and supported in a space where experts seek to meet specialized needs. Hospice and palliative care units in hospitals provide safe passage for the patients seen as dying, on the one hand, and protection for the public from "cross-contamination," on the other. My hospice colleagues observed wryly that local oncologists seldom referred patients to hospice until they were too weak to come to the office, an example of how such patients have dropped away from the legitimacy of social exchange (Baudrillard 1976).

Thus, a tension exists between safe places that support a dying situation such as hospice and palliative care and the wider social invisibility and dismissal that adheres to these places. The characterization of this seclusion as "privacy" may suit most patients and families perfectly well. But to leave it there leaves several questions unanswered: (1) How does this line-drawing between public and private, and between rescuable and dying, occur? Who decides which persons with serious illness are really dying, and by what criteria? (2) Why must such lines be drawn? How does the culture of the United States both benefit from and reinforce such removal of the dying experience? (3) How might the answers to these questions help illuminate the marginalization of the hospice experience?

Based on both my research and my clinical experience, I locate the hospice question in the U.S. interest in rescue. Rescue has become the gold standard for the delivery of acute care in the United States, and this priority profoundly affects dying situations that occur in the hospital. The quest for more time alive provides the market for the worthiest of commodities. Howard Brody's "rescue imperative" (1992: 91) and its corollary of stabilizing patients frame the care of U.S.'s dying patients, both inside and outside of hospice. To bring rescue to the forefront in this discussion rearranges familiar health-care categories.

When seriously ill patients in hospitals who are not recovering are determined to be "officially" dying, they are demoted from a first-class, rescuable status to a second-class, unrescuable status. Although dressed in clinical, scientific language, and thus supposedly an objective determination, this critical transformation is accomplished through practices in the hospital that I describe as a "ritual of intensification." Examining these ritual behaviors brings dying patients out of the "ghetto" of hospice and terminal illness and returns their problems squarely back to the land of the living. Making this line-drawing exercise that relegates dying patients to second-class status visible and challenging also allows us to reimagine its outcome.

The rescue imperative that characterizes U.S. hospitals did not emerge in a vacuum or out of positivistic scientific imperatives. Anthropology offers a lens through which we can see hospitals as institutions that evolved with specific social histories. Three strands of U.S. culture are particularly relevant to the argument of this book: ideologies involving technology, individualism, equality, and heroism; the growing instability of the concept of death itself; and the pivotal role that hospital clinicians play in drawing lines.

U.S. Ideology

Americans are enamored with drama and technological display and with the idea of triumph over adversity, dependence, and vulnerability. The popularity of body trauma television programs is a symptom of public fascination with the quick reversal of bodily misfortune through technology (Jacobs 2003). A fraught term in the social sciences[1], ideology is a useful concept with which to analyze life and death in U.S. hospitals because it rationalizes the striving toward socially acceptable goals, connecting moral understandings and representations of hope with politics. It is also a classic concept for describing the way societies rationalize gradations in social rank (Timmermans and Berg 2003). The common presumption that the United States is a single-class society is part of an ideology that blurs class and other distinctions and binds nationalism, positivism, and heroism with technology. Ideologies are often broadly shared among groups, but they serve the interests of an elite; they maintain the status quo while claiming to represent the world "as it really is."[2] This book shows how, in U.S. hospitals, prevailing concepts of egalitarianism and rescue disguise the distinction between first- and second-class patients and how those distinctions are made. The positivist ideology that technology and medicine represent operates with a view that the world "as it really is" justifies the drawing of class lines.

Critics may view technological progress in medicine as a double-edged sword, but patients and their families are almost always true believers (Eisenberg 1996: 163; Jacobs 2003). Rescue from calamity fits neatly with an ideology of overcoming adversity. In his classic treatment of death denial, Ernest Becker asserts that "society itself is a codified hero system, which means that society everywhere is a living myth of the significance of human life, a defiant creation of meaning" (1973: 7, 58). Although Becker's claim is perhaps hyperbolic in scope, it underscores the U.S. enthusiasm for heroism and triumph, indicating that both individual and societal success will depend on how well death can be denied.

These values have been a prominent part of national identity over the U.S.'s short history. Victories over the wilderness, outer space, and bodily limits in sports are seen as emblematic of the country itself. According to exceptionalists such as Seymour Lipset, binding heroism to national identity is unusually important in the United States. Because ideology rather than a common history brought the country into being, U.S.'s ideology sets it apart: "Americans are utopian moralists who press hard to institutionalize virtue, to destroy evil people, and to eliminate wicked institutions and practices. They tend to view social and political dramas as morality plays, as battles between God and the devil, so that compromise is virtually unthinkable" (Lipset 1991: 22).

The battle against death is the ultimate morality play. Even in U.S. funeral customs, to embalm and display the corpse as sleeping peacefully emphasizes the illusion of a "proper, fulfilled life" rather than the reality of death and putrescence (Metcalf and Huntington 1991: 210).

The instrumentation of medicine in flashy technology has particular meaning for U.S. society and its interest in overcoming rather than submitting to the inevitable. The fact that the health-care system costs more but obtains poorer outcomes than other industrialized countries is well documented, and some policy analysts such as Thomas Bodenheimer believe that technology accounts for a disproportionate share in these costs (2005: Part 2; California HealthCare Foundation 2006; Reinhardt, Hussey, and Anderson 2004). Such sobering international comparisons continue to travel under the public radar, while the media concentrates on stories of individual victories over calamity, dependence, and death. To reinforce the connections between technology and overcoming is to fortify salvational yearnings (Comaroff 1984; Good 1994). The willingness to be taken in by technology's dazzle is more robust for Americans than for Europeans, for example (Nye 2001: 104).[3] Publicity regarding medical breakthroughs now saturates the news media, reinforcing the idea that quality in health-care is directly related to the amount of technology applied. Dying patients who are nonrescuable share their less-compelling status with other patients whose maladies—mental illness, disability, chronic illness—are not amenable to instrumentation.

This culture of heroism and rescue is based in individualism. Because crisis readiness is prioritized, it appears that the medical system is designed to respond to every (otherwise self-reliant, unfettered) individual (Gordon 1988: 36). Such an idea of individual freedom cannot exert cultural dominance, however, unless it is equally available to all persons (Bauman 1992: 112). Anyone can call 911 and expect a response. But rescue, both as a figurative ideal and an embodied network, actually helps maintain the unequal health-care system. The universality of intent, perceived to be at the foundation of emergency rescue policies, stands in stark contrast to the widely documented disparities in overall U.S. health-care (Agency for Healthcare Research and Quality 2008; Becker 2004). Likewise, even if clinicians believe that they provide equal treatment at the bedside, perceived equality at that particular place does not address the social structures that both make people sick and present insurmountable obstacles to obtaining quality medical attention promptly (Farmer 2005; Zussman 1992: 40).

Self-reliance is a core U.S. value; pervasive fear of its opposite—dependence—proves the rule (Hsu 1972: 248). This attitude might explain the distaste for and invisibility of regarding routine care-giving in the United States described by Peter Lawler:

> We [Americans] think all human beings have an equal right to work and no right not to work. And we think that to be free means not to be dependent on others or constrained by them. We are against all forms of servitude and dependence, and we often see no real difference between paternalism and despotism. . . . Our goal is not to care for those who are suffering and dying—to help us live well with our natural disabilities—but to work hard to reduce and eventually eliminate the amount of suffering and dying in the world. (2004: 1)

Lawler implies that providing good care and saving lives are mutually exclusive, and so they have become in terms of national priorities. Rescue allows society to perform heroic acts that intrude on one individual at a time, and then only in case of catastrophe. Chapter 2 describes the development and implementation of rescue and individualism in U.S. medicine.

Universal Rescue Destabilizes Death

When the newly dead can sometimes be quickened by chest compressions and early defibrillation, death and dying are destabilized. Insofar as cardiopulmonary resuscitation (CPR) stands in for universal health-care in the United States and hospitals take their response readiness seriously, human finitude itself can appear to fade. By effectively omitting death as a foregone conclusion, rescue and stabilization strengthen the hero project that Ernest Becker identified as central to death-denying normalcy in the United States. But if natural physiological limits can occasionally be overcome, then restrictions on the use of rescue must also be found and justified. A new requirement has arisen with U.S. technological prowess and its universal application under rescue circumstances: the invention of a cultural exercise in line-drawing, a ritual for separating the living and rescuable from the dying and unrescuable, the first class from the second class.

Rescue efforts in the United States receive open, continuous support from technology, economics, cultural ideology, and the hope for salvation. By contrast, dying is poorly defined and happens in the shadows (see Chapter 3). To be admitted into hospice and receive its benefits, patients must relinquish a measure of social legitimacy in the (nonhospice) world they know, the one that privileges rescue. For these reasons, persons in the United States should not expect to receive both full attention to every physical threat to survival *along with* provisions for a comfortable dying situation when the time comes. These options do not carry equal weight, making the line-drawing much more difficult than is generally known. Further, to express or elicit these preferences through an advance directive or in some other form assumes a level of control and orderliness that may not travel in the same company with serious illness and death. It is up to the clinicians in charge, with their power as society's representatives, to mediate these differently weighted values at the hospital bedside.

Clinicians as Culture Bearers of Rescue and Comfortable Dying

My research in two U.S. hospitals examined practices around dying, situated in the environment of rescue as a social and ideological mandate. As sociologist Daniel Chambliss (1996) points out, patients and families in hospitals wrestle with issues vitally important to the shapes of their lives, including life itself. For clinicians, these struggles and the compassion they bring to them are simply what they encounter as a part of coming to work each day. How do the workplace routines and priorities inflict themselves on such life crises, and vice versa?

Nearly everyone in a hospital has brought the national culture and ideology of the United States into the hospital with him or her. The hospital is not a world unto itself but a part of the social "mainland." Meanwhile, each clinician reflects the particular culture of the hospital and even the unit where he or she practices, so that an iterative process occurs between the culture of the hospital and that of the society (van der Geest and Finkler 2004: 1998). But which society? The "mainland" understandings of technological care, best practices, and the social contract must be mediated through each hospital's corporate territory. In this book, I explore the role of the hospital as mediator between the macro and micro worlds of U.S. society, its economics, and bedside care. Meanwhile, clinicians at each site must be the action agents and the interpreters of the unfolding events in these life and death dramas. Clinicians are, then, unique as ritual agents displaying the particularity of the hospital subculture while also representing society as a whole (Singer 1989: 1193). Hospital practices are supposed to be evidence based and scientific, but they are also based on beliefs: a belief that health is the worthiest of goals; a belief that the consequences for wrong science, wrong belief, or wrong behavior are life threatening; and the practice and belief that "right science" can correct or ameliorate the consequences. The arena of the patient encounter becomes a "combat zone of disputes over power and over definitions of illness" (Taussig 1980: 9).

More specifically, clinicians represent public social attitudes, even as they, specialists in the domain of acute care, hold themselves apart. They (we) recognize that patients and families are naive when they believe that having "everything done" is almost always the best choice to protect their loved ones. If we foresee death as the outcome, we want orderliness in patient dying, so that the patient can be free of suffering, with loved ones close by, and with enough time to prepare so the death is peaceful and goodbyes can be said (see Chapter 3). We feel regret when the desire for "everything"—all the rescue that the hospital has to offer—crowds out the opportunity for peace and dignity around the death that we foresee as inevitable. We are often not aware that no other scenario may be possible and even less cognizant about why this may be so.

U.S. bioethics with its traditional emphasis on patient autonomy as the *sine qua non* of line drawing does not often address the multiple, hidden influences on agency, even as it has outlined the circumstances that permit the line drawing to occur in the treatment of seriously ill patients. In framing these issues anthropologically, I am able to describe and make explicit some of the forces that have been previously unavailable in the discourse.

Hospitals as Field Sites

I conducted ethnographic research in two hospitals in which I had never worked: a Catholic community hospital and a teaching hospital, both in a midsized city in the United States. I used a retrospective approach to interview clinicians about patients who had died. Before launching the major study, I conducted a pilot study in the hospital where I was working as an intensive care unit (ICU) nurse. For this preliminary work, the institutional review board (IRB) approved a method that allowed a member of the Decedent Affairs Office (DAO) to notify me every week as to where deaths had occurred. I could then seek interviews with the clinicians who had cared for the patients promptly after the death, even though I was not allowed to know patient names or numbers.

This process worked less smoothly in my subsequent research, partly because of my outsider status. (See the Appendix for further details of the ethnographic method.) Physicians were far less accessible in the fieldwork sites than during the pilot. In the teaching hospital, I visited the DAO every few days to obtain a new list of places and times where deaths had occurred. I would then visit the units and ask to speak to the nurse who had cared for a patient who had died there on a specific date. Without the patient's name, unit secretaries had to track down this information through their particular log books and records of patient assignments, shift schedules, and events. People were sometimes too busy to help with this. This exercise of unit detective work was the same in the Catholic community hospital units, but no DAO existed there to provide a list of recent deaths. It was several months before I cobbled together a reliable method to gather this information (see Chapter 2 for more details about this venture).

The fieldwork spanned sixteen months in 2003 and 2004. During this period I also worked weekends as a nurse in a third hospital nearby. In April 2003, new Health Insurance Portability and Accountability Act (HIPAA) regulations were enacted, further restricting access to patient information in U.S. hospitals. After obtaining IRB approval, I approached unit managers in group meetings and individually to obtain permission to be present on the units and to interact with their clinicians. Interview participants signed informed consent forms. Even with these protections in place, unit managers could, and some did, disallow my presence.

In the Catholic community hospital, my base of operation was the chaplains' group office, a large, carpeted room off the hospital lobby with desks and computers along two walls. In the teaching hospital, the too-small staff lounge in the palliative care unit was my home between interviews. Generally, I spent weekday mornings at one hospital site and afternoons at the other. I also attended gatherings on and off each site whenever the opportunity arose: in-service activities, training, commemorations, retreats, and meetings involving staff, bereavement, ethics, policy, and planning.

Through clinician narratives about their encounters with dying throughout the two hospitals and the pilot study, I heard about 211 patients of all ages and how they died. I used verbatim hand-written notes to record the interviews. I learned how nurses and chaplains, especially, along with a few physicians, respiratory therapists, and other providers viewed particular kinds of dying. Observations, meetings, and interviews with clinicians and administrators enabled me to trace variations in dying to differences in the corporate structures and management styles of the two hospitals as well as to the overarching cultural pressures they shared.

The community hospital was part of a Catholic hospital system with sister facilities elsewhere in the city and the country. The teaching hospital (also nonprofit) was an independent entity unto itself, academically connected to a state university. A third group of several for-profit hospitals competed in the metropolitan area along with the Catholic system and the teaching hospital. Each institution was exquisitely aware of the area's health-care market and its own fragile position within it. In a 1997 statewide comparison of hospital charges per case, the for-profit hospital system's charges exceeded those of the two nonprofit fieldwork sites in all thirty-five categories.[4] Operating margins for the nonprofits seemed razor thin by contrast, and their obligation to be stewards both of the community and of their own survival pulled them in opposite directions (see Chapter 5).

Arc of the Argument

Chapter 1 describes the difficulty of dying in an environment where rescue is the dominant mode of operation. It introduces five patients and the variety of dying situations that they encountered in both hospitals. The clinicians who cared for these patients used compassion, experience, and unit norms for guidance rather than established standards of care, because such standards were either not available or not useful. They experienced conflicting loyalties in carrying out this care. In an environment of rescue and stabilization, dying is a slippery category to delineate and retain.

Chapter 2 is about the rise of rescue and stabilization as the central organizing principle of patient management in U.S. hospitals. Through a series of shifts in health-care, stability has emerged as a ranking device in medicine, hospital triage, and in business, functioning as the bottom line for both profit and human finitude. With rescue as the gold standard of the delivery of acute health-care, heroism, speed, and good business can come together to reinforce each other as "democratizing": individualized, specialized care is offered to anyone demonstrating a need for it by their collapse. Stability and rescue become a vital bridge between the values of rationality and the yearning for recovery, on the one hand, and the productive engine of the health-care industry, on the other. Their respective power is built on the intersection of these beliefs, each of which is true to some extent, just as CPR is occasionally successful.

Having established rescue's primacy, it is important to understand how it interacts with the phenomenon of death in the United States, seen as accidental or coming at the end of contingency. Through rescue operations establishing machines as adjuncts to vital body functions, time can be manipulated. More time alive is produced; further contingencies can be explored; and the disorder of accident can be corrected. These efforts, which I call the ritual of intensification, offer the hope of not dying while maintaining social legitimacy. Such intense pursuit of any options other than death effectively distracts Americans from having to gaze into the abyss either individually or as a society, thereby aiding the hero project. If death results from the failure of rescue, it becomes a technical problem rather than an existential one. These developments have expanded the cultural distance that patients, families, and clinicians in the hospital must travel between "heroic" efforts for a patient with a future at one end of the spectrum, and an assessment of "dying" on the other. The ritual of intensification is the map that clinicians use to find their way through this territory. I show how this works by narrating the process as it played out in three patient examples.

Counter-discourses of bioethics and the revival of the death movement (hospice and palliative care) have risen up alongside rescue's dominance, but they sometimes enhance rather than mitigate dying's marginalization. Bioethics gives permission for the suspension of the ritual of intensification under certain circumstances, and the "revival of death movement"—so named by Tony Walter (1994)—defines an alternative space for the dying patient through palliative care or hospice. Neither bioethics nor hospice challenges the dominance of rescue, and both could be said to be necessary to it—providing relief valves for its unremitting tension and allowing it to continue to define the shape of routine medical care in the hospital.

But then how does death actually occur in the hospital? Because death is not out of the question in acute-care settings, its containment is highly developed. Rescue and stabilization efforts enable an interval of dying to be demarcated, separate from mainstream care, and clinicians in both hospitals can take steps to minimize its impact. Because death can occur, it should happen with as little dying as possible, as an anticlimax, properly domesticated, in contrast to the chaos of treating serious illness. The dying situation seems to be a greater threat in the hospital than death itself, and it cannot be recognized without proper sanction. In Chapter 4, I show that "right" dying happens in the expected times and places, progressing in a linear fashion, without chaos and with consensus. "Wrong" dying is out of order, time, and place, and not properly contained. These general patterns of dying and the attitudes clinicians expressed are significant because of the level of control they often exert in the situation, enabled by their skills in stabilization.

The striving for triumph over calamity, especially death, forms the background not only of rescue, but through these efforts it also fuels big business in the United States. The connections are appropriately mystified and cloaked within the hospital so as to be virtually unidentifiable (and unimpeachable) at the bedside. These forces have their own agendas, hidden from the participants but operating on them nonetheless, and almost impossible to resist because of the lure of more time alive. If death is the ultimate human problem, and if individual rescue represents the promise of overcoming, it is not surprising that escaping crisis is prized in the economics of health-care. Productivity and rescue are jointly beneficial to industry within and beyond the hospital because both emphasize speed of action. The economics of rescue are not divorced from the culture and the ideology at large, but are a product of it.

"Every medical action is a transaction," (Middleton 2004) but in the hospital where lives are at stake, the monetary values must be kept separate and obfuscated during the process of exchange in favor of medicine's broader significance to the culture. In Chapter 5 we explore this process. Americans must believe in medicine and its practitioners as pure, untouched by the toxic influences of economic gain, especially at these moments of extreme vulnerability. The hospital's technology is dazzling and stamps the individual receiving it as valuable and legitimate. The immeasurable value of life-saving is matched by the unfathomable mystery of its instruments. Meanwhile, elaborate coding vocabularies ensure that it is both quantifiable and reimbursable. No coding slot exists for palliative care, however, so dying has no grounding in the economic infrastructure. This process of values mystification lays the foundation for the discussion of trust in Chapter 8.

In Chapter 6, I describe how the connection between the hospital and the industry of rescue influences the care of dying patients. The issue of overcrowding in the emergency department (ED) and the diversion of ambulances to other hospitals is a window onto the issues of cost and throughput (a measurement of production over time—i.e., how efficiently patients can be treated and discharged) faced by U.S. hospitals. The resulting pressure affects care of dying patients in ways that are peculiar to each site's culture. In the Catholic community hospital, after the patient's rescuability is ruled out, it is easier to free up his ICU bed than it is to pin down his subsequent plan of care. One mixed unit of hospice and medical-surgical patients can accommodate any unrescuable patient without the need to specify goals of care. Clinicians here have no trouble extending open-ended intervals of time to patients who are dying. But in the teaching hospital's environments of intense rescue, the tolerance for waiting is low. Clinicians voice preferences for short, predictable dying situations, along with their fears that families will second-guess the decision to withdraw life support if death does not follow promptly. Dying is conflated with suffering, and no value apart from limiting suffering seems important once consensus about the dying has been reached. Finding it difficult to tolerate feelings of helplessness, these clinicians see themselves as being held hostage to the dying situation rather than deriving a sense of honor or privilege in being close to it, as is more common in hospice or palliative care.

In Chapter 7, I shift focus from the patient's dying situation back to the ritual of intensification, which comes in for closer scrutiny here than in Chapter 2. It is the crucial mechanism of transformation from living to dying, and I consider its general program along with the factors of practice that could lengthen or shorten it. The ritual creates order out of the chaos of serious illness for clinicians, according to the priorities and instrumentation required by rescue and stabilization. It provides the goals for the patient's clinical course and the shape for its narrative, along with a formula to resolve the uncertainty of his fate. True to form, this ritual enacts the transformation of the rescuable patient to an unrescuable status, and its practitioners often contest its operations among themselves. But rather than ending by reintegrating the patient into the social body as most rites of passage do, this ritual enables her to be cast off from it, while avoiding social guilt and without threatening the project of medicine itself. The ritual's "tipping point" of clinical decision and the testing of that conclusion with the family prove the success or failure of the ritual. At this juncture, the patient's deterioration toward death is explicitly declared to be not a crisis, not eligible for rescue interventions. It appears that this one-by-one reclassification of seriously ill situations into dying situations has become the extent of the American encounter with death.

The ritual enables clinicians who have been inflicting suffering in the name of life-saving to make up for it at the end by the intensity of the compassion they display in relieving the patient's dying. Not surprisingly, the ritual of intensification differs in the two study hospitals. Fewer ICU beds in the Catholic community hospital and the absence of interns and residents enable private-practice clinicians and nurses to take actions that are more arbitrary and less patterned than in the teaching hospital, where individuals have less personal power.

In Chapter 8, we consider the issue of trust in the U.S. health-care system. The elaborate rescue endeavor can be seen as a ritual display; an active demonstration of technology in crisis can be seen as an effort to compensate for the system's widespread shortcomings in providing basic care. The ritual of intensification seeks to establish trust, so that when clinicians impose care limits to avoid "futile" resuscitation attempts, families and patients will assent. The display of rescue perpetuates the differential in power between clinicians and patients while seeking to win their loyalty to it.

As palliative care programs have gained favor in hospitals, clinicians have a consolation prize to offer to patients and families when they want to close down the ritual of intensification. I investigate the trustworthiness of this option as it existed in both hospitals and explore its compromised position in the U.S. hospital and in the health-care system. If hospitals are urged to use palliative care to offload their expensive ICU beds, what message does this convey about the intrinsic worth of dying patients? I propose that neither the ritual of intensification nor palliative care can be ultimately trustworthy as guardians of the dying, because both represent a health-care system housed within a cultural system that cannot accommodate the experience of dying in a value system of self-reliance, individualism, and heroism.

What might be done? How can hospitals make a place for hospital dying to occur without it being subject to diminishment? To expect the dying patient herself to insist on her rights is not the answer. Looking again at the ritual of intensification, we find that instead of leading toward social incorporation in the normal way of a rite of passage, it works in the opposite direction, as a mechanism of isolation. As we consider how to reverse this process and incorporate dying persons into a legitimate social space, the variety of dying scenarios that occurred in the two research sites offers a glimpse into the daunting complexity of the issue. In conclusion, I invite a thought experiment with the concepts of recognition and witness as avenues for movement in a different direction.

The New American Morality Play: Becoming More Human

One chaplain told me that she derived no energy from the dying patient in the bed, in contrast to my own experiences sitting with hospice patients. "The heavens don't open," she said. It is common for hospital clinicians to express a preference for their own death to be swift and painless. During my time in the field, a friend in health-care challenged me to describe what I wanted to see happen for dying patients. If the patient is at death's door, why would one advocate for them to be allowed to die in their own time? What would be the reason, other than simple romanticism, to want to open up that space?

The answer is in three parts, and it comes from my experience at the bedside, anthropological inquiry, and existential reflection. As a long-time critical-care clinician, I am steeped in the culture of rescue, of death prevention. As long as the patient is comfortable by any measure that an outsider can judge, he should be allowed to take his own time, to define his own dying. To take steps that could invite death in is to side with the enemy. Further, it implies a lack of courage to share in the patient's powerlessness as we wait for death's approach. My willingness to wait is an act of defiance. Now that the end is at hand, death should not have it too easy.

Moving into a different metaphor, to abort the journey would be to refuse to learn from my patient's experience, or even to be in his company. It would also show disrespect for this voyage we have in common. Not to hasten death, but allow it to take its time means that I am open to the human condition that we share. I have no desire to add to his distress, but to allow the journey to be exactly what it will, as long as detectable suffering on his part is not an issue.

Finally, I believe that to characterize the dying situation as a generative process rather than an anticlimax or a foregone conclusion is a way to enhance our own humanity. David Hilfiker points out that to marginalize others is to become alienated from oneself (2005). In our zeal as clinicians to prove our compassion and wipe out suffering through large doses of opioids and sedation after life-support technology is gone, we are treating the dying patient as if he were, if not dead already, then as good as dead. It is too easy in the United States to dismiss the dying person, to put him out of *our* misery. In my role as a representative of society, as a party to the social contract, I want society not to do this. Further, persons who are dying present vulnerability and finitude to Americans more completely than any other marginalized group. Perhaps this is why they are so shunned. The title of the disability rights group "Not Dead Yet" indicates that they recognize an even greater marginalization than disability, aimed at those living persons socially defined by the imminence of their death. Even if the person herself loses her sense of personhood as the body deteriorates (Lawton 2000), selfhood can be ascribed and honored by those around her.

My objective in presenting this investigation and interpreting its findings is neither to arouse existentially appropriate despair over the human condition nor to call attention to Americans' pattern to diminish dying patients in the public space of the hospital. Nor is it only to represent the situation of hospital dying in an anthropological framework that may offer new insight. I submit an alternative conclusion, drawing from the insights of literary scholar Eugene August (1981) regarding endings and how they are judged. His points relate to the hero project in the United States and its denial of death and vulnerability in such a way that allows us to redefine our notions of heroism.

August draws a careful distinction between divine comedy in literature and the comedy of laughter, and he makes a case for removing the tragedy from its position as "the highest form of art" (1981: 86, 87). Divine comedies strike a tone of "high seriousness" and feature reconciliation with the gods or with a divine power at the end, after the hero has overcome his hubris and recognized his human limitations. "Starting with a mistaken notion of what it is to be godlike, tragic heroes often attempt to impose their will up on others in a way that denies their oneness with them; divine comic heroes modify pride as they discover what it is to be truly godlike, not by a denial of their humanity but by a perfecting of it" (p. 94).

These heroes' new awareness is not passive humility, but a quest to experience humanity more fully. I submit this road to heroism as an avenue to improving attention to the realm of the dying patient in the U.S. hospital, outlined with a few specifics in Chapter 9.

On a cultural level, one could imagine the elevation of the dying person to a place of honor, earned by having survived the ordeal of the ritual of intensification. The hospital could display this honor through a display of opulence in goods, services, and surroundings in the setting of excellent palliative care. Even if the patient is beyond awareness, such outlay would demonstrate his value as a pilgrim, an explorer of lands yet unknown to those still capable of an upright posture. An extravagant display of palliative care might inspire a consumer response. It could protect the patient from intrusion while providing persons ready to listen and record family stories, opportunities for gatherings, and invitations to ceremonies marking the importance to the culture (as well as the family) of this momentous event.[5] Barbara Adam reminds us that "Transcendence is always an immortality of the spirit which is constituted by our relationship to the temporality of life" (1995: 38).

Of course, it would not be for everyone. Vanstone (2004) indicates that perhaps a third of people might be interested in considering the "stature of waiting," as an alternative to exploring every contingency of more time alive. Satirist Art Buchwald was one of those people. He turned away from dialysis and chose, not death, but whatever might happen apart from his particular life-prolonging treatment. When he signed himself up for hospice care in February 2006, his death from kidney failure was expected imminently. The importance of his experience is not the remarkable eleven months that he lived after his decision, enjoying his status as a condemned but celebrated personage. No one could presume that such a boon would be part of the bargain.[6] Instead, the significant point was that he had the courage to turn away from rescue and explore his own humanity, rather than to seek to be saved from it.

Notes

1. In their discussion of cognitive archeology, Kent Flannery and Joyce Marcus differentiate between cosmology, religion, ideology, and iconography. See Flannery and Marcus (1993: 263).
2. Andrew Levine defines ideology as "a body of doctrine, more or less comprehensive, that, deliberately or not, systematically serves particular interest at the same time that it purports to represent the world as it really is." See Levine (2004: 6).
3. Nye sees this interest in technology as spanning ethnicities in the United States, with the exception of "the Amish, many Native Americans, some of the rural poor, and some of those living in communes" (2001: 109).
4. This consumer-oriented health-care watchdog organization has not made a more recent comparison.
5. Lock (2002) describes hospital gatherings after patients' deaths in Japan that clinicians routinely attend.
6. Stephen Connor and his colleagues (2007) have shown that hospice patients can often live longer than patients with similar diagnoses who are not part of a hospice program.

CHAPTER 1

Hospital Dying Situations

When hospital clinicians care for dying patients, they are often on their own, practicing with few or no specific guidelines in a way that typifies virtually no other hospital clinical practice. The move toward standardizing most of the care of patients in hospitals has deep roots. Near the beginning of the twentieth century, hospitals in the United States insisted that all patients have standardized medical records. One consequence of this standardization was that patients perceived to be from lower classes (people of color, immigrants, the poor and indigent) benefited from this more democratic treatment. Physicians treating well-to-do patients had to open their private notebooks, so that patient care methods used for the wealthy and powerful became accessible to clinicians and accountants (Timmermans and Berg 2003).

Using the critical task of documentation to manifest both equal opportunity and presumed transparency helped make it possible for U.S. hospitals to become demonstration projects for societal ideals. Medicine was a social good, and medical records, as tools of research, reimbursement, communication, and accountability, could advance that good. Standardization promoted goals of both science and efficiency in hospitals; it could reinforce the expectation that scientific advancement could be translated into ever improving health-care quality.

These progressive ideals, even elaborated and contested over time, have remained alive and well in the U.S. hospital. Quality improvement efforts, policies that make cardiopulmonary resuscitation the default for every hospitalized patient, and the movement toward evidence-based medicine are all grounded in the belief that practice should be guided by and informed by standards. Every life-saving intervention practiced in hospitals has a protocol to guide its proper implementation. Clinicians proclaim their belief that

25

practice must be guided by what is best for the patient, therefore general standards must be modifiable based on individual cases. Still, the standards are the starting place; they are what stamps health-care practice as legitimate and professional.

Delivering health-care according to set standards has served hospitals well as the means for holding back death have become ever more elaborate. Because compliance to practice protocols pervades clinical practice in U.S. hospitals, standards can serve as useful lenses to begin exploring how dying occurs there. Hospitals produce more time alive as their most valued commodity, and mortality rates are one measure of their success. If the hospitalized patient is officially recognized as dying, however, he is no longer a candidate for life-saving. To be disqualified from rescue may place the patient not only beyond the reach of that paradigm but also beyond the standards themselves.[1] Further, because rescue care is much more closely tied to reimbursement than nonrescue care (see Chapter 5), care for patients who are dying may be documented less rigorously and is rarely subject to review. What might this change in status mean for the patient, and how does it come to be?

Implications for dying and "Dying"

Subsequent chapters answer this question by examining the development of hospitals as both culture and industry. In this chapter, I explore what the dominant standard of rescue and the experience of being disqualified from rescue mean for the dying patient. First, I show that in the U.S. hospital, Dying patients who are officially recognized as such (thus written with a capital D) and are not under hospice or palliative care almost always occupy a devalued social position compared to non-Dying patients. Because acute care in the United States is thought to be an egalitarian endeavor with standards of excellence applicable to every patient, to move a patient beyond the reach of those standards, to label the patient as officially Dying, is an act of delegimization. Changing the patient's code status from "full code" (the default mode and often simply assumed) to "no code" or "Do Not Resuscitate" (DNR) (which requires clear articulation) is an example of this practice. As such, it requires ritual behavior to exonerate it, as we shall see. Once delegitimization has been accomplished, the patient and her caregivers are often completely at sea. To extend the analogy, uncontrolled wetness itself is an anathema (as every clinician knows), a signal of insidious disorder. The journey that had been clinically mapped toward stability and cure is now adrift, buffeted by circumstance, pulled under by hospital currents, navigated by arbitrary preference, and often beyond the reach of tracking, accountability, standardization, and quality. Most persons want to get back on dry land as soon as possible, to feel sure-footed and in control.

To become acquainted with the diverse dying situations occurring in hospitals is to discover dying to be a very slippery category, difficult to grasp. (I prefer the term "situation" to "process" because it gathers in persons beyond the central individual and because what is happening may not be at all linear or orderly [Kastenbaum 1978].) The persons who populate dying situations slide in and out of the hospital's focus, which is fixed on regulations, outcomes, and bottom lines. In the hospital, to be legitimate means being under the aegis of care standards, governed by some form of oversight or quality control. Because dying does not fit with the expectation of clinical spaces being devoted to improving health and saving lives, it is minimized when it occurs in those spaces, or it is swept beyond view into palliative care. The hospital reflects a broad-based consensus that dying (when clearly occurring) is supposed to be a private matter, properly left to families and not a matter of public or social concern. This attitude reflects the priorities of the larger society, and why would it not? The U.S. hospital embodies the most highly realized incarnation of the society's hopes for itself: a technological bastion standing between itself and death.

Just as every life is unique, every dying situation tells a story different from any other. The five situations of dying in this chapter fixed on the imaginary slide for our inspection serve as orientation to perplexities explored in later chapters. Mr. Diangelo[2] and Mrs. Harper, the first two cases, were patients in the Catholic community hospital. The next two patients, Mr. Gomez and Ms. Hunter, died in the teaching hospital.

Case One: Mr. Diangelo

Mr. Diangelo's longstanding lung problems made it surprising that he survived to see his 90s. He had been in and out of the hospital recently, and he was alert and responsive when he was admitted a week before. Details of his clinical course were not available, but during this admission a decision had been made to write a DNR (or "no code") order for him.[3]

During what would be the last weekend of his life, Mr. Diangelo was in a stepdown[4] unit so that his cardiac status could be monitored. On Saturday, his breathing became more labored, and the staff tried several interventions to assist him with varying success.

RN: He was on 6 liters nasal cannula plus a fifty percent face tent, and when I went in to check him, he was not doing well. His sats were 50 percent[5]—I mean he was BLUE. It had happened before at midnight, and the face tent was added then. [Now] We went up to 75 percent face tent. That didn't do the job for him. So we paged respiratory and we talked about putting him on a nonrebreather.[6] The fact was he was blue. We had to do something. The nonrebreather and the nasal cannula seemed to help. He did good with that through the day. Then Saturday later in the day he was in trouble again. The house doctor came up. The respiratory doctor was called. We put him on the BiPAP[7]—that worked. He seemed okay when the family was there.

Mr. Diangelo's requirements for oxygen and breathing support had moved from simple (nasal cannula alone) to just short of intubation[8] (BiPAP) over the space of a few hours. During that time he suffered several bouts of severe respiratory distress, and in each case the staff stepped up his oxygen support. This final step involved putting a mask over his nose and mouth arranged to create a very tight seal so that the machine's oxygen would go into his lungs without escaping out the sides. BiPAP is considered a temporary measure because of its discomfort, the patient's inability to eat or talk, and the dry mucous membranes it causes.

RN: On Sunday he was more awake, pulling the BiPAP off, even talking some. The problem was, I had four patients. I could not sit at the bedside. So every time it got dislodged, his oxygen saturation dropped. The family requested wrist restraints. So we did that. Sunday afternoon he could dislocate the mask by turning his head or moving down in the bed. When he started pulling that BiPAP off Sunday afternoon, we were constantly in there. I called the admitting doctor and he wasn't on call. The covering doctor—they didn't know him. He said he would call the one who saw him Sunday morning. I asked the doctor, "Do you want to put him in the unit?" "No—he's a no code. They don't want to intubate," so that was it. He would order Dilaudid.[9] We were afraid it would wipe out his respiratory drive. But I gave him some before I left, and it did fine for him. He was able to rest and didn't fight the mask.

On Monday, the respiratory doctor came in. That's when they decided it was okay for him coming off the BiPAP. They were ready. They were prepared.

HC: That was three doctors?

RN: Four doctors in all.

Having benefited from improved oxygenation overnight, Mr. Diangelo was more alert on Sunday morning, more aware of the mask and its discomfort, making the BiPAP a double-edged sword. Recognizing that Mr. Diangelo's increasing struggle against the mask was an unsolvable management problem, the nurse suggested an alternative plan of care: that the physician write an order to move him into the ICU. Staffing issues alone are rarely enough to buy an ICU bed, and this physician immediately rejected this idea along with the unspoken option that would do the trick: the invasive procedure of intubation and mechanical ventilation. His reason, as reported by the nurse, is telling. Rather than pointing out that Mr. Diangelo's need for more and more oxygen indicated that he was dying, or that intubation would not solve the problem, the doctor cited Mr. Diangelo's status: he was a no code—he was no longer a candidate for rescue care. The nurse's response is also revealing: "so that was it."

Elaboration regarding other possible options for caring for Mr. Diangelo seemed unlikely. Mr. Diangelo's no code status itself seemed to be the extent of his plan of care, although I heard the maxim elsewhere in this hospital that "'no code' doesn't mean 'no care.'" Now the plan dictated that the nurses cope with Mr. Diangelo's struggles to remove the mask and the staff's attempts to replace it or restrain his movements. The order for the medication that allowed him to rest had come well into the second twenty-four hours of Mr. Diangelo's respiratory difficulty. This measure initially presented a problem for his nurse, who was reluctant to do it in case it compromised his breathing. In the end, he received it because she was willing to take a gamble that it would not kill him by "wiping out his respiratory drive."

None of the four physicians who consulted on Mr. Diangelo's respiratory difficulties over the weekend was his attending physician, because that person was not on call. Staff and physicians did the best they could to relieve each episode of Mr. Diangelo's distress in the moment. But without the attending physician, it was no one's specific responsibility to evaluate the adequacy of these measures, to draw conclusions, or to take action based on those conclusions. The nurse told me that she thought that Mr. Diangelo's repeated attempts to remove the mask were indications of his wish to die, but she did not have the authority to act on that assessment.

On Monday morning, when they were "ready" to remove the BiPAP and allow Mr. Diangelo to die, his next-day nurse related the events that followed.

> RN: The pulmonary specialist came in and saw him. He spoke with the family and said we were prolonging the inevitable. When the doctor said, "turn the BiPAP off," he said to keep the Dilaudid. He didn't seem like he was in any distress. We kept the BiPAP on till all the family came. So we waited a little bit before.

The phrase "prolonging the inevitable" is an official pronouncement. With it, the "dying" that the previous nurse recognized on Sunday through Mr. Diangelo's attempts to remove the mask became "Dying," that is, certified by the physician and by the family meeting. It was also a statement about both the immediate past and the immediate future. In hindsight, it summed up the experiences of the weekend, confirming the common belief that to be dying is certainly also to be suffering. Hadn't they all seen Mr. Diangelo suffering before he received the Dilaudid? "Prolonging the inevitable" also framed a dualistic choice about Mr. Diangelo's future that now seemed to face them: either use the BiPAP to continue to produce more time alive, or remove it and allow death to occur. Mr. Diangelo's state of Dying in the here and now invited no particular care plan in itself, no set of interventions tailored to this situation, other than simply to get out of death's way.

Still, the nurse did not follow the physician's order immediately, and I asked her about the fact that she "waited a little bit."

> HC: How did you know to wait for people to come in?

> RN: It was common sense. He did not say I had to take the BiPAP off at a certain time. The daughter said, "You don't have to wait." But I said, "Take whatever time you need." I've had dying grandparents. You need time.

Mr. Diangelo was not suffering at the present moment. Informed by a personal experience with her grandparents rather than by protocol, this nurse gently redirected the daughter and managed the situation with perhaps the only tool she had at her disposal: determining when the removal of the BiPAP should occur and doing so according to her internal rhythm of "common sense." Her delay to allow the family to gather and have "time" was a care plan that acknowledged the unique stature of dying, one that deserved such attention.

HC: How did the death occur?

RN: We took him off the BiPAP. He did have nasal cannula. He expired in maybe thirty minutes after we cut the BiPAP off. We had him on the heart monitor and saw the heart rate go down. The daughter came out and asked me, "Could you check on him? I think he's passed." I listened to his chest and called the house doctor to ask his opinion. He came within five or ten minutes. The family stayed fifteen minutes after. The daughter seemed at peace. She said, "He was 92 years old, he had a good life. He shouldn't have to live this way." With the progression over the weekend, they had time to contemplate his passing and were okay with it.

HC: How did it go from your perspective?

RN: All in all it went well. The doctor said he didn't have much [respiratory] effort on his own.

The nurse's sensitivity about timing the BiPAP removal perhaps also explained her absence at the bedside. She may not have wanted to intrude, perhaps unaware that she had a valid role to play. If she had been present with Mr. Diangelo and his family, she could have assessed and interpreted the physiological changes that were surely occurring during the interval that passed between the removal of the BiPAP and his death. She did not join them in the room when the monitor outside signaled his imminent death, but waited for the family to emerge and inform her of his "passing." She followed the after-death protocol and called the physician for pronouncement. She perceived that everyone was satisfied with how events had unfolded, although Mr. Diangelo's opinion was not sought. Further time alive would seem to have brought only further suffering, and Mr. Diangelo's weakened frame had "proved" over the weekend that it could not generate respiratory effort. His death had been controlled, the family was "at peace" and did not overstay. For her, orderliness reigned: "it went well." The lack of respiratory effort "on his own" confirmed the rightness of the decision to stop trying to keep him alive.

Mr. Diangelo's respiratory status had been tenuous before the weekend, and the DNR order written soon after admission indicated that his attending physician anticipated a fatal deterioration at some point. The fact that he was still in a telemetry bed being monitored indicates some ambivalence about Mr. Diangelo's situation. By removing him from the category of rescuable, the DNR order had guaranteed what treatment he would *not* receive, but did not specify what clinicians should *do* in case his fragile stability gave way. When he went off duty Friday afternoon, the attending physician's instructions to the covering clinicians had omitted this detail. When Mr. Diangelo's needs changed, clinicians responded in the moment, according him increasing respiratory support but little relief. It was certainly simpler to manage his distress than to confirm openly the possibility that they were bearing witness to the final hours of his physical presence among them.

I did ask the weekend nurse what she might have changed about Mr. Diangelo's case, and her hindsight was more mixed than that of the nurse who cared for him the day he died.

> RN: Because he was a no code, I think he could have come off the monitor and gone to hospice. I don't know why that didn't happen.
>
> HC: Would the attending have done that?
>
> RN: I think so. Because it was the weekend and the on call doctors don't make those decisions, as you know. If the BiPAP could have been weaned off and gone back to face tent. But it became obvious that when he went on the BiPAP, he wasn't going to come off. Sometimes it works and sometimes it doesn't. But I'm comfortable with it. We did everything we could do, and it didn't work because it was in God's hands, not ours.

In hindsight, this nurse acknowledged that Mr. Diangelo's "obvious" dying (judging by his dependence on the BiPAP) could have become Dying, that is officially recognized, before Monday morning. She saw the possibility of finding a more substantive plan for Mr. Diangelo than simply getting out of death's way. Still, she comforted herself that she and others did not shrink from their responsibility to try to help him. In her narrative summation she used a bottom-line assessment: they had never abandoned him, and they could not save a life that God had chosen to take. She did not assess the quality of his care in terms of his being a dying patient for two reasons: Mr. Diangelo was not considered to be Dying until Monday morning, and the important outcome that merited attention in her mind was that he had died at all.

For Mr. Diangelo, the DNR order had not brought along a distinctive treatment plan, and the status of being unrescuable disqualified him from attention paid by an authority high enough to compose one. The staff's goal in the moment was simply to lessen his work of breathing. Certainly he was not left alone, but the care he received did not match his clinical situation. He occupied a bed, a portion of a nursing assignment, and the attention of four physicians, but his dying had no status at all. The system had no way to remedy the absence of his attending and that physician's power to alter the plan of care. Accountability or oversight for appropriate clinical practice for a patient who was dying did not enter the equation as it would have for a rescuing intervention such as intubation.

Case Two: Mrs. Harper

Mrs. Harper's unrescuable status had a different outcome. Her DNR order allowed her physician the freedom to convert her irreversible neurological decline into an actively dying state, an arbitrary action that distressed the hospital chaplain. Mrs. Harper was well known to the Catholic community hospital, or at least to certain nursing units. She had been a potter before she contracted encephalopathy, a progressive disease of unknown origin. Over several months, her illness destroyed her ability to interact and finally her ability to move. As Mr. Harper visited his wife during this period, the chaplain came to know him well. Just before she died, Mrs. Harper was on three East, a general medical surgical unit that happened to have four "hospice" beds (see Chapter 6). The chaplain began her account by saying that Mrs. Harper's doctor, Dr. T., was new to the hospital, and that "he has put two patients on morphine drips."

> CH: She was declining. She was in the ICU a few weeks ago, and Dr. T met with them and talked about withdrawal. The doc handled it poorly. He may have said he was tired of it—"Let's give it up." I know because when I talked to the patient's husband, he was open to hospice.
>
> She was transferred to the step down unit. A care manager became nasty with her husband. There was this ambiguity about what's wrong, and she encouraged him to transfer her out to a nursing home. "We don't know what to do with her, so she should leave," was the message from this social worker. "Things won't be covered." To the husband, a nursing home and a long painful death seemed like the only option. He talked to me about his financial worries. How to pay for everything. He frets easily. It started when this care manager was getting after him—not being helpful.

Mr. Harper had been "open" to the possibility of hospice even when his wife was in intensive care. She achieved enough stability there to be moved to a stepdown unit. From the hospital's perspective, at this point Mrs. Harper had received the benefit of time to work out an appropriate diagnosis and treatment. But the passage of this time did not bring certainty about what was wrong or how to fix it, and now the time hung heavy. From Mr. Harper's standpoint, his wife was still gravely ill. Now the worry over her condition was being compounded by financial stress the care manager, a hospital representative, was imposing. The chaplain indicated her belief to me that the system was railroading Mr. Harper into a decision to limit his wife's treatment and to go along with finding her a new place.

> CH: Then he got sick himself. He came in through the ER and they admitted him. On Wednesday morning he was discharged. He was at home, and the doctor called him to come in to talk about the plan of care for his wife. He came in, but the doc got busy and didn't come and talk to him. But the care manager came and talked to him—harassed him—after he's just been discharged from the hospital! I sat with him through that. Somewhere she shifted into hospice as the best choice. Holding onto every last hope would cost him too much money because of all the chaos of Medicare, Medicaid, and the nursing home.

At some point during this time, Mrs. Harper had been transferred from the stepdown unit to three East, an acknowledgment that she was stable enough not to need continuous monitoring by telemetry. Mr. Harper's own sudden illness may have been related to the stress of his wife's situation and his financial worries. The care manager construed Mrs. Harper's acute treatment as "holding onto every last hope," presumably a luxury beyond his or the hospital's means. Mr. Harper knew from the previous ICU meeting that even the physician had little optimism for his wife's recovery, and his current absence, busy or not, spoke volumes. To forgo "every last hope" and simply maintain Mrs. Harper in a nursing home would be complicated and expensive, and it appeared to be an overwhelming prospect. Hospice care now seemed like the best option. A DNR order was written.

> CH: They decided to go with comfort care. He didn't shed a tear. He was the calmest I'd seen him.
>
> He wanted her to die and go quickly once the decision was made. He'd been living with this person he couldn't communicate with. She had no output. The doc made it happen as quickly as he could. Yesterday he started her on a morphine drip, but she hasn't moved in days. She did not need it for pain. I'm watching this morphine pump into her and thinking, "She's gonna die." I hadn't seen it before—the drip. Maybe I haven't been paying attention. It's more common for the nurse to give a little tiny bit in a syringe.

The husband had no idea of what was happening. He seemed unaware this morning about her blood pressure being so low. He didn't seem to get that she was about to die. It would make him crazy to know that. Families expect consistency and protocol. He didn't question and he didn't think he had any reason to. Hospice had come in to transfer her in. They had just signed all the papers.

The clinical features of Mrs. Harper's care were beyond the chaplain's ability to assess. For example, it is unclear by what means Mrs. Harper was receiving nutrition if she was not able to move, nor how long she might have survived under hospice care. What is clear to the chaplain is that Mrs. Harper was not in a position that would seem to require a continuous infusion of morphine. She was struck by the fact that Mrs. Harper's death had been deliberately hastened by the new physician for his own reasons rather than for a reason that centered around Mrs. Harper. A hospice referral had been lined up, and she was not in pain. The chaplain recognized that starting a "morphine drip" under these circumstances was outside the norms of symptom control of giving "a little tiny bit in a syringe" when life support was being withdrawn. The chaplain then commented on why the drip was used and why no one interfered with this startling new procedure.

CH: In her day she was something. So creative. Now she's in this primal, helpless state. On three East they watched her diminish. It was heart-wrenching. Whose pain did we end? The system allowed this to happen. It may have been a bizarre sense of compassion for the husband and his situation. [As if to say] "We all feel better when we do this." It was a corporate covenant. "We'll end it. No one wants to see this sad vision anymore." I'm sure the doc didn't feel it was unkind. I honestly think he thought it was the most humane choice.

The plan that Mr. Harper had agreed to was that his wife would be admitted to a hospice program the next day, not that her death would be speeded up. The physician had not been part of the discussion. The infusion he ordered lacked a clinical basis, as far as the chaplain could see, but rather came out of his "bizarre sense of compassion." A pharmacist mixed the drip and nurses logged, hung, and supervised it as it lowered Mrs. Harper's blood pressure. The chaplain includes herself when she describes this action as a "corporate covenant," something "the system allowed" to happen, even as she deeply questions its morality, and admits that "it would have made [her husband] crazy to know that."

Unlike Mr. Diangelo's case, when clinicians were left alone to work out his care in the moment and hindsight revealed a preferable plan of care, Mrs. Harper's physician tailored her dying to match his own intentions to limit everyone's suffering. No one challenged his prerogative to take this action. For the chaplain, this new physician was introducing an action violating the norm that prohibits euthanasia, and he did so without apparent consequence. The "system" (the hospital, Mrs. Harper's slow deterioration, the anxiety about reimbursement) not only "allowed it to happen," it encouraged this action.

It is unlikely that any system-level review of Mrs. Harper's case would occur. Documentation of what transpires in a patient's final hours is typically sparse—who will read it? What purpose does it serve? Its function as an ongoing communication tool among the team has come to an end. The hard copy of the medical record (the chart) leaves the unit at the same time the patient's body travels to the morgue, making it beyond the reach of unit-based quality care audits and inaccessible to anyone lacking special permission, including clinicians. "No code" patients such as Mrs. Harper fly under the radar because their deterioration is expected and for other reasons such as lack of legitimacy and because their care omits targets and mechanisms for reimbursement (see Chapter 5). With the DNR comes a certain license, an opening for arbitrary practice, even if it is well intentioned. In a community hospital with private-practice physicians as this was, little explanation and less practice oversight may be the norm.

In the larger universe of the teaching hospital, complexity rules, and it is here that we find the next two dying situations, both occurring during the night. If a dying situation puts patients and clinicians adrift, it is even more difficult to find one's way by night, when death feels closer than it does by day.

Case Three: Mr. Gomez

The night nurse on a medical floor in the teaching hospital described the last hours of Mr. Gomez's life. Mr. Gomez was a man in his 60s with advanced cancer and multiple medical problems. He was retaining fluid and was receiving treatment from the consulting vascular team for clots in his legs. The nurse felt sure that Mr. Gomez would not survive till the morning, but she could not get the covering physician to get in touch with Mr. Gomez's wife.

> RN: I had him for several days. He was short of breath. He was so short of breath, he needed to be held steady at the bedside commode

to stand to void. His second day here, the day nurse spoke to the family. She asked if they had considered his [code] status. They both looked at her. They had no idea what she meant.

From a nursing point of view, Mr. Gomez was quite literally at the edge. It was asking too much for him simultaneously to stand upright, keep breathing, and urinate, a sign to the nurse that exhaustion and respiratory arrest were right around the corner. When the patient's condition is severe enough to show warning signs of collapse before the fact, as it was for Mr. Gomez, the patient is often already too sick to benefit from resuscitation. The day nurse knew this instinctively. Accordingly, she asked the couple if an order had been written to disqualify him from what she perceived to be the futile chest compressions that she, as first responder, might be called on to deliver. The night nurse relating this story was impressed that an eventuality that seemed so obvious and critical to the staff and to the Gomezes had never been addressed with the couple. She then went on regarding the night in question.

RN: At the start of my shift his sats were eighty-eight. I pulled him up in bed and put a face tent on him and upped the setting on it to 80 percent from 60 percent. He was not going to make it through the night.

HC: Did you talk to the docs?

RN: Not at this point. His blood pressure was tenuous, and his right foot was now cool. He was responsive, but much less than he had been. I called the docs and said, "His blood pressure is low. He has pain medication every two hours. He is not moving. He is circling the drain." The attending's note in the chart said, "Will speak to the wife about patient's imminent death." I called the cross-cover doc. I told her, "We need to talk to the family about code status." His urine output had been down. Why were we doing this? Making his last hours a living hell?

Low blood pressure meant that circulatory issues were becoming acute, undermining Mr. Gomez's ability to remain conscious and to overcome the blockages to blood flow in his leg, resulting in the cold foot. He was beginning to die, as the nurse's graphic "circling the drain" conveyed.

The phrase "impending death" in the chart indicated that the attending physician also saw the writing on the wall. But this item of documentation was not an order, and it affected neither Mr. Gomez's code status nor his plan of care. What it certainly must have influenced was the place his problems occupied in the minds of covering physicians responsible for many acutely ill patients that night—somewhere close to the bottom.

His night nurse had developed a relationship with Mr. and Mrs. Gomez after several shifts with the couple. What was happening to him was quite clear to her. When she could not get the covering physician to respond, she took the action that she felt was in her power: assess Mr. Gomez, change his oxygen delivery, keep his mask on his face, and alert the cross-cover physician regularly regarding her concerns. Her top priority at first was the same one that the day nurse expressed: his code status. As a "full code" and with his stamina dwindling, Mr. Gomez clearly had chest compressions in his future, which might be hers to deliver.

RN: Then at three o'clock I didn't like the feel of his breathing. I called the cross-cover doc again. I told her, "They are going to talk to the wife, but he is not going to make it." At 4 o'clock I didn't get a blood pressure. He took more rousing. I called the doc again. "His [systolic] blood pressure is 121 because he was roused." I knew we couldn't give fluids. They needed to call the wife and tell her, "Your husband's condition is deteriorating. We don't know how close it is, but you might want to be with him." But no. This hospital doesn't do it. They are so namby-pamby about the word "death." I was sitting in his room all night to replace the mask when it slipped off. I was writing a note and the nurse came in and said, "His heart rate is down to thirty." Then asystole. We did the whole code with the mask, intubation. It went on. After twenty-five minutes—but he was dead, dead, dead. I get so upset. They don't tell the families. How can they not tell them?

As the night progressed, Mr. Gomez continued to deteriorate. The nurse left off her concern about CPR and simply wanted the wife notified so that she could be present for Mr. Gomez's death. Either unit protocols or a personal reservation prevented her from making the call herself. She proposed the words that someone in the physician's position might use to break the news gently, without needing an official recognition of Mr. Gomez's dying state or an official change in his code status. She pinned the blame for the inaction of the cross-cover physician on the hospital as a whole, as it is too "namby-pamby" about death to tell the families. Her belief that Mr. Gomez was three times dead while the team tried to call him back indicates how far out of reach the system had allowed him to drift.

Physicians who are covering for their colleagues often try to defer important treatment decisions until the morning when the primary team returns to resume care. Tiding the patient over until "real" care could resume was the goal of the weekend physicians caring for Mr. Diangelo as well. "Keep 'em alive till 7:05" (when patients can be handed off) is a phrase that I heard from more than one person. The nurse was well acquainted with this phenomenon, and during the night she downgraded her expectations of the cross-cover physician accordingly. This physician's lack of response could have been due to the number of patients under her care and more urgent matters distracting her. Meanwhile, the nurse's frustration at her own powerlessness was palpable. Mr. Gomez was suffering, and his "living hell" became hers. She was complicit in his breathlessness, the missed opportunity for Mrs. Gomez to be present with him, the failure to communicate, and in the final, futile, and avoidable resuscitation efforts when he was "dead, dead, dead."

In the morning, when it was all over, the nurse stayed after her shift to finish Mr. Gomez's paperwork. The vascular team who had consulted on him during this admission made their rounds. The nurse heard them express their surprise that Mr. Gomez had died overnight, when, as they put it, "He was fine." Her vexation erupted in this reported exchange. The nurse said: "I tell them, 'FINE? With all he had going on? [She then enumerated all his medical problems]. If he was FINE, I'd like to see one of your patients who is really SICK!' They turned and left. I'll get fired for my mouth someday."

This nurse freely expressed her indignation. She saw herself as being as powerless as Mr. Gomez, and she took on his suffering as her own, in contrast to "those" others who are too "namby-pamby" to tell the family about "imminent death." What were the constraints that made a self-described "mouthy" nurse unable to contact Mr. Gomez's family on her own? Why did Mr. Gomez and this nurse face the wee hours seemingly bereft of resources? Mr. Gomez's dying had not been made official, but the attending's note indicated that the team surely knew it. Almost any other patient need was probably sufficient distraction to keep the average young physician from attending to Mr. Gomez that night, reasoning that "nothing" could be done for him. The responses that seemed basic to the nurse were beyond the horizon of the physician, who was making choices based on pragmatism. Their differences in perspective ramped up her frustration and moral distress. What was it about the system that fogged possibilities for creativity and collaboration among the team and allowed the nurse and Mr. Gomez to drift alone and out of reach?

Case Four: Ms. Hunter

The withdrawal of life-supportive measures has become a fairly common scenario when dying occurs in the hospital—most often in intensive care settings—but clinicians' roles in its enactment are strikingly inexplicit.[10] Once the decision to withdraw has been made, the physician may not return again to the bedside.[11] Often the nurse and the respiratory therapist carry a great deal of power in planning and carrying out the process of withdrawal and in communicating the plan to the families. In Ms. Hunter's case, we see the obstacles to such negotiation that contribute to feelings of helplessness and lack of control. Like the case of Mr. Gomez, this case unfolded during the night when staffing is thinner than during the day.

Ms. Hunter had been admitted to the medical ICU in the teaching hospital with lung problems that could not be reversed, therefore it was judged appropriate to withdraw life support. Because of her unique problems, reducing ventilatory support to allow her death would be complicated. As is the case with some ICUs, this unit had devised a protocol for "terminal weaning," a specific formula for reducing ventilatory support to a dying patient under appropriate circumstances, and Ms. Hunter was a suitable candidate. The protocol required the respiratory therapist to assess the patient and adjust the settings on the ventilator every fifteen minutes in coordination with the nurse who would be administering appropriate medications. The goal was to take advantage of decreased oxygen levels in the brain to lower the patient's awareness of the dying process without bringing on the sensation of breathlessness. It was thought that tailoring this method for Ms. Hunter would carry less risk of distress for her and her family than removing the breathing tube altogether, a more precipitous method of withdrawing ventilatory support, but appropriate for some patients. The day staff nurse caring for Ms. Hunter had begun the process of terminal weaning with the family's agreement. The respiratory therapist was making vent changes more slowly than usual in Ms. Hunter's case to accommodate her particular illness. The night nurse who followed described the sequence of events.

> RN: We withdrew care. Well, we started to withdraw. It got a little funky. We have a terminal weaning protocol. Respiratory did not feel comfortable getting rid of the PEEP [Positive End Expiratory Pressure]. The day nurse had told the resident we weren't going to pull the [breathing] tube. The resident probably thought, "Okay," and went on. She [Ms. Hunter] was on just enough support to keep her going for a while. It was prolonging it. It was definitely not good for the family. They were asking "How long?" It's hard to predict. They can have a heart rate of seventy and just—[go out]. I thought, "Let me go ahead and turn her," but that didn't work either. After

four hours, we still had her on [fairly high settings]. The family was starting to question. She seemed mighty stable. And so I explained the reason they wanted to keep her vent settings up.

Here was a method of withdrawing life support customized to the patient's situation. The day nurse had described her preferred procedure to the resident: "we weren't going to pull the tube," and he did not overrule that decision.[12] Staff was therefore in control of the process, even as they perceived it to be taking an unusually long time. Change of shift had occurred, but Ms. Hunter was still stable. The night nurse acknowledged the unpredictability inherent in life-support withdrawal ("They can have a heart rate of seventy and just—[go out]"), but she was having her doubts that the protocol was steering them in the right direction. Rather than interfere with the set plan, she used another strategy to hurry things up: she repositioned Ms. Hunter, in case disturbing her body and thereby increasing her oxygen requirements would bring on her death. She explained the procedure being used to the family.

The issue of how much time passes or should pass between withdrawal of life support and death is a point of controversy (see Chapter 4). As the clinicians present assessed the situation, it seemed that the time it was taking Ms. Hunter to die was becoming more of a problem than the comfort afforded her by following the protocol.

RN: But then the resident calls up wanting the bed. He said, "What's going on? I thought she'd be gone by now." I'm in shock. It was not my smoothest withdrawal. I think, "This is great." He says, "I want the PEEP off, pull the tube." "Now," I said, "you need to send the intern over." I was upset about the miscommunication. Even the nurse educator [endorsed] the method.

This phone call from the resident upset the applecart, even as he put into words what the staff had been thinking. Although Ms. Hunter was "mighty stable" rather than clearly deteriorating toward death, the nurse did not want to change course to remove the breathing tube. But now all bets were off. The resident's directive called into question the expertise of the staff who had been leading the family through this process for the last four hours. In the heat of the moment on the phone, the nurse chose to barter. As she had just explained the present plan to the family, the change he wanted would require an explanation from someone with physician authority, and the resident was not sounding like a sympathetic choice for this. The intern would do. What mattered now was that the goals had changed, extubation would accomplish the new goal more quickly, and the family needed to be on board with the plan.[13]

The intern did not come immediately. The nurse consulted with a different nurse educator who also felt that the breathing tube should stay in place. But she had her orders.

> RN: It was uncomfortable for me. It was not very consistent with the plan of care [we'd talked about]. I ended up telling the family, "I believe she's comfortable enough now. We'll pull the tube." They were the ones who made the decision. I'd not had a problem like that. We follow the protocol. It gives the parameters.

Following the protocol had provided a guide for navigating through the uncharted seas of Ms. Hunter's dying process. Now this tool had been usurped. The physician arrived at the bedside and appropriated the process. The new course dictated that not only should the breathing tube leave the patient, but the family should also leave the patient's room.

> RN: The doctor said, "Have the family step out [for the extubation]." I would have left them in. But the doctor wanted them out. I knew she would go quickly, and she did. I think that vent support was just enough. They could have been there all night. I was glad we had done that [extubated]. The whole thing could have been much smoother. I think the family was smart enough to realize it was the vent keeping her alive. Here we are withdrawing, and here we are five hours later. Maybe they would second-guess [their decision to withdraw.] "She's still here."

Events were moving fast, and the nurse ceded her control of the process to the higher authority. Removal of a breathing tube is not a procedure to be witnessed by the faint of heart, but the family had been steadfast thus far, something that the nurse knew and the physician did not. The swift death that followed confirmed her suspicions about the process. Now her regret shifted to the lack of "smoothness" in the course of events. Not only had the "backstage" maneuvering among clinicians threatened to unhinge the "frontstage" action of professional competence being shown to the family (Goffman 1959), but the nurse was afraid that the family themselves might have been wondering about the plan all along. Does the actual hastening of Ms. Hunter's death somehow make up for the appearance of having first delayed it by (apparently mistaken) good intentions? Along the way, no less than seven clinicians had supported the first plan: two bedside nurses, two nurse educators, two respiratory therapists, and the resident. Were the

plan's strengths or weaknesses rightly to be measured simply by the duration of Ms. Hunter's dying, or rather by assessing the patient's level of comfort? In any case, its lack of smoothness seemed to be its greatest flaw, and
the nurse's narrative to me was its only opportunity for oversight.

When competition arose for the bed Ms. Hunter occupied, the efficacy
of carefully titrating her ventilatory support became a nonissue. Her bed
should rightfully belong to someone needing rescue whom the resident
wanted to admit to the ICU. The decision to remove life support had officially taken Ms. Hunter's name off his active list several hours before, and
he no longer had any particular role to play in her care. This may have
skewed the respective value of the two patients in the resident's estimation.
It was clear that he felt the new patient should take precedence over Ms.
Hunter and the once-in-a-lifetime event of her dying. To him, the ICU bed
was a scarce resource to be rationed for rescuing. But how scarce was it?

Demand for medical ICU beds in this hospital is consistently high.
Because they are a hospital resource, unit beds are usually allocated by nursing, specifically by the charge nurse. It is her job to coordinate the timing
and placement of admissions and discharges for all the beds in her unit. The
charge nurse might have known of another more appropriate bed for the
resident's new patient. Failing this, she might have had alternative resources
at her disposal to ease the patient flow problem. That the resident chose to
bypass this system put Ms. Hunter's nurse squarely in-between the patient
she was caring for and the patient he wanted to admit. Her reaction? "I'm
in shock." Caught off guard and immediately aware of the relative status
between the two patients, she did not protest. Control was wrested from her,
speed was important, and she was under the gun to explain to the family
why the withdrawal plan was shifting to its exact opposite without telling
them that another patient needed the bed. Time had run out for Ms. Hunter,
and urgency for the bed held sway. With his new patient needing rescue and
stabilization, the resident was able to bulldoze the less important standards
of bed management, terminal weaning, nursing preference for family presence, and the second-class status of a dying patient.

In telling the story, the nurse's loyalty shifted surprisingly from the first
to the second plan, despite the fact that the resident's "shocking" new orders
may have caused her to lose face professionally with the family, and, more
importantly, may have served Ms. Hunter less well. Why? Because the terminal weaning process had outlived its usefulness. The nurse interpreted it
as prolonging the death and detrimental to the family's welfare: "They were
starting to question. It was prolonging it. It was definitely not good for the
family." The nurse said: "Maybe they would second-guess. We have family

that don't want to withdraw no matter what. When we do have family who want to [withdraw], we want to help them along."

Presumably, the family members had been relying on the guidance of the medical team, with no independent standard for judging what might be a long time or a short time for dying to take. But if the nurse saw it as "prolonging," they may have picked up on her restlessness. If the patient's death does not follow very promptly after clinicians withdraw life-supportive measures, proving the "rightness" of the decision, then it may appear to the family that the patient was not really so very sick after all, and that some other course of action is or was warranted. Such an outcome puts clinicians in a very difficult position. For this nurse, the speed of the new plan made up for what it lacked in finesse.

Managing the Dying Situation

In each of these four cases, hospital demands that privileged rescue were juxtaposed with situations in which a patient was dying. In each instance, the patient's dying posed a management problem as those in charge worked to meet whatever needs seemed most important at the time. Juggling priorities was complicated by the fact that the patient was dying and could command less legitimacy in the system. In the Catholic community hospital, Mr. Diangelo and Mrs. Harper with their DNR status escaped larger notice as they were dying. Mr. Diangelo's DNR status guaranteed that he would not be intubated, but it did not procure a comprehensive plan of care for him. Mrs. Harper's DNR status allowed her physician to exercise his compassion in the way that he saw fit: by hastening her death and obviating the hospice admission her husband expected. In the teaching hospital, Mr. Gomez's dying could not galvanize action that would bring his wife to the hospital or prevent chest compressions. The plan for Ms. Hunter's dying was thrown over by a new admission. In each case, the social contract obligating quality care had expired, even though the patient had not.

During Mr. Gomez's resuscitation attempt, every action, medication, and decision pertaining to it would have been recorded along with his response to it on a special sheet designed for the purpose, enabling careful outcomes tracking and process review. By contrast, whatever the nurse documented about Mr. Gomez's care in the chart prior to the code would generate little cause for scrutiny. If Mr. Diangelo had been intubated, details of this procedure and his response to it would also have been documented clearly in his chart, allowing interested parties to trace this journey to inform their care, to improve quality, and to generate various bills for reimbursement. As it happened, the omission of a care plan for the weekend was not articulated as a problem in and of itself. It is rare that methods of oversight or account-ability exist to review pre-death phases of hospital care. Documentation regarding peri-death events is sporadic, inconsistent, and unreliable by both physicians and nurses (Kirchhoff et al. 2004). Little about this phase may be useful for billing purposes, because little is reimbursable. Because the chart leaves the unit as soon as the patient's body travels to the morgue, the motive to document for clear communication to other clinicians is moot.

These cases show that although death may be tolerated if it shows up unannounced, its precursors are distinctly unwelcome. In dying's pathless seas, clinicians pluck out various values as they search for control, orderli-ness, coherence, and protection for themselves and their patients. Mean-while, their patients' physical presence and the beds they occupy are firmly grounded, and these often present obstacles to hospital momentum. "At sea" or "on land," dying patients are perceived to be out of place, and atten-tion needed for their distinct needs is difficult to marshal. In each case, the clinicians struggled to manage several elements in the dying situation: the patient's fluid position as a part of the system; family member reactions as a potential complication; the physical deterioration of the patient; the time (long or short) that it was taking for the patient to die; and the behavior (practice) that dying situations evoked from them.

Clinicians in dying situations often experience conflicting allegiances among the entities that enmesh them: the hospital, its policies, professional norms, hierarchy among colleagues, fidelity to the patient and family, the goals of treatment, and their understanding of what they are facing. These four cases and the fifth below show that both the responses and the results depend on the individuals involved and the circumstances in the moment, rather than on overarching standards of care, protocol, or other source of clear, external guidance. The fifth case, Mrs. Morgan, a patient in the teach-ing hospital, differs from the previous four because her case conforms to the protected, orderly process of dying espoused by hospice, even though she was not under hospice care.

In none of these cases did interaction with the patients themselves about the fact that they were dying figure in the clinician narratives, and this was not unusual. Even though choice and autonomy animate many discussions about care at the end of life, none of these patients may have been well enough to process this information or to participate in choices regarding their dying process (as hospice advertises). In fact, those patients who are able to interact and exert their capacity for choice in the hospital are by this very token much less likely to be designated as Dying, regardless of their physiological state (see Chapter 7). In these accounts, patient preferences did not come up and played no role.

Case Five: Mrs. Morgan

The narratives about Mr. Gomez and Ms. Hunter do not mention whether they were aware that their lives were ending. Unlike them, it was possible for a dying patient in the teaching hospital, even outside of palliative care, to be aware of her fate, to receive attention from both physicians and staff, and for her dying situation to look like a dying process—that is, to appear peaceful, orderly, controlled, and protected.[14] Mrs. Morgan, 48, had advanced cancer and had been doing quite well. A nurse who cared for her told me her story.

> RN: She came in with high fevers. Liver and kidney failure. We could have done something about the kidney failure, but not the liver failure. We can dialyse the kidney, but not for the liver. (They're working on it.) Once she went into acute liver failure, she only had three or four days. We were mystified. All her cultures were negative. We were giving her antibiotics prior to the liver failure. There was a family conference about three days before and they apprised her and the family of the situation and made her comfort care.
>
> HC: How did they take it?
>
> RN: They were naturally upset. The younger brother was hoping for a miracle. The husband had come to grips with it. The mother was very upset. The patient was very frightened.

Despite the mystery as to what caused of Mrs. Morgan's liver failure when her cancer seemed under control, this complication was both irreversible and incompatible with continued life. Here was an indisputable physiological breakdown with a defined trajectory, unlike Mr. Gomez who had appeared "fine" to the vascular team and whose status as a dying patient was widely known yet not officially acknowledged. No withdrawal of life support would be needed for Mrs. Morgan, as it had been for Ms. Hunter, since no such sustaining process could be applied to her liver. Because she was not in the ICU, her bed was not a particularly scarce resource, and with the clock ticking down between the diagnosis and the death, she would not be bumped. With no contingencies to explore and a finite time ahead of them, open and orderly preparation for death was the best course of action for everyone involved. It was simply the only course of action left to them. Accordingly, they "made her comfort care":

HC: What were her symptoms?

RN: We were keeping her comfortable. We gave her pain meds, anti-anxiety meds. All other meds were stopped. The family was here. We opened up an extra room for them. She got more and more jaundiced. The renal failure continued to get worse. She gradually lost consciousness. She had time to say all her goodbyes to her family first.

The phrase "comfort care" indicates the power of social construction. As officially Dying (rather than simply being a DNR or a "no code"), Mrs. Morgan was entitled to "comfort measures": discontinuation of now-irrelevant medications, interventions to relieve pain and anxiety, and the continuous presence of her family, with the luxury of an extra room to accommodate their needs. Her physiological deterioration was both unquestionable and predictable, so that they could take advantage of her ebbing consciousness to complete end of life tasks. She had a "goldilocks" trajectory, foreseeable and "just right"—long enough for family to say their goodbyes and short enough to be within the realm of hospital accommodation.

HC: Did it go well?

RN: The dying process went well. She was Hispanic and her husband was American, so the family dynamics were difficult. We did our best to keep her comfortable and allay her fears. The chaplain was here a lot. Her priest came. She was not a churchgoer for a long time. She didn't want last rites. She got them when she lost consciousness. Her mother very much wanted them.

HC: Anything you would change?

RN: The outcome! We did everything in our power to make the family comfortable and to have things work out for them. The unit response was very supportive. The doc was there all the time. That was very, very helpful. Some people are just not meant to live. You cure them of one thing, and they die of something else. It's a pretty jaded view, but . . .

Even with a course clearly charted before them, unpredictable elements arose. Mrs. Morgan's anxiety, spiritual conflict, and family disagreement ruffled the waters, but the staff had the time and the resources (chaplain, priest, physician) to address these problems. It is interesting that once Mrs. Morgan could no longer spurn last rites, they were administered to her. In dying situations, it is not uncommon for those in power to influence the situation in a way that comforts themselves, whether or not it conforms to the patient's wishes. The nurse expressed her satisfaction with the collaborative effort: "We did everything in our power." The only rub was that Mrs. Morgan died at all, a fate that was out of their mortal hands: "Some people are just not meant to live." These comments echo those of Mr. Diangelo's nurse almost exactly.

For Mrs. Morgan, a place could be made for dying in the public, living world of the hospital. She could be both a dying person and a legitimate part of a community who knew her until her death came. Many observers would identify Mrs. Morgan's case as close to what they would envision as the best hospice or palliative care. No alternative agendas interfered (out-of-control symptoms, confusion about the plan, pressure for the bed, arbitrary hastening, distracted staff, poor communication), so the family, the staff, and Mrs. Morgan herself had opportunities for making and finding meaning in the situation. Here was death that could be preceded by just as much dying as there was. An unusual level of orderliness and predictability made the dying "waters" calm and navigable. The elements of this orderliness were unanimity of understanding and purpose among the team and the family, certainty about the irreversibility of the disease process; "just right" timing, collaboration among staff members, flexibility and resources to adjust responses to patient needs, and orderly physical deterioration enabling Mrs. Morgan's interaction before she lapsed into unconsciousness. Few cases of hospital dying conform to this happy combination of characteristics, even within palliative care. Many more display the features of asynchronicity, disharmony, arbitrariness, and competing system agendas that we saw in the previous four cases.

Losing One's Place while Dying

These five cases lay the groundwork for exploring the tensions that confound dying in U.S. hospitals. They indicate that ideological precepts converge at the deathbed, profoundly affecting every person within range. They illustrate a disjunction between the universal ideal of doing what is best for every patient and the on-the-ground reality of caring for persons who are dying, those who portray the finitude that the system is organized to deny. Dying and death in the hospital are often disorderly, untidy, and unpredictable and sometimes cannot be made otherwise. But such circumstances alone do not account for the problems that they present to clinicians. Although goal-driven rescue interventions for trauma and resuscitation contain chaos that outweighs the disorder of dying, their clear purpose (and auditing mechanisms) overshadows the turmoil. It is the marginal category of dying itself that places these patients beyond the reach of accountability and its standards for measurement, as subsequent chapters show. Mr. Diangelo's attending physician might have made a comprehensive plan for him. Mrs. Harper's physician could have simply allowed hospice to take over her care. Mr. Gomez might not have been abandoned to undergo a fruitless resuscitation attempt. And alternative arrangements might have allowed Ms. Hunter to die in her own time. But even if these patients' dying situations had received more direct support, the improvements would not have been counted or noticed by the hospital itself. As outcomes and evidence-based medicine gain attention, more nebulous measurements of the process that precedes the endpoint may wither. Outcome measures for hospitals involve the death itself rather than the situation that precedes it. Standards for excellence in the care of the dying continue to evolve and be promulgated,[15] but little regulatory incentive and virtually no economic motivation exists to change practice (see Chapter 8 for discussion of reimbursement of palliative care). The central cultural agenda of rescue that permeates the hospital reinforces the tendency to gloss over death and to generalize about dying, to assume that to be dying is simply to be soaked in suffering. The way to dry up the suffering is to "make them comfort care only." Dampness is unhealthy, therefore sequestration of dying and dying persons seems appropriate. Not only does this conclusion denigrate the persons who are dying, it also suspends the need for delivering or documenting nuanced care in this domain.

Dying patients have no place in the hospital rescue scheme, yet they occupy space.[16] Besides being a management problem for the hospital, this state of affairs reflects a cultural and political problem as well. Dying patients bother the living (see Chapter 3). Their dying does not present many billable encounters, therefore there are few parameters to measure (see Chapter 5). The hospitals and the communities that support them want to believe that institutions caring for the sickest members of the population can be trusted to deliver care according to each patient's particular needs, regardless of their station in life. As a society, the United States prides itself on its ability to provide at least rescue on an equal opportunity basis to all comers, especially in hospitals. To learn that hospitals might routinely consign certain persons to a secondary status, even if done unconsciously, is startling. It represents a potential threat to the national self-image. Hospitals are a public space displaying important social values such as self-reliance, altruism, and equal opportunity like colorful balloons, held aloft by the precarious hand of good business. To publicly disenfranchise a patient from sharing in these values is not sanctioned, but it functions as a cultural necessity. A specific ritual of transformation, the ritual of intensification has evolved to accommodate this need. When this ritual is enacted successfully, the patient newly designated as Dying can be moved to a less important bed for less important nonmainstream care without guilt, in the name of privacy and respect. Once that declaration has been made, however, the patient's marginalization is assured. Without hospice or palliative care, accountability for the quality of care delivered to that patient will be difficult to find. Even if every hospital provided palliative care, death will continue to find many hospitalized patients without acknowledgment or accommodation of the dying that precedes it.

Notes

1. An exception to this trend comes from the University of Washington Quality of Dying and Death tools. See Fowler, Coppola, and Teno (1999); Glavan et al. (2008); Levy et al. (2005); and Mularski (2006) for discussions of techniques and challenge.
2. All names are pseudonyms; identifying details have been altered or suppressed.
3. A DNR order removes the possibility of cardiopulmonary resuscitation, meaning that the patient will not undergo either chest compressions or intubation in case of cardiac and/or respiratory arrest. It is a physician's order written after discussion with the patient and/or the family. Hospital policies vary as to how these patients should be designated to prevent persons unfamiliar with the patient from calling a code if they find the patient in distress. In most hospitals, all patients are presumed to want resuscitation unless this order has been written. See Chapter 6 for more explanation.
4. A stepdown unit accommodates patient acuity that falls between the requirements of an ICU and the regular floor bed, with intermediate levels of staffing and technology.
5. Oxygen saturation; normal is above 91 percent.
6. This is a face mask with a bag attached that delivers a higher concentration of oxygen than a nasal cannula or face tent.
7. Bilevel positive airway pressure, which uses a machine like a ventilator but does not require intubation.
8. Intubation is the insertion of a breathing tube into the windpipe allowing breathing support to be provided with a ventilator.
9. Dilaudid is an opioid similar to morphine but more concentrated.
10. At the time of my research, guidelines and protocols were rare. My worksite had several ICUs. Where protocols existed, they varied among different ICUs, and inquiries among the nurses in the teaching hospital's ICUs indicated that even

if nurses thought a protocol existed, they could rarely place their hands on it. Only the medical ICU had a protocol that nurses actually consulted and used actively. In this teaching hospital, a protocol for withdrawal of life support was being formulated for all the ICUs, but it was not complete by the time I left the field.

11. See Shield et al. (2005). Although this study refers to nursing homes, one can transfer the problem to those farthest from rescue in hospitals—those who are dying. See also West et al. (2005) and Back et al. (2009).

12. Controversy exists as to whether it is preferable in withdrawal of ventilatory support to extubate (remove the endo-tracheal tube) or to dial down the support given by the ventilator. See Gilligan and Raffin (1996).

13. See Chapter 6 for discussion about death as the goal in the withdrawal of life support.

14. "Tame," according to Aries 1981. See Chapters 4 and 7 for discussions of orderly and disorderly dying situations.

15. Notable developments: the International Association for Hospice and Palliative Care in concert with other organizations called for the recognition of palliative care as a human right in 2008. Also in 2008, The Joint Commission called for comment on palliative care guidelines to be part of a Certification for Palliative Care Programs. Later this certification was put on hold. See Center to Advance Palliative Care (2008a) and The Joint Commission (2008).

16. This is less so as time goes on. Between 1999 and 2004, in-patient deaths declined from 40.9 percent to 37.6 percent of total deaths in the United States (Flory et al. 2004; National Center for Health Statistics 2007), and the same trend is noted in Canada (Wilson et al. 2009).

CHAPTER 2

Rescue, Stabilization, and Speed

The science of Medicine is progressive; genius irradiates its onward march. Few other sciences have advanced as rapidly as it has done within the last half century.

—Coppens 1897: 1

Mr. Wayne, 66, died in the teaching hospital's Neuro ICU as a result of a suicide. His nurse described what happened in the brief time that he was under her care.

> RN: He was a gunshot wound to the head, self-inflicted. He was in the ER about noon and here about 3:30. We withdrew care at 4:30. He expired at 5:00. . . . There were six of us working on him at first, then just me. Dr. G was in, and we sewed up his head. He was gushing blood from his head like a fountain. . . . His blood pressure was so low, he was not getting blood flow to his organs. Then he started with an arrhythmia. I went to the resident and told him, "I'm not coding this dead guy." He said, "He's a full code." I said, "Then you need to go talk to the family again." They had been very honest with the family and told them "this injury is not compatible with life." They just needed time to soak it in. . . . His [oxygenation] went down spontaneously. There was no stabilizing at that point. The resident went in and talked again with the family, and they decided to withdraw care. I turned off the vent, turned off the IV blood pressure medications, turned off the fluids, and turned the monitor off in the room. He never breathed. The family stayed with him, but with no monitor and no breathing, they left the room. . . . It all felt futile.

The first priority is to stabilize them [for organ donation]. We see so much death here, it's the only rewarding part. . . . But he made that choice (to die). It's what he wanted. Stabilizing was just letting him suffer. It was hard, whether it was six of us or just me. I was just exhausted. . . . I was feeling guilty, afraid I wasn't caring enough. Then they told me, "The family wants to see you. They want to thank you for working so hard." I felt bad. . . . There was nothing I could have done for them.

Mr. Wayne's time in the hospital was packed with activity, interventions, drama, and emotion. His nurse understood that even though Mr. Wayne's life was fading, stabilizing his vital signs must take precedence over any other activity. If his death could not be prevented, perhaps recovery of his organs could provide "the only rewarding part." But the cascade of complications could not be halted. She had no illusions that this extravagance would buy anything of value, and she wanted to clarify her own limits pertaining to resuscitation: "I'm not coding this dead guy." Dead guy. Not "this dying guy." In her mind, Mr. Wayne was either rescuable or he was dead, or all but. What does it mean when clinicians are stabilizing persons who are close to death? How are these efforts transformed into feelings of futility and suffering? How did rescuing "dead guys" become such an important cultural activity, and whose responsibility is it to define its parameters? If one is either viable and rescuable or all but dead, what could it possibly mean to be dying in the hospital?

Mr. Wayne's tragic course, the attention his situation demanded, and his nurse's distress over the apparent pointlessness of his care occurred within a broad context of priorities in the culture and in the hospital that also influenced the dying situations in Chapter 1. What are these priorities, and how did they come to be? Their development was not inevitable and their existence is not without cost. Americans have the health-care system that suits its most powerful and profit-oriented players, but not one nimble enough to respond to the diverse health-care needs of its society. If a newly designed system is to be more responsive, reformers must reckon with the ideological values expressed by the apparatus currently in place.

The unacknowledged center of health-care delivery in the United States is death prevention (Callahan 2000). Dying as a state of being collapses and expires inside hospitals, as the hospitals themselves struggle for survival. The triumph of rescue over competing perspectives on health or wellness coincides with the preeminence of the values that sustain it. The moral obligation and valiant attempts to bring Mr. Wayne back from his suicide might not have been felt if the resources to support it were not so central to the well-being of both U.S. ideology and its economics.

In the United States, the practice of biomedicine as it is displayed in hospitals has particular cultural resonance. Because hospitals must compete with one another for staff, patients, and community respect in a market-driven system, they often tap into progressive ideals to promote themselves, helping one believe that their particular combination of heroic innovation, specialization, and tender loving care will conquer disease, dissolution, and death. These beliefs relate directly to national ideology, especially to the abhorrence of dying and dependency (Hsu 1972), so that they innervate the delivery of health-care. Rescue and stabilization became crucial ways to operationalize this ideology in the last half of the twentieth century, and the myriad forms of technology supporting rescue have grown ever more elaborated and diffuse to support it. Virtually every acute-care hospital must claim to be able to monitor, restore, and maintain hemodynamic stability to some degree, because this requirement to provide acute care dominates other possible paradigms for patient management, diagnosis, and treatment, such as those in public health (U.S. Department of Health and Human Services Public Health Service 1994: 5).

The quixotic lure of preventing death connects with the American dream and its implied promise that with work and ingenuity a better future must always be just over the horizon. Reacting to impending death with rapid rescue and stabilization has become such a dazzling, compelling, and profitable project that less glamorous health-care priorities suffer from lack of "face time." By comparison, preventive and maintenance medical efforts receive little attention and become invisible. The crisis response and its presumed universal availability reflect American interests in individualism, egalitarianism, and technological display. But this priority also drains critical resources and energy away from the ongoing needs of the chronically ill, elderly, the underinsured, the disabled, and the dying.

Especially in acute-care facilities such as hospitals, relative health and illness have been recast as *stable* and *unstable*. Crisis, rescue, and maintaining stability are the order of the day. The acute-care-driven system quantifies and prioritizes illness and treatment according to the perceived imminence of crisis and potential need for resuscitation. This schema forms a vital junction between scientific rationality and sometimes unrealistic hopes for recovery on the one hand, and the productive engine of the health-care industry on the other. At the same time, it creates unnamed and unmeasured areas of ambiguity in the hospital for seriously ill and dying patients who are neither in crisis nor completely stable, waiting in limbo for a better future that seems mysteriously delayed. The effort to realize this vision of excellence leads to discrimination against those inside and outside the hospital whose illnesses do not fit the paradigm of rescue, that is, patients whose futures would not appear rosier from the benefit of stabilization measures or the application of discrete procedures.

The ontological stature that "stable" and "unstable" possess early in the twenty-first century would be unimaginable without the discovery of effective resuscitation techniques late in the twentieth century. Cardiopulmonary resuscitation and defibrillation became a reality for the first time in the mid-1960s. An explosion of rescue-related technology and technique followed, refocusing the lens through which medicine (as the agent of society and business) viewed the hospitalized patient. The ability to exert control over hemodynamic instability has saved countless patients from premature death. It has also reinforced the reductionist tendencies of medicine, placing parts before wholes and ranking body systems according to their proximity to cognition and vital signs.

A key component to this new paradigm is speed. To rescue a patient from a condition of instability is to arrest both nature and time. If a patient appears to be unstable, he is in crisis, as was Mr. Wayne. According to the nurse, "It was frustrating. I gave him 8 liters straight in. It was futile. He was in full DIC,[1] bleeding from every orifice in his body. Even his urine was bloody. His blood pressure was so low, he was not perfusing his organs." Each of her observations signaled circulatory collapse and expressed both the need for urgent intervention and its pointlessness. Mr. Wayne was clearly dying, but not to act in a clear situation of urgency would constitute abandonment.

In cases of bodily collapse, life depends on pinpointing and correcting the hemodynamic or respiratory difficulty within five to six minutes to forestall irreversible cardiac decompensation and death. Stabilization thus occupies a different *and prior* category from other healing efforts in the hospital. Without it, diagnosis and treatment for accompanying illness or injury cannot get started. Circulatory and respiratory systems take precedence over other vital functions (such as kidney or liver failure) because their degradation or arrest brings the body to the point of death more quickly than dysfunction elsewhere. Because of the requirement for speed, most hospitals specify that patients are "full code" (that is, eligible for resuscitation) unless their physician has written a "Do Not Resuscitate" (DNR) or "Do Not Attempt Resuscitation" (DNAR) order.[2] The implementation of resuscitative measures is perhaps the only procedure that requires a specific order to *prevent* its occurrence, rather than one that requires it to be done. The default mode in the hospital, without such a countermanding order, is to rescue first and ask questions later. Mr. Wayne's nurse said: "Then he started with an arrhythmia. I went to the resident and told him, 'I'm not coding this dead guy.' He said, 'He's a full code.' I said, 'Then you need to go talk to the family again.'"

The most unstable patients require many interventions delivered simultaneously by several clinicians at the bedside, as happened with Mr. Wayne when he arrived in the ICU. For him, speed and six nurses could not get ahead of the circulatory derangement. His slowing heartbeat was the cue that the last resort of chest compressions would be needed very soon.

Rescue is the most intensive of care, and it may begin outside the hospital enacted by bystanders or EMTs in response to a 911 call. Successful stabilization "buys time" to define and correct the original cause of the collapse. Brain injury was the obvious culprit for Mr. Wayne, and every attempt to stabilize him was failing. Resuscitation efforts are more likely to succeed if they are the first response to an unexpected event rather than the last resort after a cascade of complications.[3] This was exactly the situation for Mr. Wayne, and the nurse knew it. Assuming their conditions improve, rescued patients more fortunate than Mr. Wayne may require fewer clinical interventions over time, such as intravenous medications or decreased respiratory support, and/or these can be more widely spaced. Clinicians consider these patients and their conditions to be more stable. They become eligible for transfer to a floor unit and, if they continue on their course of increasing stability, they are discharged from the hospital. Thus, the concept of hemodynamic stability exists along a dual continuum of time and the intensity of medical interventions.

Speed of application is crucial to the success of other medical interventions that have followed on the heels of cardiopulmonary resuscitation. Think of the "golden hour" of trauma, "time is muscle" for heart attack, "early goal-directed therapy" in severe infection or sepsis, "brain attack" (intervening early to decrease intracranial pressure), and "stroke alert." In each case, the rapidity of the response is at least as important as the intervention itself in saving function, tissue and lives. Without immediate intervention to correct the disarray caused by the malfunction, the patient's life and future (here synonymous) are in jeopardy. Urgency saturates all forms of life-saving.

The ability to rescue some patients from sudden and certain death and the requirement for speed are not the only ingredients making patient stability a foundational consideration for hospital clinicians in the United States. The policy of universal application compels hospitals to ensure nondiscrimination in the delivery of this most expensive care. This egalitarian posture can put the acute-care hospital's bottom line at risk. Institutional survival maps to the uncertain fate of the seriously ill. It is difficult to underestimate the significance of these tandem developments: a social insistence on equal opportunity rescue and the fact that stability has become a gauge of both physical and financial vigor. As such, the rescue endeavor forms a crucial bridge between the medical surgical work of the hospital and its viability as a business. Rescue's role in hospital business management comes not from measuring its success or failure in patients such as Mr. Wayne, but from the fact that relative stability is more quantifiable than nuanced descriptions of health or illness, making this classification a critical tool in hospital bed management. Putting basic survival first is a simpler ranking device than sorting through all the comorbidities of a chronically ill patient when beds are full.[4] Accordingly, the supremacy of rescue and stabilization extends beyond trauma care and the ED to set priorities throughout the hospital. Moving patients between intensive care and floor units is a decision of triage, of risk stratification. A patient with a higher potential for instability, someone with an dangerously low heart rate and a still-normal blood pressure, may be hurried into the ICU, supplanting the patient whose heart attack was stabilized by stent placement in the culprit vessel twenty-four hours before. In fact, optimal bed management dictates a preemptive strike, moving the heart attack patient out before another emergency occurs, so that the bed can be cleaned and the room readied with new equipment. (See the discussion in Chapter 6 of Code 100.) Even *potential* instability becomes equivalent to *actual* instability in terms of triage decisions, and the legitimacy of a claim to the limited resource, an ICU bed, is judged accordingly.

On the other end of the spectrum, more stability decreases the need for clinical time and attention, making discharge from the hospital's acute-care environment possible, whether the patient is well, cured, or healed. Therefore, stability/instability is a shorthand descriptor for the intensity of attention, intervention, and monitoring needed from the hospital and its clinicians, making it an effective substitute for a description of the patient's overall health or illness.

The key to the strength of this priority is to notice that an actively dying patient who may be officially under palliative care is *not* considered unstable. It is the linkage of instability with crisis and the urgency of time that focuses clinical and institutional attention. Patients in crisis (or who are potentially so) bring a correspondingly higher rate of reimbursement to the hospital, making them targets of economic as well as clinical concern.[5] To designate a patient as dying, therefore, is to make them essentially disappear from the hospital's democracy of rescue, so that they become invisible both economically and culturally. Undertaking such a serious social demotion requires ritual, as we shall see in subsequent chapters.

The urgency, speed, and intensity associated with rescuing patients from instability are infectious. They ensure both momentum and elaboration: momentum, because a sense of urgency and goal-directed movement from many individuals is endemic to rescue, and elaboration, because each intervention brings a subset of more expansive next steps. One thing leads to another as the process of rescue takes on a life of its own. This momentum and goal-directed care pervades even the routine work of the hospital. Maximizing "patient flow" opens up beds for new admissions. Transience and propulsion rule, an inexorable phenomenon in hospitals that Sharon Kaufman describes as "moving things along" (2005: 236). It is patient instability that defines the speed of this movement and the rescue imperative that quickens the step (Brody 1992). The rapid response used to save lives dovetails with and reinforces the economic benefit of productivity, "moving things along" with alacrity so that not just the patient, but the hospital itself may survive and thrive.

The trickle-down effect of rescue work unearths ancillary problems to be solved with every moment that the patient survives. All her underlying chronic health problems now become eligible for management as well, even if they had not been covered (by insurance or by medical attention) prior to her need for rescue. Even chronic illness becomes a crisis in periods of exacerbation, making it suddenly eligible for heroic intervention and rescue.[6]

The paradigm of stability affords clinicians and hospitals another useful feature: responding to crisis as the first priority for every patient leaves little room for social judgments.[7] This is not to say that discrimination is not alive and well in the hospital, but only that, as a rule, clinicians *intend* to deliver an equally high standard of care to every patient, without regard to its cost or anyone's social preferences. Unacceptable disparities in access, treatment, and outcomes characterize U.S. health-care, despite these good intentions. This discrimination, whether unconscious or conscious, exists both on the individual and the hospital level with devastating effects (G. Becker 2004; Bernato et al. 2005; Institute of Medicine 2003; Putsch and Pololi 2004; Schulman et al. 1999). But the standards for deploying rescue without discrimination, this particular "best care standard," are codified in hospital policy, federal law, and clinical practice, and clinicians believe they are practicing these standards.

Nurses predictably balk when told that a certain patient is a VIP and deserving of special consideration. "That's ridiculous. I don't play favorites. I give the same good care to all my patients," one colleague complained to me.[8] This stated practice coincides with U.S. democratic values as well as with the assumption that Western biomedicine is cerebral, scientific, and free of subjective bias (Hahn and Kleinman 1983: 312). Rescue may be the one facet of health-care that the system attempts to guarantee to everyone. The problem is that those with inadequate health insurance coverage must undergo physical collapse before they are invited to the medical party. In addition, the culture of rescue enacts a new iteration of social discrimination, drawing a line between the rescuable patients and those disqualified through the ritual of intensification.

In sum: stability/instability relates to rescue and crisis. It is measurable, thereby becoming a critical tool for hospital management and reimbursement. It provides momentum and clear objectives, and it appears to preclude social judgments. It reflects a hierarchy of clinical management requirements more than it describes the condition of the patient. It is both reflective of and active in a gradual shift in the focus of hospital care from "just" diagnosing and treating illness to a perpetual readiness to operate in crisis mode. How did this shift arise, and how does it influence the care of dying patients?

The display of intensity, speed, and complexity of rescue efforts such as Mr. Wayne's would appear to pass for the apex of medicine as it is understood and delivered in the United States. This belief persists despite research findings that show that the opposite is true: just like the news, all health-care is local. Regional areas featuring high medical intensity actually correlate with poorer health outcomes (Wennberg 2006). Further, to lionize such a narrow segment of health-care delivery imposes a hierarchy, with excellence in rescue becoming not only the highest, but also the most desirable standard of practice. This attitude engenders discrimination against those who are not collapsing, including those well enough to read the words printed on this page: persons with minor maladies, ongoing chronic illnesses (physical or mental), and those who are dying.

The most social value accrues to conquering the highest perceived threat. Holding back death and delivering more time alive would appear to count for much more than restoring or maintaining health. Having a health-care system that displays this priority was not inevitable. What has caused technological expertise and value in U.S. health-care to be associated with medical excellence and dramatic rescue? Why are chronic care and public health so much of a secondary concern? How did it come to be so, and what has been sacrificed along the way?

In the pages that follow, I review the reductionist tendencies in health-care delivery and how they developed by exploring shifts in the landscape of U.S. medical practice. Reductionism is not the whole story, however. It is important to notice how the increasing focus on the indispensible has joined with both intensity and speed, and how eliminating the causes of death has united the bottom lines of both physical and financial well-being.

Development of the Gold Standard: Reductionist Shifts

Several historical developments in U.S. health-care delivery converged over the course of the twentieth century to bring the rather narrow area of rescue into prominence. Medicine's understanding of disease trumped the idea prominent in the mid-1800s that biological dysfunction was traceable to social causes.[9] As an explanatory model, germ theory was more malleable and focused. It clearly supported a tendency toward specialization over generalist approaches. Such developments increasingly tipped the balance toward acuity and intensity, and more treatment became squeezed into smaller periods of time. By comparison, more diffuse, less dramatic medical needs (including public health) along with calls for incremental rather than transformative interventions, fell by the wayside.

Even though the roots of reductionist shifts existed well before the beginning of the twentieth century, it is helpful to start with the Flexner Report of 1910, which set the stage for trends that would unfold in the next 100 years. Commissioned by the Carnegie Foundation, the Flexner Report evaluated the state of medical education in the nation at a time when many physicians were traveling to Europe for their training (Flexner 1960 [1910]).The report placed an official stamp of approval on biomedicine's emerging dominance by defining the official domain of medical practice and applauding its preference for science and reductionism, thereby steering it away from social issues or ethnomedicine. It helped clear the field of competing influences, whether they were ideas or stakeholders.

The report cemented the emerging shape of American medicine with the dominance of allopathic medicine over its rivals (Baer 2001; Navarro 1976). It did this by recommending explicit connections among three entities: *physicians*, yoking them to funding through philanthropic support; *hospitals*, which could ensure the reproduction of the medical profession; and *science*, the use of research and technology to justify authority in practice. These linkages ensured that the medical elite, in service to the social elite, would articulate and dominate the shape of health-care delivery in the United States.

Shift One: Research Focus Narrows to Germ Theory and Killer Diseases

In the mid-nineteenth century, Rudolf Virchow promoted the idea that disease had social and economic origins (Taylor and Rieger 1985), but by 1900 his capacious vision had lost out to the new model of germ theory. The narrowing of medicine's focus from society to the cell illustrated a dominant assumption that "nature" was exempt from outside influences such as society, time, space, spirit, and cultural understanding (Gordon 1988; Kuhn 1996). It also portended the partnership of clinical, medical, and surgical practice with devices of instrumentation. Allopathic medical practice aligned itself with science, systematic research, and its puzzle-solving methods (Kuhn 1996: 36–39; Muller and Koenig 1988).

The Carnegie Foundation's sponsorship of Flexner's survey and report brought germ theory, capitalism, and philanthropy together in a weighty alliance. These narrower approaches to research and practice blossomed through significant financial support. One example was the "full-time plan," an idea for shaping medical practice that came out of the report. This plan disallowed consulting fees for top physicians at teaching hospitals, freeing them for research and helping guarantee the prevalence of the germ theory of disease (Berliner 1985).

In Europe, medical training was already hospital based and beginning to be specialized at the turn of the twentieth century. Germany prioritized scientific research as the basis for clinical medicine and trained many U.S. physicians, and this model became a U.S. prototype.[10] Young physicians returning from study abroad endorsed the European model of systematic research. Machines and factories now dominated production and permeated public consciousness so that considering the human body as the focus of attention and as the mechanistic object of manipulation were medical habits on the rise (Cassell 1974; Foucault 1977, 1994; Osherson and Amara-Singham 1981). Landmark successes—such as Jenner's discovery in 1796 that an injection of cowpox gave immunity to smallpox and the Curies' work with rabies—had already compelled researchers to focus on the search for similar "magic bullets." Because they seemed more targetable, these finite and malleable concepts of disease and the body made research a project that endowments and foundations could fund enthusiastically, post-Flexner.

Philanthropic dollars flowed into the laboratory, and in 1932 the first sulfa drugs were developed—then dramatically proved their worth by saving the life of President Roosevelt's son. A 1939 grant from the Rockefeller

Foundation helped Howard Florey and Ernst Chain isolate penicillin. Prior to the 1940s, acute infectious diseases such as these dominated fledgling research efforts because they were considered more tractable than chronic illness. With public attention focused on the drama of antibiotics, it was more difficult to notice that the real gains in public health and greater life expectancy before the 1940s came from innovations such as reliable public sanitation and running water and the availability of less crowded living conditions.

After World War II, federal interest in science policy brought public funding into research, galvanizing the mission of the new National Institutes of Health (NIH) and eclipsing philanthropic donations. By mid-century, with the dramatic achievements of antibiotics and the doubling of the average life span in fifty years, the social mandate given to research endeavors in the transition from philanthropic to federal funding was "Don't let us die." NIH shifted its research emphasis to noninfectious causes of death: cancer, heart disease, stroke, diabetes mellitus, and, later, AIDS. Compared to infectious illnesses exacerbated by crowded living conditions, most of these were diseases of modernity and relative affluence. The key strategy shifted from reducing deaths in populations to reducing the threat of individual death by attacking its causes in the individual.[11] In that spirit, the research projects of cancer, heart disease, and stroke established their legitimacy with burgeoning infrastructure, receiving large amounts of money early and often from NIH.[12]

Successful rescue from a life-threatening assault transforms a disease into a set of chronic problems: heart attacks and strokes turn into congestive heart failure and rehabilitation. Their less-galvanizing, open-ended manifestations command much less attention until the condition becomes exacerbated sufficiently to require another rescue. Chronic conditions are certainly an improvement over rapid, unexpected demise, but the discovery of magic bullets effective against them is elusive. Meanwhile, death-defying research is a heroic endeavor, and the infrastructure to support it is well established. Charles Rosenberg aptly describes its place in medicine: "Even if we regard it as romantic or delusive, the idealization of research and its presumably inevitable practical applications has always been a part of the emotional and institutional reward system of science—and thus of medicine" (2006: 18; and see Callahan 2003).

National pride and corporate investment now fuel the massive research endeavor in the United States. Profit potential in the health-care industry helps direct its priorities (Angell 2009; Callahan 2003). (See Chapter 5 for a discussion of technology and its connection to salvation.) The paradigm shift toward medical care that is evidence based—grounded by investigational findings of well-designed clinical trials—reinforces the emphasis on measurement and results versus process. In an environment that insists on ever more stringent standards of proof and positive outcomes, it is ironic that resuscitation's poor record of success has not materially threatened its central status.[13] In an affluent, death-defying culture, research that pushes the limits of finitude is sure to be frustrated as its targets become ever more elaborated, diffuse, and elusive, but its position at the bench will remain undisturbed.

Shift Two: Shifting Targets for Medical Attention and Intervention

Over the twentieth century, the social standard that dictates whom (or what entity) should receive health-care narrowed from the welfare of the general populace to the single patient in the bed. In acute care, this focus has compressed even further from the body in general to distinct organ systems. Such concentration of attention supports the practices needed for rescue and stabilization. This shift is inseparable from corresponding changes in the sites of medical practice discussed in the next section, but it is broken out here for ease of organization.

In the twentieth-century United States, "dirty" individuals became more troubling than dirt itself to the well-being of the populace. As Mary Douglas (1966) points out, hygiene is a critical means of structuring the social and cultural order, and the understanding of what entities were responsible for producing contamination shifted during this period. Mirroring the gains in bacteriology, the twentieth-century perspective shifted from the promotion of public sanitation in general to individual personal habits in particular. As opposed to European understandings, Americans view hygiene as both an expression of rationality and a distinctively U.S. virtue (C. Davies 1996; Starr 1982). The germ theory contributed to the importance of personal responsibility in preventing contamination by indicating that dirt alone was less important in causing disease than deficient personal hygiene, resulting in a more politically acceptable and less expensive approach to public health.[14] The virtues of cleanliness, always more accessible to people of means, moved into a more exalted dimension in hospitals at this time with the development of sterilization, a ritual that cancels pollution.

Well before Flexner made his report in 1910, a tiered hierarchy for the delivery of health-care that held most-favored recipients at the top was firmly in place. Slaves and former slaves had virtually no access to hospitals or to health-care and because of their race did not often qualify as the "deserving poor," the legitimate objects of charity (Byrd and Clayton 2000). At the end of the nineteenth century, most actual medical care was given at home, and a few urban dispensaries treated the poor. Hospitals in their early incarnations were unclean places for "unclean" people—pesthouses (for the sick without families) and almshouses (charities for the deserving poor). In these institutions, inmates often cared for each other. The public's interest in avoiding dirt and contamination as sources of disease translated into a fear of the Other, the "nonnormal," seen as potentially contaminating (Baynton 2001). The ability to project contamination outside of oneself is an antidote to fears of social and personal susceptibility, as Sander Gilman describes:

> [T]he fear we have of our own collapse does not remain internalized. Rather, we project this fear onto the world in order to localize it and, indeed, to domesticate it. For once we locate it, the fear of our own dissolution is removed. Then it is not we who totter on the brink of collapse, but rather the Other. And it is an-Other who has already shown his or her vulnerability by having collapsed. (1988: 1)

The fear of death, dependency, and of the Other coalesce as a mechanism of self-protection. "Degeneracy" as a term for the Other had become a popular concept and useful as a channel for social anxiety in the late nineteenth century (Bauman 1992: 151). Its continued utility helped fuel the eugenics movement in the first quarter of the twentieth century. Sterilizing persons with mental retardation, for instance, would presumably stop the hereditary proliferation of "degeneracy." Social "fitness" gained legitimacy from science as it simultaneously undermined social outreach (Lombardo 2008).

Eugenics and its one-by-one solution to "degeneracy" through sterilization did not seem to be an extreme measure prior to World War II. In this period, the definition and role of public health was in flux and guarding the well-being of the population was falling out of favor. Physicians were entrepreneurs in the first decades of the twentieth century, uninvolved in the emerging hospital bureaucracies. They wished to practice in residential communities with families and individual patients, an arrangement that suited both parties (Freymann 1977: 43–44).

By the 1930s, clear lines between preventive and curative medicine had been drawn in the infrastructure, even if they could not be in patients themselves, and preventive medicine clearly held secondary status. Health became embodied in having regular checkups. Physicians applauded public health efforts such as these individualized exams that boosted their practices (Starr 1982). Competition from group patient settings such as venereal disease clinics was less to their liking. The historic association of public health with social welfare tainted public health in the eyes of health-care interests that were increasingly tied to market forces. A countervailing movement in favor of public health rose between 1875 and 1930 without strong success. Public health and chronic illness concerns continued to be accommodated poorly within the now-prevailing acute-care framework (Fox 1993: 56).

With increasing medical specialization, the treatment of individual bodies gave way to the focus on separate organ systems. Hospitals were reorganized in terms of physiological breakdown, rather than by social class (see below).

Shift Three: Practice Sites of Health-Care Delivery

The reductionism of explicitly scientific, disease-focused medicine and the primacy of individuals over populations corresponded with emerging styles and locations for medical practice. In the United States, these shifts occurred in three domains: (1) It became necessary for the sick to physically move toward the care they sought rather than to expect that care would approach their sickbeds. Ambulatory (outpatient) care moved from homes and clinics to physician offices (for those who could afford it) or to emergency care in hospitals, and a proliferation of hospitals became the means to broaden public access; (2) surgical intervention emerged as the premier hospital service; and (3) hospital bed allocation shifted from social to physiological demarcations. Each of these developments deserves a closer look.

Public Health to Inpatient Care

In 1900, hospital beds were filled by persons at the margins of society, and the movement of large city hospitals from the periphery to the center of medical practice did not appear very likely. In Flexner's time, most medical care was being delivered by junior physicians outside of hospitals in dispensaries and clinics, often at no charge to the patients (Rosenberg 1987: 316). Although this practice provided challenging cases for the hospital's attending physicians to oversee, it garnered them no status and served the patients poorly. Nonetheless, the public (and some physicians) opposed this free care, seeing it as morally hazardous and encouraging abuse. Dispensaries and community care might have become the center of focus for medical care delivery, but because of the social skepticism regarding free outpatient care and the trajectory toward greater concentration, this was not to be so (Starr 1982: 182, 184).

Shorter hospital stays, higher acuity, and sentiment against widespread charity care corresponded to the new alpha: the rise of private medical interests over public health. At the time of the Flexner Report and afterward, outpatient care, too, declined in importance as clinical interests moved closer to the laboratory's hard science and the drama of the operating room.[15]

Many hospitals and medical schools closed after the Flexner Report, especially homeopathic schools and those catering to African American students (Baer 2001: 36, 39, 40). These institutions were ill positioned to take advantage of the reductionist trends in biomedical research and practice. Dispensaries with their walk-in clinic services disappeared along with the doomed medical schools. The institutions that expanded and thrived were those with the wherewithal to procure the facilities, the technology, the potential for specialized services such as pathology, and the nursing expertise to care for patients (Rosenberg 1987: 344).

Surgery as the Premier Hospital Offering

One word encapsulates the rise of the U.S. hospital's social position in the public's view: surgery. As the hospital became the primary site for the treatment of acute medical problems, surgery came to occupy a central place in every type of hospital. The divergent cultures of indirect versus direct methods of healing characterizing medicine and surgery have been recognized since the 1750s in England and France. The hospital became an advantageous location for both practices, but surgery maintained a special prestige. Today, surgical procedures are reimbursed at a higher rate than general medical care, and they form the backbone of hospital revenue (see Chapter 5).[16] Because it is both an economic lynchpin for the hospital and a mainstay of rescue, surgery has a unique place in the story of rescue's rise to prominence. Its dramatic effects make it attractive and accessible to public understanding, and its clear-cut results and boundaries make it a good fit with results-oriented medical care and U.S. interests in progress, drama, and individualism.

A more performative practice than medicine, surgery's history includes public displays of violence to the human body done in the name of treatment, often in emergency circumstances. By 1910, surgical training had moved away from the amphitheatre in Europe, but surgical lectures followed by demonstrations continued in U.S. hospitals until the 1940s (Wangensteen and Wangensteen 1978: 472). Improved ventilation and cleanliness, along with greater understanding of germs because of Joseph Lister, decreased the fear of infection, enabling surgery to move from dispersed homes to the hospital. Gradually, surgery's outcomes became more important than its exhibitionary aspects, allowing surgeons to transfer its corrective powers from emergencies to elective procedures. The technological requirements of operating rooms began to dictate hospital design, and hospitals gained legitimacy through their association with surgical success (Rosenberg 1987: 343). As its power became dominant in the hospital setting, surgery brought along its heroism, its faith in progress, its clear-cut boundaries, its spectacular results, and its one-by-one care. As a strategy for personal enhancement, surgery's prestige continues to grow (Rothman and Rothman 2003).

Surgery both reflects and replays American ideology. During the nineteenth century, surgeons were seen as civilizing, democratic heroes. The wellspring of this high virtue was the backwater of the body where, surgeons declared, "darkness was giving way to light and civilization was taming the 'primary terrors' of pain and suffering."[17] This impression of subjugating was doubly reinforced in the South if the person undergoing surgery was black, as the sufferers of surgical learning and experimentation often were (Savitt 1982). The language of the frontier and its heroic submission was self-consciously used to describe surgery in nineteenth-century documents, but it is not lost in the late twentieth century. The persistent prestige of surgeons is evident in Charles Bosk's observations during his 1970s research into surgical mistakes. "As my research progressed, I was struck by the almost primal awe my friends and acquaintances had for surgeons. Normally sophisticated urban dwellers . . . would literally beg for details about what surgeons were really like, about what went on in operating rooms, about what their doctors were really like" (1979: 210). The popularity of recent "body dramas" in television programing (Jacobs 2003) is further evidence of a public fascination with surgeons and even a return to the voyeurism of the surgical amphitheater.

Elective surgeries are the most lucrative for hospitals, but it is the link between surgery, trauma, and the ED that enhances the dramatic persona of surgery in the imagination. The association of rapid intervention to better outcomes from injury has given rise to benchmarking trauma-response levels for hospitals, which carry prestige for attracting potential patients and staff. To achieve Level One Trauma Center status requires a costly infrastructure along with high on-call payments to surgeons, and this cachet is expensive for hospitals to maintain (Taheri 2004).

Hospitals Enabling Wide Access to Advanced Care
Hospitals now classify patients and their care according to stability and by the primary body system affected. Just as workable CPR is a very recent invention, the categorization of patients along medical rather than racial or class boundaries is also new. It reflects the shift of the site of medical attention and intervention from the particular body to its parts.

The evolution of hospital types during the twentieth century reflected social demarcations, even as some hospitals brought diverse social classes into close proximity. As hospital insistence on standardizing medical documentation had an equalizing effect (see Chapter 1), some hospitals brought different social classes closer together for physician convenience and to improve medical education (Starr 1982: 171–172). But patients did not actually mix by race in the first two-thirds of the twentieth century. Black patients were often treated in halls and basements if they were admitted to white hospitals at all, a pattern of marginalizing medical care for African Americans rooted in slavery (Byrd and Clayton 2000; Smith 2005a).

After World War II, a priority toward health-care emerged in the national consciousness. Postwar optimism and growth sought to correct the inequalities in the hospital system as part of a vast expansion in health-care delivery. On the heels of a successful war effort, the government sought to alleviate the afflictions of its populace by investing resources on two fronts: medical research (expanding the impact of NIH) and local hospital construction. The idea was that by building new hospitals in every community and tying the funding support to provisions for the needy, the nation's expanding productivity would provide the resources to take care of the nation's health-care without resorting to "socialized medicine," anathema to the now-powerful American Medical Association (AMA). This approach illustrates a popular political stance toward systemic inequality in the United States: it is best to grow your way out of it. The 1946 Public Health Service Act (Hill Burton Act) provided assistance to 6,900 hospitals in the next three decades. It expanded and upgraded the number of hospital beds and improved access to hospital care in rural areas.[18] The mid-century passage of this legislation confirmed several facts about health-care: widespread social inequality existed and needed correction; a belief that the best, most advanced health was the most concentrated in its methods (i.e., research-based, surgical, customized to the individual, and located in the hospital); and a confidence that growth in the latter would solve the problems of the former.

We have explored concentrations that occurred in three material, visible practices in health-care in the twentieth century: research, medical treatment, and sites of practice. Two intangible shifts in the perceptions of time accompanied these operational adjustments. Shift Four involves intensity and time *compression*: stuffing more activity and intervention into smaller segments of time. It involves the move from waiting and watching, a conservative approach associated with passivity rather than action, to more aggressive care. Intensity becomes the order of the day: trauma care, war, speed, triage, ER, ICU, CPR. Here we see that clock time is the enemy because it is finite, running out, and cannot be reversed (Adam 1995: 39). Time is something to fight, the immediate obstacle to be overcome, in order to insert the corrective interventions needed to hold back death. Rapid defibrillation transforms sudden death from a final statement into a reversible syndrome, contingent on the application of rescue. The catastrophic event discloses or induces hemodynamic instability, but it need not be allowed to define the outcome—correction is available, if it occurs swiftly and intensely enough.

But clock time is also something to fight for, and Shift Five explores the use of technology in the hospital to "buy" time.[19] A larger quantity of time alive is what rescue in hospitals produce, fighting against time to buy time, indifferent to its quality. Bare survival is the minimum victory required for all others. Technology for instrumentation and treatment *expands* time. Time stops (through the ritual of intensification, see Chapter 7) in service of procuring the future, starting with more time alive, the product that the staff of the Neuro ICU attempted to deliver on Mr. Wayne's behalf. Life lived in the hope of simply obtaining more time alive is of greater value, presumably, than any moments lived without the promise of an unlimited future.

Shift Four: Using Intensity to Compress Time: War, Drama, and Rescue

The shift to greater intensity in rescue harnessed into service the rising obsession with speed in the struggle against death. *Fighting for survival* became the new understanding of what it meant for Americans to overcome adversity in the area of health-care. Perhaps this change from conquering the "frontier" through the scientific advancement of the middle decades of the twentieth century resulted from experience with four major wars. Certainly a preoccupation with the imagery of war implies death, drama, and heroism. Obituaries of deceased cancer patients frequently cite the valor of the fight waged against cancer. Stories of American heroes of health-care resonate strongly, such as organ transplant recipients and Lance Armstrong who overcame cancer in 1996 and raced against time on his bicycle to unparalleled victories. By contrast, Christopher Reeve, the Superman rendered utterly dependent in 1995 by a spinal cord injury, faded out of the spotlight because such profound dependency was abhorrent to a people obsessed with self-reliance.[20]

Battlefield experience itself had a very real impact on clinical medicine, especially in rescue and triage. Here was the most profound social disorder and violence, reflected in multiple acute and life-threatening injuries to the body. These disruptions compelled greater intensity of treatment, spawning entire systems designed to enable rapid intervention. Each successive war in the twentieth century brought a deeper understanding of shock (the hemodynamic response to injury), new surgical techniques, the importance of antibiotics, and most of all, the impact of time on the patient's outcome. Medical and surgical intervention moved ever closer to the lines of battle until helicopters made swift evacuation to trauma teams on hospital ships possible (Gabriel and Metz 1992; Wangensteen and Wangensteen 1978). Survival rates from initial injury continued to improve, showing that speed was nothing less than a life and death matter.

No widespread effort was made to transfer this knowledge to civilian application at first, even though urbanization, automobiles, and affluence had amplified civilian trauma. A National Academy of Science publication "Accidental Death and Disability: The Neglected Disease of Modern Society" published in 1966 helped focus medical and surgical attention on trauma. At this point, the drama of rescue in the field began to be explicitly transferred to U.S. everyday experience and to public expectations of appropriate medical care (e.g., rapid evacuation to treatment areas with skilled staff able to intervene immediately to correct the effects of the traumatic insult and save lives). Also in 1966, effective cardiopulmonary resuscitation became a reality with the invention of the defibrillator, so that "sudden cardiac death" could eventually be classified as an illness rather than an outcome. As the most troublesome afflictions such as cancer were proving to be more intransigent to research efforts, events in the domain of trauma care could not help but transform the orientation of hospital medical practice and the expectations of the public, much as the discovery of antibiotics and the rise of surgery had done in the first half of the century.

With successful rescue came elaboration. By the 1960s, intensive care and its technology demanded that hospitals adjust physical design and retool nursing skills. Now that mechanical ventilation, cardiac monitoring, and defibrillation were available, coronary care units proliferated in U.S. hospitals, even though their efficacy in reducing morbidity and mortality was not proven (Waitzkin 1983). Various centers of power in the country collaborated to build the necessary infrastructure: academic medical centers, philanthropy, corporations, medical device manufacturers, federal legislation, and research.

The 1970s brought federal support for a national vision of field rescue through the 1973 Emergency Medical Services Systems Act, which would build a system that would presumably make emergency health-care available to everyone (Beachley 2002). Building on the life-saving potential of CPR and the efficacy of rapid, coordinated intervention, attention to the trauma victim caught the national imagination. The neighborhood fire station became the model for rapid response among the local citizenry, the resource for rescue from both fire and physical collapse. Under the direction of surgeons, hospitals incorporated a specialized, intense response to trauma, beyond general emergency care and separate from surgical care. Both CPR and trauma care required rapid, coordinated, and intense response for the patient to stand a chance. Stability linked up with trauma care, becoming a model for patient care in general. Robert J. Baker noted in 1978 that certain "facts of life" in emergency care would become pervasive, predictions that have proved correct: "Categorization and regionalization are facts of life in emergency medical services delivery, as well as in other, less visible areas. It is imperative that all concerned physicians realize that as yet untouched health care segments will be treated in a similar way in the future" (p. 1134).

Pressure to deliver intense rescue interventions with excellence and speed came to define many academic medical centers. The ability to do so is benchmarked and advertised. Level One Trauma Centers typically feel pressure to maintain this status, reflecting the prestige and heavy expense of providing cutting-edge, salient (because it appears dramatic and heroic) medical care to all comers, even the "undeserving poor," that is, those who are most often affected by traumatic injury.

Rescue may not always involve trauma, and trained bystanders can perform CPR and defibrillate patients. It is trauma's urgent link to surgery and to technology as the strategy of rescue that compels the hospital to be "rescue headquarters." The trauma patient's injuries may require that several surgical teams work on different parts of the body simultaneously, again highlighting speed and intensity as the most efficacious standard of care. Not until the surgical team transfers the patient to intensive care is resuscitation considered to be complete (VonRueden and Hartsock 2002).

Shift Five: Using Technology to Expand Time: The Instrumentation and Display of Life Support

Using public health techniques to prevent infection in populations or medicines to reverse infection in individuals has a quiet and unassuming character that belies the significance of their effects. They operate behind the scenes, and their exact mechanisms are not directly observable. But a mechanical ventilator that supports a single patient's breathing and requires a dedicated technician to operate it provides a dramatic, tangible display of scientific achievement that holds back death. The connection between visible procedures and measurable results is logical and obvious to the instrumentally minded public in ways that treatment with medications is not (Moerman and Jones 2002). Technology is heroic, offering hope of corporeal salvation.[21] Americans appreciate technology's display because it affirms their national self-image as achievers, problem solvers, and conquerors of adversity (Nye 2001: 104). For these reasons, specific inventions that could reverse death and support vital hemodynamic systems have energized research toward the technology of rescue. They have transformed acute care, making it possible to reverse or slow the effects of heart attacks and acute respiratory failure so that they may not be immediately fatal. The invention of the mechanical ventilator in the 1950s enabled the ultimate rescue: transplantation of vital organs from one human to another. The 1968 AD Hoc Committee of the Harvard Medical School established the criteria defining irreversible coma, framing a particular kind of death as appropriate for this purpose, enabling the death of one person to be transformed into the rescued life of another.[22] The staff of the Neuro ICU hoped that such an outcome might be possible in Mr. Wayne's case, but he could not be stabilized.

In the eighteenth century, physicians' access to the technology of forceps made the services of midwives less desirable in the minds of many prospective patients, because they lacked access to these instruments of progress (Ulrich 1990). Quality in medical care continues to be associated with the display of technology through rescue and the maintenance of vital organ systems. As Lisa Day observes, "For patients and their families, critical care can be perceived as a sort of 'black box,' where patients are expected to enter, be subjected to whatever device is needed, and emerge alive and healthy to rejoin their communities" (2005: 552). Besides the ventilator and the defibrillator, elegant machines set up at the bedside may supply episodic or continuous support to kidneys, blood, heart, (replacing its electrical and/or pump functions), and nervous system, together with continuous readouts of the patient's internal environment. Along with the personnel to tend them, these technological advances provide tangible, auditory, and visible evidence of a significant commitment of resources dedicated to the welfare (in terms of more time alive) and presumed legitimacy of the individual patient.

By the end of the twentieth century, the reductionist trends in American health-care delivery built on the drama of research breakthroughs, surgery, and war had come together in life-saving technologies focused on individual hospitalized patients rather than in more diffuse interests such as population-based health problems, maladies that did not respond dramatically to interventions, chronic mental or physical illness, disability, or (with the exception of hospice, see Chapter 3), the needs of the terminally ill.

The United States is the only industrialized nation without universal access to basic health-care, yet its use and dispersion of technology in health-care exceeds all others. These two factors help explain the high cost of U.S. health-care, its poorer outcomes, and the burden of this framework on the poor (Bodenheimer 2005; Fuchs 2005; Reinhardt, Hussey, and Anderson 2004). How can this occur? How can stability of individual organ systems become the health-care priority that eclipses all others in the hospital and elsewhere? One portion of the explanation comes from understanding rescue as an egalitarian enterprise, a form of equal opportunity medicine. The concept of rescue brings together several powerful ideas popular in the United States, such as "best" with "technically intense," "most advanced," "universally available," and "capable of postponing death." Penetrating all of these values is the insistence on customized, individualized care. Hence, rescue becomes a distraction from and perhaps even a replacement for efforts to deliver health-care more generally—it's so dazzling. It seems at once to promise, display, and deliver the future in the form of salvation from death for anyone in dire straits. We now turn to this enticement.

Universal Availability of Rescue and Stability

Recall that in 1946, building more hospitals was seen as the solution to the disparities in health-care, averting the threat of a nationalized health system. The Hill Burton Act was a federal mandate underlining the old link between hospitals and the care of the indigent. From this mandate came the requirement to provide treatment first and ask questions about payment later for patients in crisis. Certainly the passage of the civil rights legislation in 1965 and Medicare and Medicaid provisions the following year seemed to reiterate the federal government's attitude toward correcting disparities in a dramatic expansion of the postwar legislation. Rescue, especially the norms surrounding its deployment, continued this egalitarian stance. But in hospitals, the impact of rescue itself as a phenomenon has made a new and different kind of disparity operational, one that emerges from the fact that rescue and stability cannot be allowed to stretch into infinity.

When successful techniques for CPR were discovered and named in the 1960s, the American Heart Association advocated that lay rescue groups learn it, rather than physicians only. In 1969, the first paramedic nonphysician units formed independently in several cities, a uniquely U.S. approach that broadened the responsibility for rescue from the medical enclave to everyman (Eisenberg 1997: 131–133, 213, 224; Nurok 2001).

Once the American Heart Association and the American National Red Cross threw their organizational weight behind CPR and invested in national education campaigns, they implied that the postponement of death was everyone's responsibility. Every American could and should participate in attempts to reverse sudden death. Life-saving thus became a conditioned reflex, part of the popular fascination of "real-life" TV and movies. Because of the concerted activities of emergency organizations, the popular press, and, eventually, juries in courts of law, CPR and defibrillation became the legal standard for care for sudden cardiac arrest outside the hospital.[23]

Clearly the need for speed trumped not only demonstrated expertise but everything else, including efficacy and considerations of social worth. Here was the perfect combination of individualized care with the illusion of egalitarian accessibility, so important to the national self-image. If the message of CPR at its inception in the United States was that any bystander could save a life, certainly no hospital could be exempt from this responsibility. If rescue from crisis was the new requirement and the norm, hospitals had to adjust, and they did it quickly and quietly. Not only did their personnel need to be able to deliver first Basic Life Support (and later Advanced Cardiac Life Support) techniques to any patient showing signs of cardiac or respiratory arrest, but patients had to be housed according to their distance from or their potential for resuscitation and stabilization, not according to race or class. It is not difficult to believe that the combination of effective CPR and the Great Society legislation of the mid-1960s had a startling effect on institutional policies toward egalitarianism in patient treatment. David Smith (2005b) writes of this period:

> In contrast to the civil rights struggle in the 1950s and 1960s to integrate schools and public accommodations and to ensure voting rights, hospital desegregation received little public attention. Most of the changes took place quietly behind the scenes, and during this period, involved only a handful of lawsuits, several brief public local demonstrations, and a couple of headlines. (p. 248)

By the end of the 1960s, desegregation of hospitals was complete, even in the South, and it went down swiftly and in virtual silence.[24] At the bedside, the ideology of rescue is incompatible with a practice of discrimination in the traditional sense.

Now that critical care had been invented, triage *on the basis of the patient's clinical condition* could be the new "impartial" discrimination. Clinicians could believe that this framework was socially value-free and that they were doing what was best for every patient.[25] As rescue became more elaborated, institutions could be classified according to their ability to rescue, to respond to trauma (Beachley 2002: 8–9). This transformation united triage, treatment, evacuation, (transport) with the concept of first responders, as in fire; public health, which used to be defined by individual physical examination, now included rescue from crisis and stabilization for the nation's population.[26]

CPR made emergency care more elaborate and much more expensive. Private hospitals felt more pressure to transfer ("dump") less desirable patients to public hospitals after minimal emergency treatment, and the 1946 Hill Burton Act was not robust enough to prevent this practice. In 1986, the passage of EMTALA (the Emergency Medical Treatment and Labor Act, widely known as the "anti-dumping law") eliminated this option. Now hospitals that received Medicare funding had to provide "stabilizing treatment" for every patient with emergency medical conditions. No longer was it possible to transfer patients who were undesirable from the hospital's point of view to another facility without rescuing them to a stable situation first.

Likewise, almost every hospital is and must be prepared to deliver cardiopulmonary resuscitation and advanced life support to any patient who needs it at any time. The universality of this expectation comes perhaps less from the requirement for immediacy than from the understanding in the United States that rescue is an egalitarian obligation, the best care that can be offered, and the last, best hope of salvation from death. Clinicians in the hospital know how spurious this hope is, and this awareness is a burden. Policies for carving out an exemption from resuscitation with a physician's order awaited the maturation of the bioethics movement in the 1970s and 1980s. By 1988, the Joint Commission for the Accreditation of Hospital Organizations required hospitals to have DNR policies (Chambliss 1996), and many had them much earlier.

The point is that the intensity and display of rescue and its high stakes (holding back death) make it seem at once like rescue-and-stability is both the most advanced and the "most important" work in health-care, especially to hospitals and their workers, and to the public, who watch body trauma programs on television. Its supposed equal application in emergencies makes it appear to be democratic. These associations are powerful and difficult to break, because they are all true to some extent.

We have seen that the ability to deliver hemodynamic stability to patients and save their bodies from crisis and imminent death is a relatively new development in medicine. It has assumed a centrality in the space of U.S. health-care that would belie its youth. Mr. Wayne's family could be comforted after his death in knowing that everything was done to arrest his suicide. Rescue has become the gold standard of health-care delivery because it resonates with ideological interests in heroism, technology, individuality, and universality as well as the dramatic overcoming of death. In doing so, it joins with longstanding predilections toward reductionism and hierarchy in medicine, cementing its position. Besides the fact that it delegitimizes patients who are not immediately eligible for rescue (persons with mental illness, the chronically ill, the officially Dying), this orientation creates states of ambiguity between life and death in the hospital that the society, the hospital, and the clinicians are not prepared to address. This ambiguity is complicated by postmodern understandings of death and by a counter-discourse regarding "a good death" in the United States that we will explore in the next chapter.

Notes

1. DIC is disseminated intravascular coagulation, a life-threatening blood disorder.
2. DNR is often characterized as DNAR (Do Not Attempt Resuscitation) which emphasizes the procedure's poor record of success compared to other standardized medical procedures. As more physicians in the United States are taught to question patients about their preferences for resuscitation on admission to the hospital, it remains to be seen whether CPR will remain the default. Assumptions about resuscitative measures vary between the United States and England (see Mello and Jenkinson 1998).
3. This is a major reason that Mr. Gomez's day and night nurses wanted the DNR order to be written for him (see Chapter 1).
4. Scoring systems such as the iterations of APACHE have been developed, but have proved too cumbersome to use rapidly (See Apolone [2000] and Sprung et al. [1999]).
5. This is a double-edged sword—see Chapter 5.
6. Kaufman (2005: 97, 98) differentiates between a heroic pathway for hospitalized patients, and a revolving door pathway. The stable/unstable paradigm includes both.
7. See Zussman (1992: 36, 40–41). For Kaufman, patients and families' ethnic variation predicted nothing regarding how death occurred. "It is the structure of the hospital system itself—along with the politics of hospital staff practice, that, more than anything else, affects how death is made" (2005: 333). My findings were similar.
8. Another colleague corrected this impression. He told me, "We have one standard we use for all our patients, but we try harder for the patients we like."
9. Rudolf Virchow, per Taylor (in Taylor and Rieger 1985). His ideas may be reemerging in new form as indicated by the public television series *Unnatural Causes* (California Newsreel and Adelman 2008) and work by the World Health Organization Commission on Social Determinants of Health (Commission on Social Determinants of Health 2008).
10. See Berliner (1985) and Callahan (2003) for discussions of these developments; see also Rosenberg (1987).
11. This strategy has been identified by Callahan (2000) and Bauman (1992: 138).
12. An excerpt from the NIH legislative chronology is illustrative:

August 31, 1965—A supplemental appropriations act resulting from recommendations of the President's Commission on Heart Disease, Cancer and Stroke provided an additional $20,250,000 (shared by NCI, NHI, NIGMS, and NINDB) to intensify and expand support of research in the three major "killer" diseases (P.L. 89–156). (National Institutes of Health 2007)

13. See Timmermans and Berg (2003) for an in-depth discussion of the impact of this new-found medical "religion." See Blackhall (2006) and LeBlanc (2006); LeBlanc questions CPR's prevalence. The counter-argument offered by career clinicians in resuscitation research is that the field is still in its infancy, and recent developments in cooling the post-resuscitation brain illustrate this point.

14. See Starr (1982: 189–191). The moral implications of "healthy" personal habits and the betterment of society is repeated in the twenty-first century as well with the idea of "personal responsibility" for maintaining one's health as a strategy for reducing the general demand for health-care services, costly to the society.

15. It has gained legitimacy only recently as a cost-effective substitute for inpatient care, as the acuity of illness required for admission has ratcheted upward.

16. The growth of such procedures as angiography has blurred the boundaries between medicine and surgery, enabling dramatic, targeted interventions to solve medical problems without general anesthesia.

17. See Lawrence (1992: 30). As Brieger writes, "Surgeons performed great and noble deeds that required bravery, boldness, nobility, fortitude and strength, all attributes of the hero as well" (1992: 224).

18. "Please note that the community service obligation is different from the uncompensated care provision. The community service obligation does *not* require the facility to make *nonemergency* services available to persons unable to pay for them. It does, however, require the facility to make *emergency* services available without regard to the person's ability to pay" (HHS 2005, emphasis in the original).

19. Barbara Adam explains this aspect of clock time as "decontextualized and disembodied from events. Content of time is irrelevant" (1995: 90).

20. Yet Reeve continued his quest to overcome spinal cord injury both personally and by raising funds for research. Certainly he gained the admiration of many as he fought back as well as he could. My point is that the profound dependency of his condition unfortunately made his heroic efforts less media-worthy. The difference in public adulation accorded to these two iconic figures embodies Hsu's (1972) essay on U.S. self-reliance and its twin abhorrence of dependency.

21. See Good (1994: 83–87) for discussion of this view of medical care.

22. See Lock (2002) for a thorough discussion of this phenomenon, in particular the nonresponse of Americans to this development as opposed to the Japanese.

23. See Timmermans (1999) for the development of this phenomenon.

24. "To Savannah black doctor Collier, the really amazing thing was how swiftly and completely the whole segregationist edifice collapsed. White doctors, said Collier, 'acted like it was never any different, like segregation had never existed'" (Beardsley 1987: 272).

25. This approach is a clear distinction from the situation described by Sudnow as the "wait and see" attitude of physicians at "County" when patients were thought to be seriously ill or dying (1967: 99).

26. This policy was confirmed in 1985 by the Committee on Trauma Research (Committee on Trauma Research, National Research Council, & Institute of Medicine 1985).

CHAPTER 3

Configuring Dying and Death

Entry to the hospital is an unmistakable signal of human vulnerability to patients and their families. Whether or not crisis seems at hand, they worry over the current difficulty (or at least inconvenience) while focusing on their hopes for a better future. Coping with trouble in this way lifts the burden of personal worry as it maps to progressive ideals in the United States. It is an expectation that adversity will be met with intensity and technological display, anchoring visions of tomorrow's progress in today's energy and ingenuity. Waiting through the present uncertainty is nothing compared to the better future waiting just over the horizon, ensured by yesterday's track record of success.

Death is a dreaded, unexpected outcome, but to imagine a loved one *dying* within those walls is even more outrageous. If dying indeed represents a different level of threat than death itself, how might these two conditions relate to each other in the hospital? Since the discovery of effective methods of resuscitation in the 1960s, three phenomena have arisen to address the menace that death and dying represent: the ritual of intensification, which is the dominant discourse in and of the hospital; bioethics; and the revival of death movement. These cultural efforts to parlay with dying and death exist in cooperation and in tension with each other.

Death versus Dying

Tony Walter describes hospice and palliative care jointly as the revival of death movement (1994), whose advocates often refer to the desirability of a "good death." In fact, this phrase usually refers the situation that immediately precedes death, a "good *dying*." It is important to tease these concepts of dying and death apart to distinguish the kinds of threat they pose to the

79

individual and to society. But it is difficult to keep them from snapping back into each other, as we shall see.

The concept of personal finitude (death) is so dangerous that it is forbidden entry into the everyday business of life. As a reality one might anticipate, one's own death is rarely on the table for discussion in the hospital or elsewhere. It seems either too soon (surely more contingencies will exist to be pursued), or, like a bolt from the blue, impossible (and foolish) to anticipate. Even the robust advance-care planning movement (part of bioethics) would imply that preparation for one's incognition is more important than preparing for one's actual death. It is quite socially acceptable for middle-class Americans to urge each other to complete advance directives in the hopes that their autonomy survives their interactional deficits, and much less common to plan for earthly departure or for the dependency that will most likely precede one's death.

If personal death is an abstract, unreal notion, it is usually polite enough to keep its distance. To be actually dying is even more horrifying because it inserts death into the familiar territory of living, tarnishing the self-reliance project with doubt. Expending energy and cultural resources on rescue and stability has not quite succeeded in destroying death, but it has made dying disappear almost completely from public view.

Death as Contingency and Accident

The two modern conceptions of death interlock with rescue and stability: death as contingent (always in the future and not quite real) and death as accident (sudden, overwhelming disorder that banishes the known).[1] Both ideas preclude preparation or individual responsibility, and neither is permitted to threaten the daily heroic project of self.

Death as Contingent

Zygmunt Bauman describes how the strategy of chunking death down into its separate causes has made it appear vanquishable.

> The truth that death cannot be escaped "in the end' is not denied, of course. It cannot be denied; but it could be held off the agenda, elbowed out by another truth: that each *particular* cause of death (most importantly, death which threatens the particular person—me; at the particular moment—*now*) can be resisted, postponed or avoided altogether. Death as such is inevitable, but each concrete instance of death is contingent. Death is omnipotent and invincible;

but none of the specific cases of death is. (1992: 138, emphasis in the original)

Finitude is faced down by specialization into infinity. When serious illness strikes, empirical medicine reinforces the illusory isolation of the individual and the contingency of her death by filling the space at the bedside with technological "life," the armamentarium designed to exorcise contingent death (Foucault 1994: 198).

Death is not only contingent, it is also private and individualized and must remain so. As long as one lacks clear foreknowledge of death's aleatory time or cause, and because death's presentation among middle-class Americans often occurs away from public view, it need not penetrate everyday consciousness.[2] Contingent, individual death can and *must* be denied, on both a personal and societal level (Becker 1973). If death is now contingent, individual, and isolated, then interpretation of its meaning appears to be separable as well, a problem only for those immediately affected by it, rather than for the society at large. In the meantime, fighting the causes of death becomes the meaning of life for individuals in modernity.[3] Health becomes the stand-in for salvation, with medicine as its intermediary (Comaroff 1984; Good 1994: 87). Poor health becomes reframed as a character failing of those individuals who are unwilling or unable to muster the resources to live the politically correct healthy lifestyles (Seale 1998: 78).

When death is contingent, a viable future for the seriously ill person still seems graspable, only just beyond reach. The prospect of continuing with the present difficulty into the foreseeable future can seem unbearable, unless the alternative becomes no future at all. Focusing on the time to come and planning for future events are activities associated with self-esteem and social legitimacy (Baudrillard 1993; Cassell 1991).

By contrast, to have no meaningful future must mean "as good as dead," as the nurse in Chapter 2 referred to Mr. Wayne as "this dead guy." It certainly enacts social death. To be classified as Dying in the hospital is an act of stigmatization, as David Sudnow observed in the attitudes of physicians during his research:

From the physician's standpoint, a case ceases to be medically interesting in the comatose, predeath stage. Once "palliative care" is instituted, diagnostic enthusiasm becomes less sustainable. The care of such patients is considered as essentially a matter for nursing personnel, and physicians lost their interest in the patient. When that point is reached where the likelihood of an improvement of condition is considered negligible, the activities of diagnosis and

consequent treatment lose, for the intern and/or resident in training, one of their key functions, namely, their ability to allow him to
demonstrate his technical competencies and engage in semiexperi-
emental learning ventures. (1967: 91)

Sudnow's description still rings true. The intervening decades since he
investigated hospital behaviors have brought expanded capability to support vital organs, making death appear even more contingent than ever.
What persists is the social disinterest in patients whose contingencies and
futures have run out.

Not only has contingency made death unreal, it has helped move death
out of public view. The phenomenon of death has lost its overt cultural significance (Callahan 1995). This idea brings us closer to the cultural (in)sig-
nificance of death as accident. Death has meaning now only as an accidental
intrusion into human life (for everyone except those immediately affected),
and is therefore meaningless in itself. Octavio Paz asserts that by making the
workings of nature plausible, science and medicine have removed the super-
natural from death. Without the option of blaming death's disorder on the
gods, the possibility of restoring order through reconciliation with them was
also removed. "This reconciliation, whether illusory or not, had a specific
virtue: it inserted misfortune in the cosmic and human order, made the exception intelligible, and gave the accidental a meaning" (Paz 1969, 1974: 111). If
individual death now represents "only" a personal problem rather than a tear
in the social or cosmic fabric that requires mending, the cultural responsibility for providing interpretation is removed. With death distant from daily life,
it appears as a rare interjection, "accidental" because of its sudden peculiar-
lity. Death and accident are conflated and reinforce each other.

And what of the true accident? Mounting today's sophisticated trauma
response means that the search for cultural interpretation is subverted to
the immediate drama of "correcting" the disorder caused by the accident
and winning back a future for the victim, as the staff worked hard to do for
Mr. Wayne. Action and instrumentation around the injury come first, followed by a search for liability and efforts at prevention. Investigation into the
accident's meaning is no longer a responsibility of society at large. The boil-
ing energy that mobilizes such a pragmatic response to trauma is revealing.
Modernity's failure to eliminate the arbitrary makes the accident (and therefore death itself) more terrifying and repulsive (Paz 1969, 1974). As such, it
must submit to technological correctives as punishment, even as we redouble
efforts to subdue its terrorism through prevention. No other public effort to
confront our ultimate vulnerability or to atone for it seems necessary.

Particularly egregious accidents often bring media attention demanding containment, if the victim carries enough social status. Reassurance of a future for others, if not the unfortunate victim, is the first order of business. Because accidents are nothing less than an offense to rationality, instances of accidents resulting in death are a broad social concern. "It matters little whether death is accidental, criminal or catastrophic: from the moment it escapes 'natural' reason, and becomes a challenge to nature, it once again becomes the business of the group, demanding a collective and symbolic response" (Baudrillard 1976: 165).

Rescue and stability have taken center stage as societal and symbolic instruments of correction of the accident, applied whether it is a true accident or simply individual death as an accident of fate. Should the victim be rescued alive, then the hospital becomes the site of this moral drama and its management (Good 1994: 85). To overcome adversity with technology and intensity defeats the reminders of human vulnerability. Such is the impetus behind the valorization of rescue and its infrastructure.

To summarize, the concepts of death as contingent and death as accident both fit with the idea of corporeal salvation and the need to restore a jeopardized "future" to the patient. Both are distractions from facing the reality of death itself, either on an individual or cultural basis. Conceptualizing death in these two ways enables the routine, broad-scale "denial of death" essential for the project of illusion and heroism to be maintained (Becker 1973).

Death as Contaminant

Death in any form is socially contaminating. Hospitals routinely hide death from the public. The morgue is often located in the least visible portion of the physical plant, allowing funeral directors invisible access; transporters move the dead ("expired") on shape-disguising carts through private hallways and elevators.

Ironically, the fact of mortality (and the statistics it generates) is critical to evaluating hospital performance, according to the Institute for Healthcare Improvement.[4] But hospital administrators may still hide deaths and the fact of them from themselves, just as polite society keeps its distance from the physical reality of death. When I encountered an administrator doing exactly this, his attitude prompted me to explore the tensions between dying and death. Here is what happened.

My research design required that I learn where and when deaths occurred within days of their occurrence so that I could locate clinician informants while their memories of the dying were still sharp. Fortunately for me, the teaching hospital had a Decedent Affairs Office that produced daily statistics for administrative tracking and state reporting purposes, easing this part of my task. But the Catholic community hospital had no such staff and no uniform process for documenting and overseeing deaths in the institution as they happened. It took several trips down blind alleys before I found a fairly reliable mechanism for obtaining "fresh" death information from the Risk Management Office, and even these records did not include deaths in the ED.

At one point, I went to a highly placed informant for help. I described my problem and my efforts to solve it. I suggested to him that my difficulties in discovering timely information about deaths in the hospital might indicate a lack of interest. If so, I thought this practice would contradict the hospital's mission statement that explicitly mentioned the care of the dying, and said so. In his answer he was not confused about the difference between dying and death. He said, "You're asking me about dead patients. That's different. They are not a part of our mission. It's like waste management. I can tell you that we take care of it, but I can't reproduce exactly how each piece is handled." But he knew who did have this information, and we walked over to a managers' reception to find the risk manager who had just completed an analysis of the after-death process. Before that person arrived, he spied another administrator who was enjoying the refreshments. He asked him, "If I wanted to get information about patients who died, where would I go?" Between bites the other administrator replied, "I don't know. I don't like to think about death." We then found the risk manager, who gave me access to the information I needed.

The Western separation that the administrator invoked between the dying who are "part of our mission," and the dead as "waste" (evidently requiring a month's margin of safety to track) was startling and disturbing. I could not shake my suspicion that his assertion did not hold water. Could it be true that institutional policies regarding the "disposal" of the dead had nothing to do with the hospital's care of the dying? Several weeks later I asked a chaplain to comment on such differentiation, being careful not to disclose what I had been told.

HC: What does it mean if the hospital doesn't pay attention to the death statistics, except monthly? Does it have any impact on the dying process?

CH: It has an impact on bereavement care. At my old hospital, we had weekly reports of death, so I could send out bereavement cards. It feels very willy-nilly to me here. It was so much tighter there.

The chaplain's recollection implied that the "tight" business mechanisms of her previous hospital included efficient notification of hospital deaths given to the chaplain's office. Because she could generate time-sensitive work products that demonstrated the hospital's compassion, she felt in control. In her present circumstances, the hospital's "willy-nilly" practices prevented her from meeting the performance standard that she preferred.[5]

As a representative of the larger culture, the administrator's differentiation placed the dead firmly outside of his realm of concern, perhaps a sign that his secular unease with death overcame a traditional Catholic interest in (at least) the soul after death. The force of rejection in his remark rattled me a bit; perhaps my speculation about the hospital's mission to the dying had stung him. Whatever else it might have meant, his delineation between dying and death certainly indicated that he was highly sensitive to the danger that putrescence poses to the social group, easily pinpointing the death's polluting effects (Douglas 1966: 125; Metcalf and Huntington 1991).the clear bright line that he drew between those with legitimacy and those without it was an attempt to contain a threat that exists in four domains: the problem of the periphery, the definition of death, the difficulty of differentiating between the living and the dead, and the definition of the relationships between them. I examine each of these in turn.

The problem of the periphery is the problem of borders. Mary Douglas reminds us that "[A]ll margins are dangerous. If they are pulled this way or that the shape of fundamental experience is altered. Any structure of ideas is vulnerable at its margins" (1966: 122). A strategy to limit the problem of the periphery is to declare that such close-on edges do not exist: dying and death do not bump up against one another, causing potential overlap, but are cleanly separated. One is either alive and valued or dead and waste. Indeed, because of the ritual of intensification discussed below, it is very difficult to identify and hold onto a patient who might occupy the dangerous marginal space between living and dead in the hospital.[6] But if there are no patients at death's periphery who are dying, where would the hospital's mission to the dying be located?

The definition of death, our second domain, has been problematic since vivisection informed anatomy studies. It became even more troublesome in 1968 (and thereafter) when brain death without cardiac death was deemed acceptable for the purpose of organ donation. In comparing U.S. transplantation practices with those of Japan, a country where brain death is still very controversial, Margaret Lock has concluded that the moment of death is unavoidably a social construction rather than a physiological point in time, making problematic the working consensus that patients must be declared dead before organs may be removed (the "dead donor rule") (2002: 361). The "dead donor rule" in transplantation continues to undergo fervent discussion as better stabilization methods lengthen the list of potential recipients desperate for whole organs (Gawande et al. 2008; The President's Council on Bioethics 2009). Applying the "dead donor rule" in practice is complicated by the coexisting policy of universal resuscitation in the hospital so that death cannot be accepted as fact unless all attempts to revive the patient have failed. Because the definition of physiological death is not immutable, the administrator's assertion that a clear bright line is visible between the territory of dying and that of the dead is not convincing.

The problem is further confounded by the third domain, the difficulty of differentiating between the living, the living who are dying, and the dead. Rescue has complicated efforts to set living patients apart from patients who are either dead or dying. As long as the outcome of serious illness is in doubt, patients occupy a gray zone.[7] Certain specialty hospitals maintain patients in persistent coma, bringing about a form of "life" not seen prior to the invention of the ventilator (Kaufman 2000). Disability groups such as Not Dead Yet advocate especially for patients with severely impaired neurological function, lobbying against a particularly Western habit of disregard.[8] Neurological dysfunction is an all too frequent unfortunate outcome of otherwise successful resuscitation, and it is the fear of being kept alive in this condition that motivates many persons to fill out advance directives. The fact that many clinicians and lay people confuse DNR orders and advance directives in practice indicates that severe brain impairment and death can be conflated in the minds of the public.

Even when we are certain that persons are truly dead, it is not clear that our relationship with them is ended, which constitutes our fourth domain. How do individuals and social entities negotiate an appropriate connection with persons whose physical presence no longer animates their world? Many societies emphasize a dynamic social relationship with the dead that evolves over time, and they use ritual to mark transitions in the "soul's career."[9] Living out this understanding in daily life contrasts sharply with a Western attitude that consigns the dead to a static wastebin, where they will surely stay dead and remote forever. Any possibility of a relationship would seem to concern only the few who felt a need to maintain an ongoing relationship with the noncorporeal loved one, certainly not the society at large.

Looking at the dead from the standpoint of quality brings a pragmatic approach. A lack of interest in the dead, in death, or in patients now dead must surely derail the hospital's mission to the dying. Even if timely bereavement cards were the only gauge of success, the administrator's assertion to the contrary fails. The event of death may not put patients beyond the hospital's mission. The proof lies in the fact that a patient's state of Dying may only be confirmed retrospectively (i.e., only by the death that follows it). This is why evaluating quality around care of the dying (the hospital mission) would need to begin retrospectively with a mechanism for reviewing the deaths themselves. Various medical and surgical services in U.S. hospitals typically conduct their own regular morbidity and mortality reviews ("M&M rounds") critiquing specific missed opportunities, instances in which different decisions might have brought a more favorable result to patients who died. Using this principle to enact a similar review of Mr. Diangelo's last weekend in the Catholic community hospital, for example, would be instructive. If his finitude and death might be accepted as inevitable (a proposition made easier in view of the DNR order the attending had already written for him), then the focus of evaluation could shift to the care delivered. Was it appropriate? What obstacles to clinical foresight might have prevented a better plan of care from being formulated and carried out? "An old aphorism among reformers is that 'you can't improve what you don't measure,'"[10] and measuring requires caring about specific aspects of the patient's clinical journey.

Enacting a mission to the dying requires identifying who these patients are (not so easy in a rescue environment) and claiming their care as a specific set of responsibilities. Despite a mission statement that explicitly mentions the dying, the Catholic community hospital illustrated an aversion to "owning" patients who are dying. It is by no means alone in this sentiment. Even though pain for any patient is to be assessed as the "fifth vital sign," it is rarely anyone's responsibility to evaluate the quality of attention or palliation that a patient receives, especially after a death has occurred. A factor complicating such review assisted the administrator in his desire to unhinge the living from the dead: as the body is transported to the morgue, hard copy medical records are moved off into storage. As patients travel through the hospital, their charts must accompany them. Accordingly, the deceased patient's records are locked away from the living at the same time that transporters move the body to the morgue. Chart retrieval and review is time consuming and might reveal little about the care given in the last phases, documentation around death events being particularly spotty.[11] Even the monthly M&M rounds meant to instruct physicians about opportunities for rescue fell by the wayside in the unit where I worked because the preparation for it required such labor-intensive chart review. Efficient methods for evaluating the care the hospitalized patient received in the last days and hours before death would require dying to become a status deemed worthy of both reliable documentation and scrutiny.

Meanwhile, Americans expect the hospital to be producing more future for the patient by killing off death and the effects of accident. Technological support of contingent body systems buys more time alive, time for a miracle, even in fatal illness. The speed and intensity of rescue and trauma care serve as strong societal antidotes to the caprice of accident. When death is not killed, it is at least isolated and sealed off from everyday life. Bauman links this strategy to the social practice of associating dangerous and contagious disease to the Other, groups that are not and cannot be "self" (1992). Isolation therefore serves a critical cleanly purpose in the social project of the denial of death, as Mary Douglas has argued. Bauman connects attitudes regarding death to the social rejection of "degeneracy," a powerfully imprecise term that represents any reminder of ultimate human powerlessness. The ideal life to which Americans aspire would resonate with self-reliance, spurn dependency, and be odorless (C. Davies 1996; Hsu 1972). Echoing Douglas, Bauman is explicit: "Hygiene is, let us repeat, the product of the deconstruction of mortality into an infinite series of individual causes of death, and of the struggle against death into an infinitely extendable series of battles against specific diseases" (1992: 155).

In what way is death especially menacing to Americans? Emphasis on individualism, self-reliance, and difficulty in acknowledging personal or social limitations make death a particularly potent threat to the heroic project (Hsu 1972). Seeing it as contingency and accident ensures that any death one hears reported can be applied to others only. Most of the time, death in middle-class America seems infinitely separable from self. In fact, it is *dying* that presents the true threat, the label that Americans are most reluctant to confer on themselves or one another.

Isolated, individual death may appear as easy to put aside as it did to the hospital administrator, but because of the role the hospital plays in U.S. life, death in that setting remains a cultural concern. Should the disease or injury process prove irreversible,[12] the blame for it must be placed squarely on the individual's intransigent body for refusing to submit to the rescuing interventions of civilizing medicine. The blame must not appear to fall on those hygienic activities themselves, or worse, on some inherent mortality of the human condition.

Ritual of Intensification

But death *does* occur in the hospital, although patients and clinicians point themselves so firmly in the opposite direction. When death comes, it must be shaped so that it will fit into prevailing norms. Clinicians use a *ritual of intensification,* an obligatory redoubling of their efforts, to first fight and then elucidate the inescapability of this patient's particular situation of finitude.[13] With it, death may be characterized as an accident of the patient's body, of circumstances beyond the control of the best of what medicine and society can offer. It is, after all, a surprise to find that the contingencies of hope no longer exist and that this particular individual is mortal *now.* An explanation is necessary. The ritual of intensification presses on while clinicians search for a plausible excuse to attach such a stunning result as dying firmly to this particular patient's physiology.[14] This effort preserves the integrity of the medical project as it rubs up against the margins of death. The ritual maintains the illusion that death comes only as the accidental convergence of this particular set of circumstances. The rest of us might still be exempt.

The ritual of intensification exists in tension with two other discourses: bioethics in the U.S. and the revival of death movement, discussed later in this chapter. Bioethics has supplied the philosophical permission to close down the ritual along with the patient-centered vocabulary (autonomy, privacy, the right to refuse treatment) that disguises the dismantling of social concern around dying itself. The revival of death movement manifested through hospice and palliative care offers possibilities of specialized attention, if a time and space for dying can be opened at least privately.

When asked about the medical care they want in case they cannot speak for themselves, many patients say they want "everything done to save my life. When there is nothing more to do, just keep me comfortable." This purports to be a statement of preferences that reflects public expectations of the U.S. health-care delivery system, but in a hospital structure organized to rescue and stabilize patients, it is a recipe for extraordinary ambiguity. Non-clinicians are not aware of this eventuality (Kaufman 2005: 58–60). The "me" of the statement (so clear to the patient) is hard for biomedicine to define because its representatives focus on parts of bodies and organ systems in their quest to rescue whole persons. People write advance directives for themselves, not for the separable organ systems around which biomedicine arranges itself.

Because of the cultural belief that death is contingent, unpredictable, and therefore unreal and because hospitals are the ultimate battlegrounds for delivery from death, hospital admission brings action: assessment, stabilization, and treatment, by law. Usually these efforts are successful, so that in a hospital's several thousand admissions per year only a few hundred will end in death. Should initial treatment efforts be inconclusive, that is, the patient neither improves nor dies, the next step is the *ritual of intensification,* based on his particular physiological configurations as they present themselves through subsequent hours, days, and weeks. Clinicians stabilize blood pressure, place intravenous lines, treat infection, perform surgery, move the patient in and out of the ICU, and manage large and small complications. The assumption or the directive that "everything" should be done brings an open-ended elaboration leading to an undefined, liminal period of unknown length and description, with almost no possibility of planning or preordained control by anyone. To classify a whole being as terminally ill requires a pronouncement that seems inappropriately global when discrete body functions continue functioning with support, extending time alive. The ritual of intensification buys or produces more time alive in the hopes that healing may still occur, making a place for the miracle, for the patient's condition to "turn around." As long as this promise of the future is applied to the patient, her eligibility for the plethora of stabilizing interventions remains intact.

The ritual of intensification takes on a life and impetus of its own. This is a gray zone of ambiguity, but it is not stagnant. It changes as the demands of the culture, the hospital, and the persons involved at the bedside interact with time and its passage.

Outlines of the Ritual of Intensification

The full exploration of the ritual of intensification comes in Chapter 7, but it is helpful to understand its outlines now as the premier social response to death and the peril it presents to the heroic project. Momentum and time influence the character of the ritual. At the outset, its activity represents an enthusiastic demonstration of compassion and communal altruism on behalf of the person made vulnerable by illness or accident. Everyone witnesses this confirmation of the patient's worth, his validation by view of participation in social and economic exchange (Baudrillard 1993, 1976: 263–264). Both public and private constituencies seem to suspend time in the present, looking to the future and recovery that the ritual will deliver. Staving off death is the definition of legitimacy and of endorsable, reimbursable care in the hospital.

Nancy Johnson and her colleagues describe this moment as the start of a therapeutic narrative among the family, the clinicians, and the patient (if he is able to participate) that begins with indeterminacy and "the maintenance of competing plot lines, each with a different ending. Hope lies in the possibility of a desired ending" (Johnson et al. 2000: 279). In this stage of liminality, the benefit of the doubt regarding the future is usually accorded to the patient.

The patient's physiology does not always cooperate with a clearly positive or negative trajectory. Illness and injury are chaotic. Maintaining stability as a first priority allows the assumption to persist that given enough time and support, the body will heal itself in cooperation with sophisticated technological innovations. At this point, care given by humans, medical inventions, and the "true" nature of the body are all in sync, fighting the "unnatural" invader of illness or injury. Late in the ritual of intensification this relationship will be reversed, so that the disease becomes naturalized and the instrumentation is constructed as the invader (Johnson et al. 2000: 279). Robert Steiff, describing his own disquiet around his mother Susan Sontag's final days, quotes Diane Meier, a palliative care physician expert:

> [Meier] spoke of "the denial, the kind of winking that goes on, where, yeah, we all know the patient's going to die but we're all going to pretend like there's hope, so we're all going to go through these rituals because that's what we believe the patient wants. In the meantime the patient is watching the doctor who is offering this treatment and clearly thinking to himself, if the doctor didn't think it would work, he or she wouldn't offer it, but what the doctor is not saying is that the odds are minute and that he is trying to be responsive to the needs of the patient for hope. It's like a minuet. It's surreal." (quoted by Robert Burt 2009: 40)

This "surreal minuet" occurs because of the operation of time on the participants. When recovery remains unclear day after day, enthusiasm wanes. Minus a clear predilection in the patient's body toward recovery, the perspective shifts from the glass being half full to being half empty. Clinicians, and perhaps the family, may sense that ritual of intensification is not leading to a clear endpoint and that something different needs to happen. How does one go about closing down the ritual when ambiguity reigns? The need for a shift and the problem it presents has occupied clinicians, ethicists, and other contributors to the discourse, and it is illustrated in the three examples below. Part of the problem is that the ritual is instrumental rather than celebratory. It transforms the patient's social status negatively, so that its closure lacks the motivational aspect that elevation or ceremony might confer.[15]

At this point it is helpful to see examples of the ritual of intensification to illustrate the exquisite balancing that stability and rescue make possible, confounding prediction when contingency rules and patients are "not allowed to die but [they are] too frail to recover" (Kaufman 2005: 178). Just as in the cases presented earlier, each of these patients eventually died, and clinicians told me their stories soon afterward. These examples reveal the issues that led clinicians to believe that the ritual of intensification had outlived its usefulness. Unlike the accounts in Chapter 1, these narratives do not portray a state of dying, either officially or unofficially. The act of hindsight and its imposition of order do not rob these accounts of their lived uncertainty.

Examples of the Ritual of Intensification

Mrs. Homan was in her early 50s when she died in the Catholic community hospital's ICU after six weeks.

> RN: She had emphysema (chronic lung disease). Dr. A. told her "if we put you on this vent, likely you won't live without it" and she wanted it. She had [a compromised immune system, pneumonia, and chronic digestive problems as a side effect of medication that required surgery, and malnutrition]. She had bouts of sepsis and gastro-intestinal bleeding. She never got better. The family wanted everything done. We tried multiple times to wean her from the vent. Multiple times.

Mrs. Homan was a relatively young woman undergoing repeated rescue and stabilization efforts with gastro-intestinal complications and sepsis after her initial treatment for pneumonia. According to the clinicians caring for her, time and contingency had run out, and they wanted to close down the ritual of intensification. The "multiple" attempts to wean her lungs from their need for life support proved to the clinicians that recovery was not in the cards for her, so in their minds, continued ventilation was postponing her death. When the family did not agree, clinicians pushed hard using an ethics consultation to convince the Homan family to go along with a plan to withdraw life-supportive measures.

Mr. Mendez in his late 50s died in the Coronary Care Unit at the teaching hospital. His nurse told me that Mr. Mendez had come in with congestive heart failure. While on a floor unit, he collapsed and required CPR. Clinicians placed a breathing tube during resuscitation and transferred him to the coronary care unit (CCU). Most likely because of the poor perfusion his organs received during this collapse, his kidneys, liver, and especially his digestive tract failed to function in subsequent days. Nonetheless, he improved enough to have the breathing tube out and to spend part of the day out of bed in a chair.

> RN: He watched the game. I had him up in a chair, positioned to try to get his gut moving. He was miserable. Never comfortable. His belly. I would give him ginger ale and ice chips and anything he wanted. It was sucked right back out the [naso-gastric] tube, so it

didn't matter. He was never comfortable. I asked his wife, "Was he depressed?" No, it was his baseline. He was never very talkative, affectionate. I would joke with him. He watched the game. He never seemed very comfortable. He went out to the floor, then Wednesday he coded on the floor. Then he came back to us. The family decided to withdraw support. He was just not there anymore. So before, when it was all so acute [we kept doing things]. When they [the family] realized this was a terminal event, they decided to withdraw [life support].

During this one hospital admission, Mr. Mendez went in and out of the ICU environment, always presenting a mixed picture. Despite the failure of several organs and two episodes of CPR, the nurse recalled that "other things were getting better" or "looking up." In her mind, the ritual of intensification was justified "when it was all so acute." Not until "he was just not there anymore" did it seem appropriate to call Mr. Mendez "terminal," a "realization" that made the family the agents of decision rather than the clinicians. These events occurred over a two and a half week period.

Mrs. Turner was a 73-year-old who died in the surgical ICU at the teaching hospital. My informant was a physician resident. Mrs. Turner had come to an outside hospital after a fall, sustaining a collapsed lung. The chest tube placed to reexpand her lung had gone awry. Like Mrs. Homan, Mrs. Turner's chronic lung disease before this acute episode made it difficult to wean her from the ventilator. Upon transfer to the teaching hospital she suffered two episodes of dangerously low blood pressure, perhaps signaling sepsis, a bloodstream infection. Clinicians started intravenous drips to support her blood pressure, administered IV antibiotics, and performed a bronchoscopy, a bedside procedure to examine and wash out the lungs. The physician told the family that Mrs. Turner's prognosis was poor. They decided that she should not be resuscitated, and a DNR order was written for her. Mrs. Turner improved enough to make the blood pressure medications unnecessary, and the family wondered whether the DNR was still appropriate. The physician explained that medical interventions would continue, and this assurance satisfied them. The turning point came not from Mrs. Turner's condition, but from a comment made on rounds and a declaration of poor neurological function from neurosurgery.

MD: On rounds the chief said, "Don't keep giving this family hope." So I talked with them. I reviewed antibiotics. We thought she would do better. We weaned off the pressors. She was normotensive and normothermic (normal blood pressure and no fever). But she was not any better. We caught the infection in time. But we can't get her better. I never saw her move anything. We got a neurosurgery consult. They said she had brainstem function only. I let the family know that this would go on forever. The son said that the last thing she wanted was this.

In her narrative, the resident described "going back and forth" and "making no headway." Even though CPR had been ruled out by the DNR order, stabilization efforts continued while she sought an explanation for Mrs. Turner's lack of recovery. She pressed on, despite the fact that her chief did not support her efforts: "Don't keep giving this family hope." The chief recognized that families interpret a high level of attention from physicians as a reason to maintain unrealistic expectations, an example of the "surreal minuet."[16] This remark redirected the resident's focus from diagnosis and treatment for Mrs. Turner to difficult conversations with the family. Mrs. Turner was in this second hospital for eighteen days.

These three examples illustrate the ambiguity and uncertainty that the ritual of intensification addresses. Because these patients were not recovering in a straightforward way and suffered recurring but treatable complications, clinicians continued to wrestle with each one, maintaining stability while they explored every contingency and "played every card," as one nurse put it. Lack of clarity was everywhere. In each case, it was not a change in the patient's physiological condition that triggered the change in the care plan, but the crossing of an invisible threshold of time.

Because the final outcome of these cases is known, it is tempting to project it backward and wonder why the clinicians did not see the writing on the wall. To do this is misleading and unjust to the people who lived through the unfolding chaos and practiced in good faith. But to look closely at the last days of persons who died in the hospital compels one to wonder if at some point before death they might have been officially acknowledged as persons who were Dying, and what this confirmation might have meant in terms of adjusting their plans of care. The nature of those adjustments continues to garner discussion and debate, but it is remarkable that comparatively little attention accrues to the cultural ramifications of changing their rescuable status. The official designation of Dying (or the more common euphemisms such as "irreversible" or "comfort care only") means that the communal, democratic responsibility for the patient is officially ended, even though the patient continues to occupy a legitimate space of public focus in the form of a hospital bed. Such an anomalous position requires ritual to enact and redeem. In no other way can a rescuable patient become disqualified for first-class care and thereby become transformed into a second-class citizen in the eyes of the hospital.

Mrs. Homan, Mr. Mendez, and Mrs. Turner were all in the ICUs of their respective hospitals. For Mr. Mendez and Mrs. Turner, the ritual of intensification closed down successfully, each was designated as Dying, and life support was withdrawn. To clinicians, theirs played out as tidy, untroubling deaths. In Mrs. Homan's case, the ritual failed. Because it did not lead to consensus among the participants, no sanction could be found for a change in her status. Her life support continued for days through an ethics consultation, family disagreements, and physician weekend absence, while clinicians increased her sedation and pain medication. Mrs. Homan's final days disturbed her caregivers greatly. The ritual had convinced *them* of the need to change her status, but the family's preferences held sway because of the credence given to the bioethical principle of respect for autonomy, a counter-discourse discussed below.

The ritual's work of determining the patient's status is usually more riveting than the events that occur between its close and the actual death of the patient, a period that seems settled and predictable by comparison.[17] Clinician narratives often displayed the orderliness of hindsight, as if the ritual's denouement and its aftermath might have been foreseen. In other stories of dying and death such as that of Mr. Gomez (Chapter 1), no resolution emerged. No sigh of relief was shared among all the players that because the patient was dying, the care plan could authorize efforts to limit suffering to the heart's content. Often the Dying became an anticlimax, a coda that marked the end of the ritual of intensification, rather than the end of a life. The ritual of intensification may often identify the end of exploring contingencies, but it does not create a new space for what might follow.

Important counter-discourses based on individual rights have emerged to challenge the dominant position of the ritual of intensification in the hospital. They influence the latter portion of the ritual of intensification, how it is dismantled, and the framing that clinicians use to describe this process. These discourses also influence cultural ideals about the management of a "good death."

Counter-Discourses to the Ritual of Intensification

In the generic statement of patient preferences mentioned earlier, rescue and stability are reflected in the wish to have "everything done to save my life." Two major counter-discourses exist in the United States, but their influence on public thinking about these issues is difficult to measure. Bioethics has insisted that the question about preferences itself be asked (codified into law through the Patient Self-Determination Act of 1990), and the revival of death movement has made "Keep me comfortable" a goal with teeth. Both of these discourses do affect the ritual of intensification, however. Bioethics provides the tools to define and contest the ritual of intensification, although without challenging its dominant cultural position. Similarly, the revival of death movement points to and elaborates the dying situation as a space worthy of attention, and in doing so presents a protest and an alternative to the ritual of intensification. Like bioethics, it also fails to stand up to the ritual's cultural sovereignty.[18] Both of these discourses emerged in the United States at about the same time as the discovery of successful methods of CPR in the mid-1960s.

Rescuing and stabilizing individual bodies by attaching machines to them seems corrective and life-saving to many but horrific to others, especially if the machines are used to "prolong" life whose quality is open to question. Both discourses, bioethics and the "good death" or "revival of death" movement as Tony Walter calls it (1994), were founded in support of primacy of individuality and choice, but they contest the U.S. valorization of more time alive as the most important goal that a society should champion. Bioethics has given philosophical permission to bring the ritual to a close in some cases and it has supplied rubrics that are so culturally salient (e.g., a patient's right to refuse treatment) that professional codes of ethics such as the ANA Code Ethics cite them and national regulatory agencies such as The Joint Commission police them. The revival of death movement has argued that continuing aggressive care in patients who are dying creates a situation that fails to honor the individual and deprives that person of choice. Although the influence of palliative care initiatives in the hospital is recent and still unfolding, its hospice-acquired concepts of dignity, relief of suffering, and the idea that dying can be brought under submission to the individual are intuitively appealing. The option to offer hospice or palliative care often forms the backdrop for "shifting the narrative" of the illness as the ritual of intensification is negotiated (Johnson et al. 2000).

Bioethics

Born in the consumer movement, bioethics addresses a broad range of concerns aimed at empowering the vulnerable individual in health-care settings of treatment and research (Rothman 1991). Its proponents have offered rationales and defined principles of negotiation that clinicians, families, and patients rely on when they argue against producing more time alive at any cost. The individualism of traditional bioethics resonates with national ideals of freedom as it validates the person "lost" in the search for contingency.

Bolstered by egregious abuses such as the Tuskegee syphilis study and media attention to court cases such as Karen Ann Quinlan and Nancy Cruzan, proponents of bioethics have had far-reaching influence in the hospital in the development of informed consent requirements, DNR orders, advance directives, permission for withdrawal of life support, and The Joint Commission requirement that every hospital have a mechanism for ethics consultation. Its influence is global, but bioethics is very much a phenomenon rooted in U.S. life, strongly tied to the explosion of technology and ready access to resources able to maintain hemodynamic stability without cure (Callahan 1995). The custom of hospital bioethics to focus attention on point of care dilemmas sidesteps the corporate, economic, and system influences that may be at work (Chambliss 1996; Farmer 2005; Guillemin 1998).

Speaking of the history of U.S. bioethics, Jeanne Guillemin critiques this bedside focus and points out that by omitting broader domains, bioethics has let (at least) physicians off too easily:

> The conceptual narrowness of the ethics enterprise assisted the physician in avoiding the onus of the social, which for decades in medicine has been associated with the threat of socialism and even of socialized medicine. Such apprehensions are more than linguistic. In a nation that prizes pragmatic action, the recognition of a social order of problems fairly dictates broad-based solutions that threaten the individual. The problems that bioethics ignored were, among others, the bureaucratic structure of hospital organization, the capitalist expansion of medical industrial complex, disparities of income and life chances between rich and poor, and gender inequities, as if these more sociologically defined areas were without important moral dimensions or consequence for practicing physicians. (1998: 62)

Not only has the focus on the individual left the bioethics perspective with large blind spots, but by framing the ambiguity of prolonged, serious illness mainly as a crisis in decision-making, it has influenced the shape of dying in the U.S. hospital in three ways: (1) bioethics concentrates on the unique, individual aspects of any particular ritual of intensification rather than addressing itself to the systems issues that will almost always be in play, such as the access to palliative care and the covert influence of reimbursement policies; (2) by focusing on the precariousness of the position now occupied only by the patient, bioethics downplays the vulnerability, finitude, and humanity that the participants hold in common; and (3) the consummate struggle to chart an ethical course through life-threatening ambiguity leaves participants spent. Often little stamina remains after the final course is set, thereby reducing the opportunities to engage in making meaning around the dying and death to come.

Bioethics has not addressed the need to prepare persons for the moment when physicians will tap them to make vital treatment decisions for loved ones who cannot speak for themselves. Advance directives may help if they are available, but if patient circumstances do not reflect what is on the page, they are unusable (Fagerlin and Schneider 2004). The need for sensitivity to ethnic variation in the supposedly universal values of truth-telling and patient autonomy in decision-making has been noted by researchers and commentators, but the need for "moving things along" often trumps such nuance in the hospital.[19] Bioethics does not address the momentum that the ritual of intensification projects, nor does it notice the differing understandings of time and linearity among the patients and families, clinicians, and the hospital. Anthropological tenets indicate that specific group practices evolve to match unmet social needs, and they offer theoretical perspectives that allow us to examine how this happens.

Clinicians are able to use their understandings of bioethics to justify their assignment of the patient to the nonrescue category. When clinicians are confident that the family's interest in continuing the ritual of intensification is postponing the patient's death, such as in Mrs. Homan's case, their perception of benefits versus burdens permits them to advocate for life-supportive treatment to stop. Mrs. Homan's family did not agree, and an ethics consultation was called. In the cases of Mr. Mendez and Mrs. Turner, nurses cited patient autonomy through substituted judgment (e.g., "the last thing she wanted was this") as the ethical justification for limiting aggressive treatment (see Chapter 7 for further discussion of the "tipping point" in the ritual of intensification). Clinicians hold the power advantage in these negotiations and, as unwitting representatives of the public and the hospital's interests, they may be unaware that their good faith is not completely clear to families under stress. Families may see discontinuation of treatment as abandonment or murder (Kaufman 2005: 50).

With one notable exception (the Rule of Double Effect), the attention of bioethics at the bedside ends as the ritual of intensification shuts down and the "dilemma" is resolved.[20] Bioethics does not routinely address how the final approach of death might be orchestrated, nor whose values should hold sway. It does not acknowledge the space that opens as the ritual of intensification winds down, nor does it suggest possibilities for creativity. Recommendations for managing this period of life come from the revival of death movement.

Revival of Death

Although the ritual of intensification is surely about individualized care, the patient's self becomes lost within it, subjugated (temporarily) for the greater goal of more time alive. When hope for this outcome is also lost and there is "nothing more to be done," the recategorization of the patient as Dying removes him or her from the sphere of public concern. Philip Mellor and Chris Shilling argue that contemporary social life has privatized the experience of death during the period that religion's influence over a pluralistic public has contracted and self-identity and its identification with the body have expanded. The removal of the signs of public legitimation of death makes "the challenge of death to modern people's sense of reality unprecedentedly radical" (Mellor and Shilling 1993: 413). How can one face this challenge without the benefit of this modeling by one's society? Can the self be rediscovered and meaning made at the end of life? The answer is emphatically yes, according to the revival of death movement, even in the absence of cultural accompaniment to dying in modern society decried by social observers such as Daniel Callahan (1993) and Clive Seale (1998). Hospice philosophy and practice promotes the possibilities for exploring meaning in the context of life that is drawing to a close. Reacting to the perceived domination of medicine and the loss of self-determination at the end of life, the revival of death movement has bolstered individual self reliance in coping with the approach of death. Tony Walter describes this phenomenon as the means toward realizing the twentieth century ideal of "an emotionally satisfying, rather than a spiritually efficacious, death" (1994: 22). It is fueled by the authority of the self as it is expressed through relationships, interactive choice, self-improvement, and self-disclosure.

The revivalist movement sees death in the hospital as medicalized, bureaucratized, and male, the essence of rationalism that makes the individual an object rather than subject. The revival of death in general and hospice care in particular seeks to recover the individual while emphasizing process and context. Hospice is associated with spiritual (usually Christian), middle-class, and "feminine" values. The revival of death serves as foil to the rationality of medicine realized in rescue, and the two neatly embody

Stanley Tambiah's schema of world-ordering ideas: causality (the scientific ordering of reality) and participation (relations of contiguity and shared affinities) (1990: 105–110). It is not surprising, then, that the origins of the revival of death movement coincide with mushrooming of medical technology after the discovery of successful resuscitation methods, as they complement each other so well.

The revival of death movement carves out a space for meaning making, for what is not measurable, and for an agenda ruled by the needs of the patient, her body, and her family. It pays homage to the postmodern ideal that the individual is entitled to control over self and body until the very moment of death. Because so little guidance for doing this now exists in the public sphere, hospice provides "expert" advice as to what the "good death" might be, combining autonomy and affirmation.[21] Critical expertise in pain management and symptom control, fueled in large part by the revival of death movement, has freed the patient and family to live and attend to each other in the dying situation rather than to be consumed by its agonies. Ironically, these new understandings have received far less public attention than advances in rescue-oriented medical technology. With control of distressing bodily symptoms, the patient and family (with the aid of the caregiving team) may work toward realizing progressive ideals of meaning and growth in dying, such as accomplishing what Corr, Nabe, and Corr (1994) term the "tasks of dying," or living out Kübler-Ross's (1976) understanding of death as "the final stage of growth."

If one abjures the technology associated with more time alive sometime before all the contingencies have been explored, the ritual of intensification and its need to "move things along" falls away. To so renounce the production of the future brings a reorientation to the present. For hospice and palliative care, time containment is not the major goal. The pressure of linear time divisions can give way to process time, the time for social relations and "care work." It is quite a different sensation to allow one's perception of time to flow from the needs of persons in need of care than from the dictates of the clock (K. Davies 1994: 281).

In the revivalist understanding, the patient's dying is allowed to unfold in its own time and way, guided by an expert view of the "good death," while caregivers demonstrate what Paul Ramsey called "solidarity in mortality," an entering into the limitations of the humanity they share (1970: 129). Meaning and dignity are found in watching the time unfold, rather than working for or against death's arrival. In its intention neither to hasten nor prolong death, hospice seeks to make social death and physical death coincide in time.[22] The "revival of death" movement appears to promise a measure of freedom and customization by naming a dying process, celebrating it, allowing time to make meaning, reacting to symptoms, and providing interpretation along the way. This is the irony of hospice's hope work: patients must relinquish their belief in an unlimited future, and their hope that more time or more therapy will produce a cure in order to participate in the more romantic hope for a "good death," a practice of positivism that sustains the moral order.[23]

The appeal of this alternative view of dying can be seen in the steady growth of hospice and palliative care in the United States. The social impact of revivalist ideas rose to the level of federally mandated funding in 1983, bringing a "hospice benefit" to Medicare beneficiaries. Before this (1974–1982), hospice programs relied solely on donations and grants. By 2007, hospice programs were caring for 38 percent of deaths. Of these, 81.3 percent of patients were Euro American, 9 percent African American, and 9.7 percent other or unknown, indicating that hospice's appeal has stayed close to its predominantly white, middle-class roots. The percentage of nonwhite patients has increased, but the hospice demographic will need much more diversity to match that of the population as a whole (Connor et al. 2004). The multiple requirements for implementing hospice home care (a safe structure, a telephone, a designated caregiver, and persons willing and able to provide the labor intensive work of nursing a patient near death) can discriminate against those without these resources, even though admission is usually not denied for inability to pay. Distrust of the health-care system and history of discrimination figure into different patterns of hospice use by African Americans. Hence, the health-care disparities and access issues endemic to health-care delivery in the United States are also manifested in hospice care.[24]

In recent years, especially since the landmark 1995 SUPPORT study's clear documentation of poor care for dying patients in hospitals, palliative care has brought revivalist principles into the hospital setting in ways that hospice, with its stigma of mortality, could not. Palliative care emphasizes the control of symptoms in serious illness along with end of life care, so that it may insert itself before the patient is designated as Dying. It has a rationalist association for physicians, and board certification reinforces its medical legitimacy.[25] These advantages may still have limited effect in a health-care environment that encourages dichotomous thinking by excluding the reimbursement of curative therapy under the Medicare Hospice Benefit (Lynn 2004: 21; Morrison 2005; and see Chapter 7).

Other than the continuing gains made by palliative care, the revivalist discourse has not gained a visible foothold in the hospital. Hospice practice occurs most often in the very private space of homes, beyond the gaze of most hospital clinicians, a fact that increases its attraction for those who gain access to it, but also keeps it isolated, so that it need not intrude on public life. In this way it performs an important cultural service. "Much of the activity in hospice care involves the bandaging or mopping up of leaky bodies, containing contaminating fluids and maintaining a separation between the hygienic life world and the disintegration of the flesh. In fact the word 'palliation' derives from the Latin 'palliatus' meaning 'covered', 'cloaked' or 'disguised'" (Seale 1998: 119).

Palliative care may be presented to hospitalized patients and families as a reasonable, compassionate alternative when clinicians seek to close down the ritual of intensification. But because of the simultaneous motivation to move the patient's care out of the mainstream and the dismantling of technology's instrumentation, it may appear as abandonment—and in some senses it is. The family must often make a difficult trade: to choose palliative care effectively removes them and their loved one from conventional legitimacy in the hospital and the public realm. They must give up their hope for an unlimited future (a socially acceptable good) and accept the imminence of mortality along with symptom control and targeted support (a more equivocal social good). Even to disclose mortality is seen as abandonment in many societies (Blackhall et al. 2001; Gordon 1990; Seale 1998: 178). One of the chaplains in the Catholic community hospital revealed the equivocation in palliative care: "There's this energy to move into palliative care. When we can't help people anymore, then we have to. We set goals. The system is geared toward goals. We have to be *doing*. When we're not clear—With the palliative care pathway, we have a name for doing nothing."

Accrued time in the ritual of intensification burdens clinicians with the realization that "we can't help people anymore," an acknowledgment that the original goal is lost. Palliative care may be "nothing" in comparison to rescue and stabilization, but its name conveys the legitimacy belonging to a real plan. The chaplain's comment was a telling description in the Catholic community hospital. Although it had a six-page palliative pathway, the expertise of palliative care patient management did not exist within its walls. The hospital's concerted efforts to organize a palliative care program during the period of my research generated no bedside results in the sixteen months I was there.

The consistent opportunity for getting patients' troubling symptoms under good control is not yet a reality in the U.S. hospital, whether or not the patient is dying. Clive Seale's "leakiness" observed in the dying person's body can bring profound self-deprecation (Lawton 2000: 94). A further disappointment comes from Julia Lawton who cautions that the "craft of dying" offered by hospice may not materialize due to the strong cultural association of the self with the body. As dysfunction mounts, the self shrinks. In Lawton's fieldwork, she observed that patients' sense of self dissipated as they lost their agency and capacity for movement. This dependence of the psycho-social on the physical bodes ill for hospice's efforts to promote autonomy and control at the end of life. Many seriously ill hospitalized patients lack consciousness, whether this state is induced by clinicians or part of the patient's condition, making the sense of self that hospice promotes difficult to realize and uphold.

The revivalist model of the so-called dying process assumes that it can be bracketed well before death, ignoring the muddiness introduced by the ritual of intensification. Its ideal picture projects a conscious, voiced patient surrounded by loving family and friends. When the patient is beyond speech, it is not hospice but bioethics that seems interested, although in a very narrow way. For bioethics, the lack of voice or consciousness before death (whether physiological or induced) becomes a site of struggle to define autonomy and choices about further treatment, rather than a place to wonder about creating meaning before death. In fact, the very discourse about autonomy and choices skews the perspective, turning the gaze away from the reality of death to the act of decision-making and the need to redeem it (Drought and Koenig 2002).

The revivalist discourse offers a conceptualization of the time before death by naming it and drawing attention to it as a logical way to complete a life that has been accustomed to entitlement and control. In doing so, it asserts the subjecthood of the seriously ill patient lost in the contingencies of acute care. In this way, it becomes the perfect foil for the ritual of intensification, providing a customized haven of order and linearity in contrast to the chaos of managing complications. The trajectories of few illnesses truly conform to this ideal, however, especially in the hospital. The movement suffers from further drawbacks. First, it deploys no comparable display of validation equal to that offered by the ritual of intensification; second, despite palliative care inroads, a clear declaration of terminality is usually required for referral to hospice or palliative care, a step that physicians are often reluctant to take (Christakis 1999); third, the patient must agree to forego both the search for more time alive and/or public interest to right the wrongs inflicted by the accident; fourth, for home care, the patient must be stable enough to survive the transport and must have a caregiver and a safe location for care; fifth, to reap the most benefit, the patient must still be conscious, able to interact, and have people available to listen.

Despite these drawbacks, the revivalist discourse is a powerful ideal well-suited to self-reliant middle-class Americans who want to define death "on our own terms" (Moyers 2000). It is also a voice that maintains the importance of honoring both the person and the process of death among those who are privileged to participate, a critical wedge argument challenging the disappearance of dying and death from modernity.

The meaning of death in modernity concentrates on the contingency and unpredictability of its presentation. Cultural interests in death avoidance fuel the ritual of intensification in the hospital to push the envelope of contingency and correct the physical and societal disorder of the "accident." Dying becomes a tricky category. Expired patients may not have received "care for the dying," because the label would have been a form of disapprobation. Expired patients' charts may be as distant from quality-review initiatives as their final outcomes were from the goals of acute care. Counter-discourses of bioethics and hospice influence how clinicians make a case for closing the ritual, providing a "good death" and thereby serving the hospital's primary interest in "moving things along" (Kaufman 2005). In the next chapter, we explore how these forces play out in both orderly and disorderly hospital dying situations.

Notes

1. Daniel Callahan has come to a similar conclusion (2003: 68).
2. See Mellor and Shilling (1993). Of course, in many urban neighborhoods, young people grow up expecting to meet a violent end at any time.
3. See Bauman (1992: 140). Bauman does not differentiate among individuals with or without access to health-care.
4. See Institute for Healthcare Improvement (2003a). A typical measure of overall hospital quality is delay of death, indicated by mortality and other measurements (Lynn 2004: 93).
5. These findings indicate that the "path" of info/statistics regarding dying/death/dead within hospitals is likely to be internally determined rather than standardized across institutions.
6. Problems of prognostication (Christakis 1999).
7. "Zone of indistinction," as Sharon Kaufman (2005) calls it. "Indeterminacy," according to Nancy Johnson and colleagues (2000).
8. See Lock (2002) and Fadiman (1997) for critical studies of this attitude. Fins (2009) comments on the attitudes absorbed by a physician in training regarding brain injury.
9. The newly dead in Berawan culture are menacing, but they are also the pathway to communication with the long dead (Metcalf 1982: 109). But perhaps the most striking feature is that the corpse is treated in ways that seem to deny that it is dead after all: it is talked to, offered food and cigarettes, and even, on one

occasion, spoon-fed. What these gestures express, in the most direct manner conceivable, is continuity (1982: 45).

10. Bach, Schrag, and Begg (2004), Lynn (2004: 139), and Teno (2004) have advocated the use of mortality follow-back studies to overcome constraints to research on dying patients, although such data may not generate meaningful results.

11. See Kirchhoff et al. (2004). An informal review of charts of deceased patients from my unit supported these findings; Glavan et al.'s (2008) results were more promising, while indicating the labor-intensive nature of the work. Electronic medical records could ease this burden.

12. Although this term is often used as if it were an unequivocal marker of dying, the Society for Critical Care Medicine has been able to differentiate between "weaker" and "stronger" irreversibility (Society for Critical Care Medicine Ethics Committee, American College of Critical Care Medicine 2001).

13. An explanation regarding the ritual of intensification as ritual can be found in Chapter 7.

14. Jane Seymour notes the contrast between "bodily" and "technical" dying, and that nurses identify the former before the explanation is in hand (2000). See Chapter 7.

15. Metcalf and Huntington (1991: 96) differentiate between celebratory and instrumental mortuary rites.

16. See Kaufman (2005: 102). It also recalls the "surreal minuet" engaging physicians and families that Diane Meier described above.

17. Even most of Kaufman's cases concern the difficulties of decision-making and "moving things along" rather than the process of dying that comes afterward.

18. I am grateful to Barbara Koenig for this insight, in a private conversation.

19. For discussions of ethnic variation, see Blackhall et al. (2001), Dula (1994), Waters (2001), and Dula and Williams (2005). For "moving things along," see Kaufman (2005).

20. It is perhaps surprising how infrequently broader cultural conversations such as physician-assisted suicide, the difference between "Killing and Allowing to Die" (Sulmasy 1995) and cases such as Terry Schiavo receive explicit attention at the bedsides of particular patients, at least in my experience.

21. See Walter (1994: 123, again echoing Hsu 1972). The tension between the "expert" opinion of hospice and the individual's self-expression concerns much of Walter's exposition.

22. Walter notes that this is the "fashion," and that hospice and the euthanasia lobby promote opposite means of accomplishing this end (1994: 51).

23. See Walter (1994: 135). In contrast, Julia Lawton notes that hospice patients who felt well enough to participate in a day care program exhibited a distinct unease with references to the future, preferring to focus on the present and the past (2000: 67–72).

24. For discussion as to differing views of hospice and palliative care by African Americans, see Dula and Williams (2005) and Crawley (2005).

25. This attempt has been unsuccessful, and palliative care certification is being taken over by Board of Internal Medicine (Stephen Connor, personal communication).

CHAPTER 4

Death with as Little Dying as Possible

> One can speak of an amortal society. There are no dead around; only the memory of lives that are not there. The ordinary person suffers from the inability to die.

> —Illich (1995a: 1653)

The hospital administrator quoted in Chapter 3 wished to insert a clear bright line between those who are dying and those who are dead. His attempt at demarcation is more effective if the two entities being separated are the public and death. As industrialized society has made it possible to confine death *to* the hospital and also *within* it, the distance between the living and those who might be dying is increased (Mellor and Shilling 1993). The hospital space protects the general public from the bedside and vice versa; clinicians caring for patients represent society and act as its agents (van der Geest and Finkler 2004). As such, they carry out the mandates of society, whether they are aware of it or not. It is not surprising that the spaces of the hospital where the open-ended altruism of life-saving occurs exhibit greater cultural endorsement than other spaces. In these spaces, highly trained individuals solve diagnostic puzzles (Kuhn 1996), enact procedures, and perform technological displays such as intensive care, surgery, and angiography. Other clinical spaces such as rehabilitation, psychiatry, or palliative care units may appear more humdrum by comparison, deprived of the potential for a dramatic turnaround. They command a lower rate of reimbursement, or none at all. Here the activities of chronic illness and dying may play out, unlit.

It is not death but dying that poses the greater menace in the hospital. Writing contemporaneously with David Sudnow about hospital dying in the 1960s, Barney Glaser and Anselm Strauss noted that "Dying must be defined in order to be reacted to as dying" (1968: 242). Because the designation is so culturally stigmatized, it now requires the ritual of intensification to make it possible. Without it, death in the hospital is rarely preceded by Dying. Patients who appear seriously ill may not die before patients who appear more stable (Fox et al. 1999: 1644). This unpredictability is a problem. In the Catholic community hospital, presumably healthy elderly patients can be admitted for a benign complaint only to collapse and die, despite attempts to revive them (see Mrs. Jennings, below). Patients who were very seriously ill in the teaching hospital, perhaps on life support and waiting for organ transplantation, are not treated as terminally ill. This is not to say that clinicians are blind to a patient's deterioration, but that a threshold of requirements must be met for the official change in status to occur. Physical death may or may not be one of them. Mr. Mendez suffered cardiac arrest several times, but not until "he was not there anymore" was he admitted into the Dying category. Only when the chief halted his resident's zeal and Mrs. Turner's neurological devastation sealed her fate (a common benchmark, see Chapter 7) was she seen officially as Dying.

Clinical behavior shifts significantly when consensus is reached that the patient is Dying, indicating that if death must occur in the hospital, it should (and often does) happen with minimal dying. Clinicians want this final interval to be manageable, free of chaos, and subject to their control. In relating a cancer death, one nurse's summation was telling. When I asked her "how it went," she said,

> RN: I've been involved in a couple that have been very dramatic. Family members laying on the floor, "I can't believe he's gone." This was quiet and peaceful. There was a sitter who had been with the family a long time. She was in the room when he passed. He was not alone when he went, and it was a good thing.
>
> I truly think that—nobody wants to be around dying people. But if you can help them find closure and go peacefully—

Her comments indicated that from her perspective, it was good for dying to be peaceful and accompanied rather than dramatic and subject to acting out. She felt that "closure" and "peace" could perhaps redeem a situation that "nobody wants to be around." One ICU in the teaching hospital placed labels on the doors of patients for whom a DNR order had been written. If such a patient suffered an arrhythmia, the green sticker would serve as a warning to staff who might otherwise rush in to defibrillate. At all other times they also reminded staff continuously of the patient's lack of legitimacy in the prevailing system of rescue.

> In a meeting about ICU protocol, the ICU nurse made a very interesting comment. She related that the husband of a patient who had been made a DNR and had a green sticker on her room said that he noticed that the nurses don't go in the rooms as often with the green stickers—this one and the one across the way. He'd been counting. (excerpt from field notes)

Clinicians are largely unaware of the hospital and cultural agendas that influence their practices as they move patients to more "suitable" (nonpublic, nonrescue) beds and/or administer medication so that dying is peaceful and death is prompt (see Chapter 7). Several "situations" of dying (to call it a "process" suggests that it is both internal and linear when it is neither [Kastenbaum 1978: 227]) exemplify patterns that conform to clinician expectations of order and minimize social exposure to dying, according to the two hospitals.

The time and complexity of negotiation that establish the patient's second-class status through the ritual of intensification is so resisted and so wearing on the participants that the period of Dying itself becomes an anticlimax. Opening up the process of dying so that meaning might be made according to revivalist ideals requires training, energy, time, attention, skill, and commitment. This effort receives consistent, reliable sanction only in the more secluded reaches of palliative care. It is a common misperception that patients must already be Dying or at the "end of life" to be admitted to hospice or palliative care. This idea is fueled by the Medicare Hospice Benefit requiring a physician to declare a patient's lifespan to be shorter than six months for its activation.[1] Despite programmatic efforts to displace this fallacy (see Chapter 8), the difficult work of appending the label of Dying must often occur before the referral can be made. Dying itself, therefore, has little cultural advocacy in the trenches of the battle for more time alive. If dying becomes Dying only with such difficulty in the hospital, then how does death actually happen?

To be dying in the hospital is to be placed in the category of Other. In Deborah Gordon's study of women with breast cancer in Italy, she found that keeping the dreaded diagnosis a secret was a strategy for retaining the patient's social standing.

> The strong association of cancer with death, suffering, and hopelessness in much of Italy, coupled with the tremendous power attributed to naming and "sentencing" makes nondisclosure a major

mechanism for keeping the "condemned" in this social world, and keeping death, decay, and suffering in the "other." It is the social reality that is dominant here, such that informing a patient of cancer can be tantamount to social death. (1990: 275)

Gordon's description of retaining membership in Italy's "social world" trumps the U.S. imperative to acknowledge the physiological presence of cancer in the autonomous self. But the "death, decay and suffering" must still be excluded somehow.[2] In the U.S. hospital, to be officially Dying carries a social stigma that is similar to naming breast cancer in Italy. If death is successfully consigned to the abstract through contingency or to the bolt from the blue in the everyday life of many Americans, it would appear that little social meaning need be made of it. But to be *dying* is to bring death close on to life's business, risking its contamination. In the hospital where it is accepted that death will intrude sporadically despite its banishment, dying is a traitorous activity. Even when it is thoroughly vetted through the ritual of intensification, dying retains its spurious character, staining the patient in the eyes of polite society. To be rescued or eligible for rescue confers all the legitimacy of accepted social exchange, and an ambiguous prognosis carries most of it; but to declare that in this particular person's case death will not be treated as if it were premature is to drop the patient out of public social concern. It is an anathema to do this according to the egalitarian ideas of the United States.

The problem is that dying itself is untidy, unsettling, and loathe to be contained. Boundaries of closure and peace must be imposed on it to ensure that it does not offend. Clinician reactions to dying in the hospital reflect cultural understandings that to control disruption is a moral exercise. A "good death" in the hospital (outside of palliative care) means that the dying will be orderly and that death will be timely. The presence of life support and the ritual of intensification often allow the convenience of planning ahead, of imposing discipline on the dying situation (Kaufman 2005: 32). Dying (if not death) should wait until all the lab results are in, family meetings have been held, and consensus is reached. When life-supportive measures are withdrawn, Dying can usually be well-behaved, seen and not heard. A peaceful death should arrive promptly enough to "prove" that life support had only been delaying the "inevitable" and no longer serving as the means to produce more time alive.

Hospice principles, too, assume that dying can be domesticated and that events will occur in a linear sequence. First, life's finitude must attach itself recognizably to a patient at the conclusion of a valiant struggle, and there must be enough time left for hospice or palliative care to be called. The experts in symptom control and dying can then move in, claim the space, and re-create it. If all goes according to plan, the stigma of dying then disappears as the patient is embraced by a group where he "belongs," no longer of concern to the public culture. It is up to the group in charge of the patient to determine how and whether dying is perilous for him. In palliative care, the patient's individualism in dying can be encouraged; in the greater culture, which includes the hospital proper, it must be minimized.

Disorderly Dying and Death

Clinicians' understandings of what comprises an orderly, manageable dying situation and what does not may have little in common with the perceptions of the patients or the families. It is the clinicians who hold the power to name and determine the components of time, sequence, location and access to the bedside. Their control of the turf persists, even as closure of the ritual of intensification mandates that the (now) Dying patient is no longer a public concern. Dying is supposed to be a private matter. But the hospital is often a difficult place for patients and families to reclaim their agency and direct such private events, even if they are prepared to navigate this "nowhere land" of dying, as one chaplain called it. Clinicians themselves may be no better equipped, but as agents of the society, they may value orderliness as a higher priority than family concerns, even if the latter are discoverable. Clinicians' sense of purpose enables them to inject this private matter with societal concerns even unconsciously, so that no party is fully aware that it is happening.

Still, dying and death can go astray for clinicians in a number of very disturbing ways. Lack of consensus about the care plan is frustrating. If the patient is dying and the care plan does not reflect this, moral distress is common among nurses and lower level physicians (see Chapter 7). Even if the family and the team agree, dying and even death is fraught with pitfalls. Death can be "wrong" for the patient (too young, not sick enough to die); clear but often unacknowledged errors occur (examples were a "filleted trach," instances of euthanasia, an error in identifying a driver's license preference for organ donation, paralytic infusions not stopped prior to withdrawals of life support); or persons exhibit "wrong" behavior (families not available or acting out; coworkers inappropriate; plan of care unclear; chaos). Clinicians caring for patients with brain death feel the outcome is flawed if death occurs without organ donation. Occasionally, clinicians doubt themselves, their own abilities, or reactions.

Two major derangements regarding dying and death are disorders of time and place. Deaths that occur while patients are in the elevator or on the commode are upsetting. By contrast, a chaplain told of an elderly woman who died in her wheelchair while her companion was conducting her through the hospital searching for her doctor's office. The chaplain found them, noticed that the patient was dead, and escorted them to the emergency room. This event aroused very little interest, as the woman was no one's responsibility at the time that she died.

Death is also disordered if it comes at the wrong time. Patient management requires anticipation of unlikely contingencies, and surprises are disliked. Patients who die at shift change, who are found dead, who die with turning, or before the family arrives die at the "wrong" time. "Right" dying occurs when patients do not "linger" after life support is withdrawn, codes (resuscitation efforts) do not go on too long, and patients do not die too soon for palliative care to be involved. What once was called the death-watch is uncomfortable for persons accustomed to goal-directed activities (Vanstone 2004: 43–51). Pressure exists to minimize one's exposure to such helplessness.

Orderliness is the other side of the coin. Clinicians express satisfaction when dying occurs with the team, family, and patient in agreement; families make appropriate choices; the patient is transferred to palliative care; dying is peaceful, with no chaos; the patient's physical symptoms seem controlled; family is present; and they themselves receive support from coworkers. In other words, there are no surprises. These attributes emphasize control and minimal disruption of routine necessary to maintain normal operations rather than openness to possibility (Kastenbaum 1978: 227).

Orderly Dying: Consensus

Dying as a "situation" is more orderly for clinicians if it is either named or unnamed, that is, if it comes either as a surprise to no one or else to everyone. Consensus, then, is the first level of order, and the ritual of intensification is the means to achieving that unanimity. The management of the interval between the achievement of consensus and the patient's actual death is felt to be a distinct anticlimax, especially if the patient is unresponsive. Patient awareness of their own dying process before the fact, a basic assumption in the revivalist ideas of good dying, occurred in only 3 percent of the 211 total cases.

What follows is a description of four dying situations that appeared orderly to the clinicians involved, with consensus as the determining factor: resuscitation attempts, withdrawal of life support, good dying in palliative care, and brain death with organ donation. Lack of consensus can result in profound disorder, bringing clinician suffering with it. Discussion of the latter is reserved for Chapter 7 as part of a more detailed exposition of the ritual of intensification.

Orderly Dying 1: The Surprise Collapse

At the same time that resuscitation protocols are designed to restore heartbeat, circulation, and breathing, they are also a classificatory device. Simply to lose any or all of these vital functions when clinicians are unprepared for it cannot qualify as death in the modern hospital, even though death has been so measured for millennia. The ultimate contingency of CPR must be applied to the disorder of sudden death, and it must fail for the patient to qualify as truly dead. This social agreement has been codified into some state laws. Codes preceded approximately 23 percent of deaths in the study (but not all of these were unanticipated).

Rescue is what hospitals are designed to do. Mock codes and Advanced Cardiac Life Support training give opportunities for rehearsal, and official sanction is everywhere. But schism exists, and the appropriate code status for a patient is a frequent point of contest in the ritual of intensification. Clinicians justify CPR most readily for young patients, those with few or no comorbidities, cases of sudden collapse rather than gradual deterioration, and for neurologically intact patients. These conditions coincide with patients who are "not disabled" and "not dying." Greater clinical disagreement occurs regarding CPR for the old, the frail, the sick, and those with cancer or with impaired consciousness.[3] *Expected* codes may be extremely distressing to nurses, who as first responders often try to get the physicians to change the patient's code status to DNR to head off the requirement to perform chest compressions on patients who already look "bad," or whose quality of life appears poor and likely to remain so. One floor nurse in the Catholic community hospital reflected on her successful intervention to obtain a DNR order before she was required to perform CPR on a patient she thought was dying.

> RN: Unfortunately we beat dead horses. Imagine if the patient is at all aware. Codes are such a frightening scene—a mob scene. They descend on the patient. Furniture is moved, there's no time to be nice about things. We're slapping stickies on [the chest] to run

[heart rhythm] strips. Anesthesia is looking down the throat for intubation. From my standpoint, I prevented that from happening, since it wasn't going to change the outcome. . . . Fortunately many of our patients come in and code status has already been dealt with. When not, I've been afraid that someday I might meet these people in some hereafter somewhere. I don't want them to say, "That's the woman that beat on my chest." You've got to live with yourself.

This nurse's remorse over CPR emboldened her to overstep hierarchical bounds if necessary to create order and prevent pointless suffering. Codes have special significance because they are both public, announced over the hospital paging system and requiring several clinicians taking turns at chest compressions, and brutal, often breaking ribs. Resuscitation attempts may last a few minutes to more than an hour, diverting numbers of staff from their responsibilities to other patients. Outcomes for in-hospital CPR vary based on skill of the rescuers and underlying co-morbidities (see below). Ironically, those who suffer sudden collapse *are not often considered to be dying* if spontaneous circulation returns. The contamination of the brush with death can be canceled out by the triumph of rescue.

Perhaps if CPR enjoyed the efficacy of treatments such as cardiac stents or the early days of antibiotics so that some large proportion of patients survived the onslaught with minimal side effects, it would not be a point of contention. But such is not the case. Despite the mistaken impression of overall CPR efficacy implied by body-trauma programs, the true success rate is both surprisingly poor and difficult to measure.[4] Expectations on the part of the public and some clinicians are unrealistically high (Jones, Brewer, and Garrison 2000; Roberts, Hirschman, and Scheltema 2000). Recall that Mr. Mendez survived two codes but did not recover to leave the hospital. Acknowledging CPR's relatively poor record of patient survival, an administrator of Emergency Medical Services (EMS) stated:

> The benchmark [for measuring CPR success] is changing. I like to ask, "Survival till when? What is a failed outcome?" Resuscitation is still in its infancy. What is it and what should it be? How do we define successful resuscitation? EMS is a practice, an exercise. We optimize skill for the people we can help. Even if this [present case] is futile, you're honing your skills for the next person, for whom it won't be. So it's worth doing. Maybe in thirty years we'll do it all differently.[5]

This respected field rescuer objected to measuring the value of CPR by mortality statistics, even though outcome data fuel the popular paradigm of evidence-based medicine. In his view, even useless CPR attempts have value in "honing skills for the next person," and judgments of its quality require a broad perspective. Even if statistics indicate that CPR is often ineffective, the alternative of doing nothing in the face of certain death seems not to be acceptable, a phenomenon that neither he nor the poor survival numbers address. Public confidence in the effectiveness of CPR, backed by media depictions of general success, advances the rescue enterprise (Diem, Lantos, and Tulsky 1996; Timmermans 1999: 83–84).

Another reason to persist in rescue despite its poor record is for the social gratification it provides. When individual crisis happens, the community proves to itself that its response is prompt, thorough, and egalitarian. Mrs. Jennings, a woman in her late 60s, came into the Catholic community hospital with an abdominal complaint. The physician prescribed a diagnostic colonoscopy for the following day. She had been drinking a liquid to clean out her colon when her collapse occurred. The nurse told the story.

RN: It was totally out of the blue. Usually I have sixth sense about these things. This was not the case. It was totally unexpected.

HC: How did you know she was dying?

RN: She was alert and oriented as you and me. She was drinking Golitely for a colonoscopy the next day. Her husband was standing in the hallway and he said, "I wish someone would come look at my wife." Her eyes were wide open, her pupils were dilated. She was the color of that khaki-colored jacket. The "I'm dead but I'm still breathing" color. She was not responding. Her breathing was shallow and rapid. She had a pulse. But in 30 to 45 seconds that was gone. Her breathing slowed down. I told him, "We'll have to code her." He said, "Can I go home?" I told him, "This is serious. Maybe you should go to the waiting room." He said, "I can't handle this. I'm going home." The code was called. Twenty-five people converge on her. We work on her for one hour. They'd get a rhythm, they'd get her back briefly, they gave drug after drug. Forty-five minutes into it, I get a phone call from a woman with a foreign accent. I ask, "Who am I speaking with?" I ask, "Is the patient's husband there?" She says "Yes," I say, "I need to talk to him." I tell him "They're working on her. She's on a ventilator, it's serious. We're preparing to transfer her to the ICU." He said, "Do the best you can." They called the code (off) fifteen or twenty

minutes later. The doc called him and told him. It was not like it
was [expected]. There were no signs ahead of time, no shortness of
breath, no chest pain. Totally unexpected.

This was death as the Accident, coming without warning to someone
"as alert as you and me," patently *not* dying, and entitled to a total communal response. Because her death had arrived out of order, it could not
remain unchallenged. Rescue was called for. When it failed, Mrs. Jennings
could be declared dead with a clear conscience. People had "done the best
they could" on her behalf, regardless of the inefficacy of their response. Few
situations carry such a powerful opportunity for the testing and exoneration
of heroic altruism. Serving the cause of rescue consumed everyone's attention except Mr. Jennings, whose shock drove him from the scene.

In describing a different case, a CCU nurse in the community hospital
expressed pride in her unit's orderly practice during codes, usually tumultu-
ous activities.

HC: How did it go from your standpoint?

RN: It went very well. Codes are very good in here. People are
very experienced, they know what they're doing. Calm and under
control. Very experienced. We all kick into action. We fall into
a rhythm. As things happen we yell it out, "3:05, another epi."[6]
Someone is writing everything down, even though the pharmacy is
recording. Especially if things are going from intubation to [place-
ment of central intravenous] lines. Someone starts documenting. I
was running the monitor and checking different rhythms several
times. She had a jagged rhythm. After thirty minutes you start trying everything you can do.

In the teaching hospital, clinicians also expressed conformity to the
algorithm *(we did everything step by step)*, but seemed to take codes as
more mundane. They attended to the features of a code that differed from
the "norm." The registered nurse said: "We worked on her for forty-five
minutes. It was the longest code I've ever experienced. They couldn't do
anything. Every time we'd get a rhythm, it would fall out after twenty or
thirty seconds. We could never really revive her."

Orderliness in codes was not synonymous with efficacy or skill, but it
added to a perception of existential control in the face of mortality. This
is not to say that clinicians were unmoved by patients' deaths, but that
there was satisfaction in doing a difficult job as a team. Clinician narratives

described the convergence of personnel, unity in their efforts, working in synch, many simultaneous roles, and effort that persisted over time.

But what happens to this unified societal concern afterward? All the intensity disappears immediately when the physician "calls it," and the crowd of clinicians, unified by the emergency, rushes out of the room to catch up on neglected duties involving other patients. Only the chaplain may be left with the body to notice the significance of what just occurred. One chaplain at the Catholic community hospital described the phenomenon: "He called it, I turned around and there was no one in the room and the covers were pulled up! It's like turning on the light and the roaches scurry away in all directions."

What this graphic description conveys is the code's naked destruction of the space that remains when the clinicians hurry off to other tasks: overhead lights blazing, trash cans and needle boxes overflowing with the detritus of used central line kits and discarded sterile garb, bloodied gauzes, alcohol swabs, clamps, and needleless syringes scattered on the bed and the floor. The flat board placed between the unrelaxed patient and the mattress (required for effective chest compressions) and the useless endotracheal tube protruding from the mouth make it look as if succor had never come near to this patient.

In fact, the proven dead must be relinquished immediately in the name of the pressing needs of those still living, who had been abandoned when it was necessary to try to snatch the newly dead back to life. A chaplain in the pilot study reflected on this circumstance after a code. He spoke aloud about the wisdom of introducing a new element into the postcode dynamic by proposing a moment of silence—an idea suggested to him by a palliative care physician. He considered the personal fortitude that it would take to try this:

> CH: The code was routine in many ways. Sometimes the family is present, sometimes not. I've become more intentional about staying with the code until the pronouncement [of death] and staying with the doctor. Or if the family is there, staying with them. I did think about Dr. B's comment to give people a moment of silence to honor what has just happened. I was thinking, "How would that work here?" You'd need a chaplain gutsy enough to say it. I think it could be very powerful for the medical staff. I know if I did it, I would hear about it. Which is not necessarily bad.

The peculiarity of social convergence to save life and then the scattering when life is gone recalls the idea of death as a matter for the wastebin, making the now-abandoned body congruent with the trash in the room. A call to collective commemoration would sharpen the humanity of both the patient and the staff, dulled respectively after the code by death, failure, and disappointment. But to interrupt the staff's unspoken dispersal would be a radical, public act, as both the chaplain and Dr. B recognized. The factor of speed at both ends of the code illustrates the complementary aspects of rescue and productivity. Homage to public meaning is at its highest in the imperative to rescue (announced over PA at Catholic community hospital, in every instance) and at its lowest when the code is declared (privately) to be over. For clinicians, unease is a personal matter, to be attended to sometime later when things calm down.

The attempt to rescue patients when they collapse provides consensus, satisfaction, and synchrony for clinicians as the agents of society. A situation of dying may be thereby happily avoided, regardless of the outcome for the patient. CPR is not the only gateway to life-supportive interventions, however. Many patients acquire breathing tubes, blood pressure support, or cardiac pacing without first undergoing cardiovascular or respiratory collapse. When the ritual of intensification closes down, these supports must be dismantled to introduce official Dying.

Orderly Dying 2: Dying by Arrangement, or the Withdrawal of Life Support

Even though clinicians have nationally set algorithms to follow, codes can seem extremely chaotic while they are in progress. By contrast, the withdrawal of life support is almost entirely free form. Yet, it also feels orderly to clinicians for several reasons. First, it follows the deliberate closure of the ritual of intensification so that the sense of relief that comes with consensus and the end of uncertainty persists into these final activities. Second, by comparison to the intensity of aggressive treatment, its pace is far more relaxed. Third, it is a more private interval, often orchestrated by the nurse, less prone to interruption, and more subject to his control. Finally, with "comfort care" now the primary rather than the secondary goal, the nurse can administer symptom relief to her heart's content, perhaps for the first time in this patient's clinical course.

Withdrawal of life support preceded death in 23–26 percent of the cases in my fieldwork, and it is a rising phenomenon in the hospital. In a 1998 prospective study of ICUs in the United States, 38 percent of deaths were preceded by the withdrawal of life support (Prendergast, Claessens, and Luce 1998). In contrast to codes, there is often no formalized training in best practices nor are there protocols to serve as resources.[7] In what order should one dismantle the instrumentation that was individualized to the patient's needs? What dosages for pain and sedation should be given, if any? These and other details usually depend on practitioner judgment. The entire procedure may be negotiated among the clinicians (nurse, respiratory therapist, physician) and perhaps the family involved, and/or clinicians work independently. Clinicians often learn procedures from each other, from anecdotal reports, and through their own experience. Perhaps no other aspect of hospital clinical practice may be so practitioner dependent, vulnerable to inconsistency, unsupervised, and poorly documented. This phenomenon also makes it overtly parochial and cultural, entirely subject to clinician and hospital agendas.

Withdrawal of life support in an ICU is the most straightforward and orderly dying situation for clinicians because it is bracketed as a separate procedure enacted at the end of the ritual of intensification, after the patient has been openly declared as terminal. It conforms to linear expectations. Clinicians can and do exert control over its unfolding. "Only when death is named and expected, when a space for *waiting for death* has been created, can families characterize the death of their relative as 'good' later on" (Kaufman 2005: 201, emphasis in original).

Recall Mr. DiAngelo who had been placed BiPAP for his respiratory distress over the weekend. On Monday morning, the decision was made to discontinue this method of supporting his life. With Dying officially in place, the staff could manage the when and the how to a significant extent. Accordingly, the nurse kept the mask in place, delaying the withdrawal (and the onset of instability) long enough for the family to spend time with him.

One nurse in the teaching hospital described the dying of 72-year-old Mr. Sanders, who was not recovering after his last surgery for a digestive problem. By now Mr. Sanders was no longer talking or interactive. A family meeting occurred, resulting in a plan to withdraw his life support. Specific physician orders may be written for each action, but they are often left to nursing discretion. Especially in the teaching hospital, ICU nurses exercised their own judgment over these matters, as they did in Ms. Hunter's case until the resident took things over (see Chapter 1). Mr. Sanders' case illustrates the agency of the nurse in the situation and unit reluctance to set limits on individual practice.

> RN: It had been discussed before I got there. When I came on in the morning they were waiting for the last of the family members to get there. They were all in support of letting him go. It was surprising.

You get so many dysfunctional families in here, that can't deal with it. So many people here I work with who are not normal. It was probably pretty normal. [I'm just not used to it.]

The nurse told the family that they expected Mr. Sanders "to go pretty quickly," after the life-supportive medications were taken away, but it can be very difficult to predict precisely how individual patients will react to these measures in the moment. The nurse told me that she systematically turned off all the drips that were supporting Mr. Sanders' blood pressure. At the same time, she doubled dosages of the pain medication and sedation drips. She said: "He was hanging out with a blood pressure of fifty over thirty for 15 to 30 minutes. So we turned down the vent settings and so he passed. We didn't want his family to be there a long time wondering, 'When is he going to go?' We were not wanting to lengthen the experience for them."

In this case, the nurse set up the expectation that the withdrawal and the dying situation would not take long. When Mr. Sanders did not die immediately after her initial actions, she removed Mr. Sanders's breathing support: "We turned down the vent settings and so he passed." She expressed her desire to hurry things up in terms of compassionate consideration for the family, just as the nurse in Ms. Hunter's case had justified her newly accelerated dying. If Mr. Sanders' nurse had seen the procedure as patient-dependent and open-ended, an element of meaning making might have been introduced. But the fear that the dying will go on too long is a frequent concern. Her narrative continued.

HC: So everyone was there? Was the chaplain there?

RN: The chaplain was there.

HC: How did it go?

RN: It went well. There were a few tears. Everyone gave him a kiss. Said their last words. Then they dispersed. It was pleasant to be with them and hear all the good things they had to say about him.

HC: When did they do that?

RN: Everyone wanted to touch his hands and give a kiss when they came in. One or two spokespeople for the family said, "We're ready." I don't think they were really aware of what I was doing in there. They weren't aware of when I turned off the vasopressin. Some were boohooing and others were talking.

I confirmed with the spokespeople that I'd turned off the medications as we'd talked about. I let the chaplain take over, and I monitored from the outside.

In this portion of the narrative, the nurse indicated that she had discussed the plan of withdrawal with the family before she started, and she allowed them to spend time with Mr. Sanders beforehand and as she turned off the drips. Because the nurse did not alert them, the family did not know, as she did, exactly when the interval of active dying had begun. Its starting point was in the front of her awareness, but she could not know what it might mean to the family. As did many of the nurses in these narratives, she tried to stay very much in the background with her actions, wishing the family's major interactions to be with the chaplain, the patient, or with one another.

HC: Do you have a protocol for doing this?

RN: No. I brought back information from a class I went to. But the reaction was, "We don't want cookbook nursing." It's so personal. People do so many different things. I'm not sure it would go over. One thing I learned in the class. A point of interest. Not turning off the vent at once, but weaning it down and turning up the morphine at the same time. But I brought it to our nurse educator, and she said "Enh." (Nixed it.) I don't think we have a problem with anything we're doing now. People go peacefully.

This nurse had attempted to introduce information she obtained from an educational experience, but her unit resisted efforts at standardization, or even opening up the topic for discussion that might improve practice. Her observation "it's so personal" indicates that this domain does not lend itself to standardization that more public aspects of clinical practice do. Her rationalization for accepting the ruling of the group was that idiosyncratic practice was good enough; "people go peacefully." In an environment that lionizes evidence-based medicine in other areas of patient management, holding fast to local understandings regarding the withdrawal of life support is unusually protective behavior.

For Mr. Mendez and Mrs. Turner (Chapter 3), the ritual of intensification ended with the pronouncement of their irreversible neurological devastation. Their deaths resulted from the withdrawal of life support (often referred to as a plan to "withdraw," "withdraw care," or "withdraw support," abbreviations that reveal unconscious attitudes). In the nurse's account of the process for Mr. Mendez, several things did not go smoothly. The respiratory therapist in charge of the ventilator insisted that the physician "by law" had to be the one to disconnect his ventilator. Neither the nurse nor the resident felt in a position to challenge his assertion, so they complied. A nurse with less experience was also involved who was unaware that a stepwise reduction in the blood pressure infusions was not necessary in the case of withdrawal.

HC: So how did it go from your perspective?

RN: The resident was good with the family. It went rather smoothly.

HC: Is it unusual to have the doctor there?

RN: It's the law. [He has to be the one] disconnecting the tube to the vent. Respiratory therapy said, "No, it's the law, a doctor has to do that."[8] I've never heard of it. Well I've heard rumors. I never thought it was for sure. He could do everything else, but a doctor had to do that. The doctor was not familiar with that either. He said, "Okay." The respiratory therapist sounded like he knew what he was doing. We don't do that much [death with withdrawal] because usually they move out [after extubation] or they die on the vent. Very rarely do we have families wanting the vent off.

HC: Did you wean the dobutamine (heart medication by IV) or turn it off?

RN: I told her, "Just turn it off." It was at ten or five. I think she halved it. I think it was the nurse not realizing. We turned off the pacer and weaned off the dobutamine. The doctor disconnected the vent, and we extubated.

HC: Then what happened?

RN: We put him in a pajama top. We had the wife and the son sit with him until he passed away. When I left here his heart rate was thirty. He looked so peaceful. He looked the best I'd ever seen him. He had looked so miserable. I hadn't realized it until I saw him then. The wife and the son were in the room.

We had the chaplain come. Each of the family spoke. I was [sniffing]. It's funny to see how families are. They held hands with us. They thanked us. That was nice. A couple of them said prayers after the chaplain. That was nice. I thought they did real well.

The nurse's impressions were that Mr. Mendez was comfortable, the family was present and did well, and it was a moving, meaningful experience that included the staff. Neither the disagreement about who should disconnect the ventilator nor the fact that they were making up the procedure as they went along detracted from her impression of orderliness and satisfaction.

Like Mr. Sanders and Mr. Mendez, Mrs. Turner also was unresponsive by the time the family and the team decided to withdraw life support. Here the nurse orchestrated the arrangements, explaining that the ventilator would be removed, she would be breathing on her own, and she would put her on medications "to make her work of breathing easier." Her account of the withdrawal differed from the physician's, who believed that Mrs. Turner's lack of pain was achieved using very low doses of medication. The nurse increased the infusion of pain medication (Fentanyl) and began an infusion of Midazolam (trade name Versed), a sedative. When the family told her they were ready, she said:

RN: I started putting the pieces together. I watched from the outside. I watched the monitor. It took about twenty minutes. Before she passed, they were watching the monitor. I came in. They had been focusing on the monitor. I'm not sure they understood any of the numbers up there. I came in. I told them, "She has passed." The doctor came in and spoke with them briefly. Today I found out they'd had quite a few deaths in the family the last two years and it was too hard for them to stay. I said they could stay as long as they wanted.

HC: What were the meds? Do you remember the doses?

RN: The Fentanyl was on when I came on. At 100 mics (micrograms per hour), and I started—I gave a bolus of five of Versed and left it at five. I turned the Fentanyl up to 300 mics, and she was a small woman. Not moving very much!

HC: Did you extubate or turn off the vent?

RN: She had a trach. I put the trach collar on over to the plug in the wall. I turned it on. I offered the chaplain several times, and they were not interested.

HC: How did it go?

RN: Well. I was glad they were all there. They all had a part in that decision when to do it. There was nothing in her appearance that showed she was suffering. It went very smoothly. There were tears, but they were not overly emotional or kind of out of control. They were here two hours prior to, twenty minutes till she passed, then waited five or ten minutes after they left. The chaplain gave them the bereavement packet. They didn't stick around.

The nurse's impressions emphasize the consensus around the decision, the family's presence without being "out of control," and the patient's lack of suffering. These are indications of her satisfaction with orderliness. The purpose of the medications she told me was "to stifle the guppy breathing." This phrasing was different than what she used with the family, and it indicated that she wanted to preempt any appearance of struggle. It is possible that her wish for orderliness ensured Mrs. Turner's quick demise. She also mentioned that this was her second withdrawal, and she felt guilty because she wasn't touched by the experience. "It was all in the course of the day there."[9] The physician's account differed from the nurse's, indicating that she did not know or remember the exact doses the patient was receiving, but she also said, "She had no pain." She was also not present in the process until after Mrs. Turner had died. Dignity and lack of suffering were two major themes in the discourses of clinicians around goals of order for this process that echo Sharon Kaufman's findings. "Talk of dignity, suffering, and quality of life circulates widely in American society in general, and it permeates hospital culture, organizing the ways staff and families think about patients and what should be done" (2005: 207).

Orderly Dying 3: Good Dying in Palliative Care

The medical surgical unit in the Catholic community hospital has twenty-four beds, four of which are "hospice" beds. These are located at the far end of the unit in larger than standard-sized rooms, appointed with curtains and arm chairs convertible into small beds. Patients in these rooms are meant to receive hospice-like care, but they are not managed by a hospice program. The staff around the hospital is well aware of these four so-called hospice beds on three East, and the unit itself is particularly associated with dying. The staff on three East feels that the rest of the hospital "dumps" their dying patients on them, even as they pride themselves on their care of the dying.

In the teaching hospital, an actual palliative care unit has been set up with specialized staff who wish to care for dying patients exclusively, viewing it as a privilege. They are eager to admit dying patients and fight to justify continuing their hospital stays (see Chapter 8). They are uncomfortable caring for nonpalliative care patients. A palliative care nurse stated, "It's hard to change gears like that. We don't fix vital signs here. If the blood pressure is low, we don't fix it. It's hard to remember [how to handle other patients]. It gets confusing. We're so used to abnormal things. It becomes normal."

Nonetheless, the cases that they related to me bear little resemblance to the ideals of the revival of death movement. Many of the problems of disorder that plague nurses on other units occur here as well, such as families' chaotic behavior, errors in process such as inappropriate orders, timing, and the difficulty with families second-guessing the choice to forego aggressive treatment. But in the palliative care unit, these problems occur without the overlay of forward momentum that pervades the hospital as a whole.

For most patients, the ritual of intensification is complete before their admission to the palliative care unit, as it is in cases of withdrawal of life support.[10] The relaxed attitude in the palliative care unit about time intervals is remarkable. If the patient is "lingering," then efforts to justify her stay on the basis of acute care rather than custodial care become an issue for the case manager, but concerns about it are not transferred to the bedside or expressed in nurses' behavior. Clinicians routinely describe patients who reside in the unit for days rather than minutes or hours, and families are encouraged to create ways to participate in the journey. Sheltered within palliative care, physicians, physical therapists, and chaplains along with nurses embrace this interval of dying. A nurse described Ms. Stevens, a young woman with a failed bone marrow transplant.

> RN: She had lots of family. Her sister was the primary caregiver. She was in bed with her all day long. The family did all her personal care. They changed her, positioned her—we didn't do anything. She had the thermometer on the pillow above their heads, and periodically she would take out and shove it under her arm.

Here expansive dying is encouraged. The predictable trajectory, supportive staff, and protected space allow the freedom to choose, to customize care, and to be fully accompanied in the way that middle-class revivalists envision as a "good death."

Recall Mrs. Morgan from Chapter 1. Although she was on a floor unit, the staff's joint participation modeled the ideals of the palliative care unit and exemplified the orderliness of "good dying" in palliative care. The nurse indicated the decision to close the ritual of intensification for Mrs. Morgan with the phrase "they made her comfort care." The ritual of intensification plan makes the patient into a different entity, one who is unrescuable. The phrase illustrates the lack of agency ascribed even to a conscious patient. Here was a dying process that was difficult for everyone, staff, patient, and family, but it was not made private, of concern only to the immediate family.

It conformed to the ideals of the revivalist movement because of the open awareness (Glaser and Strauss 1965: 79–106), consciousness of self and the presence of others open to the situation, ability to interact in its context, and the presence and interaction of family and staff. Most interestingly, the death remained in public view, rather than consigned to a particular set of caregivers (Walter 1994: 59), an unusual occurrence outside of palliative care.

Orderly Dying 4: Progressing to Brain Death

The neurosurgery unit of the teaching hospital receives patients with trau-matic brain injury that the Catholic community hospital rarely sees. If patients do not die from the injury itself, it can leave them neurologically devastated with infinitesimal chance for meaningful recovery. Swelling in the skull over the next several days can become severe enough to cause death by neurological criteria, or brain death. Such patients may qualify as whole organ donors, an outcome that these clinicians hope for. Recall the nurse's comments regarding Mr. Wayne in Chapter 2: "The first priority is to stabilize [for organ donation]. We see so much death here, it's the only rewarding part. We're big advocates for it here. I've seen so much of it."

Devastating brain injury plays havoc with the regulatory systems of the body, so the first job is achieving and maintaining hemodynamic stabil-ity. For Mr. Wayne and those with similar injuries, the goal may not be life and eventual recovery for the patient, but enough blood perfusion so that the organs remain viable. For one patient, all the arrangements for organ donation had been made when cancer was discovered, eliminating him from consideration. The nurse stated, "The transplant surgeon was really ticked off. I wasn't here, but I can just imagine. You treat it differently if they're not a donor at all. You don't treat as aggressively to keep all the organs perfused."

Clinicians express this pragmatic, means-to-an-end attitude in the phrase "progressing to brain death" in describing the tragic cases that may portend more time alive, but only for someone else. They derive satisfac-tion from caring for patients who have been declared dead but for whom stabilization efforts continue because workup for donation is in progress. Procedures of preparation often take hours before the patient, the "dead" donor, is transferred to the operating room (OR). Until that time clinicians' bedside care need not classify the patient as either dying or dead, but pro-ceeds as if the patient were heavily sedated and on a ventilator.[11] The fact that this is a very ambiguous form of death does not appear to trouble the clinicians who describe it. Brain-dead patients who do not become donors (and therefore require the withdrawal of life support) comprise a far more disturbing outcome for them.

One hospital policy in particular lends legitimacy to the idea of "progressing to brain death." When patients come to the teaching hospital's ED with a devastating neurological injury, a specific protocol is triggered in anticipation of the need to request whole organ donation, in case brain death might be declared a few days after admission. The policy recognizes that if the family has been continuously and deliberately supported throughout the tragic ordeal, the chances improve for a positive response to the request. To meet the dual need to (1) provide strength to families struck down by tragedy and (2) maximize the opportunity for organ procurement, the hospital protocol stipulates the following: particular chaplains who have received training from the organ procurement agency rotate a 24/7 on-call responsibility to be available solely to these families. Chaplains, who may be otherwise marginalized in acute care because their role in "hard medicine" is questionable, get a boost. With a crucial part to play in medical rescue, they gain a portion of its cachet, which enhances the standing of chaplains in the hospital overall. At the same time, the hospital tangibly demonstrates its support of brain death as an acceptable, public, heroic death. The combination of the Accident and altruism transforms one kind of dramatic, disorderly death into a victory for the public good.

Death must be accepted as an occasional fact of life in the hospital, as it may not be in many other modern settings. Dying is more difficult for clinicians to tolerate. Unconsciously, they seize opportunities to impose order and containment on dying situations. Clinicians described the foregoing deaths as orderly and satisfactory, but that does not mean that they conform to revivalist ideas of the "good death," nor to the bioethical proscriptions against hastening death. This is not to say that families and patients are displeased with the course of events, but their preferences do not often play a deliberate role. Dominating priorities in favor of rescue continue to marginalize the care for the dying, even when clinicians are unaware of this influence. A patient's state of dying is difficult to identify in the hospital and even more difficult to support.

Although the discourse around end-of-life issues (the now-common phrase that allows dying to enter into hospital conversation while denying its existence) continues to expand, little of this commentary addresses the hidden economic pressures of time and momentum. Exploring how the agendas of rescue and speed operate covertly to disenfranchise dying patients in the hospital is the subject of the next two chapters. Nursing literature probes the phenomenon of moral distress around end-of-life decision-making, but without addressing the unintended consequences of its relief when permission to limit suffering arrives. With the closure of the ritual of intensification, if clinicians feel that they are back in control, with everyone on the same page, and with the ability to administer pure compassion at the last, patients and families with minimal preparation for dying in the hospital may or may not be well served, as will be explored in Chapter 7.

Notes

1. See Morrison (2005) for a thoughtful discussion of this major issue affecting hospice admissions.
2. See Aries (1981: 568) about the "dirty death."
3. These parameters match those for longer or shorter durations for the ritual of intensification. See Chapter 7.
4. Outcomes vary by many factors and locations; Rhea et al. (2004) list the percentage of survival in the United States as ranging from 1.7 percent to 21.8 percent. Hazinski et al. (2005) report a worldwide average of 6 percent. Abella et al. (2005) report a rate of hospital discharge after resuscitation as 10.4 percent. Researchers have not reached consensus on the terms used to report cardiac arrest. Establishing enough uniformity to enable realistic comparison is a task that continues to occupy various international work groups (Task Force of the International Liaison Committee on Resuscitation 2004).
5. Indeed, new approaches to resuscitation are yielding better outcomes. Techniques that emphasize circulation to the brain ("cardiocerebral resuscitation") are proving that the ABCs of basic life support have been wrong to emphasize airway and breathing before circulation (Garza et al. 2009; Kellum, Kennedy, and Ewy 2006).
6. "Epi" is epinephrine, the premier medication used in resuscitation.
7. See Hansen et al. (2009). In the teaching hospital, I attended a series of meetings to establish such a protocol. Guidelines exist; see Prendergast and Puntillo (2002) and Truog et al. (2001).
8. The state law regarding health-care decisions does not speak to this issue.
9. Nurses' regret at their own lack of feeling was feeling itself. Nurses and physicians often expressed strong positive and negative feelings reflecting their own investment in the course of events. See Oberle and Hughes (2001) for the effects of witnessing suffering.
10. The palliative care unit staff often reported that they received patients from ICUs after life-supportive measures had been withdrawn, but the methodology of the study did not capture these patients. Place of death was the entry point. When life-supportive measures had been involved and were withdrawn prior to the patient's transfer to the palliative care unit, the study design did not discover this.
11. For an excellent discussion of the ambiguous status of brain death and the brain-dead patient, see Lock (2002).

CHAPTER 5

"Every Medical Action Is a Transaction": Rescue as Industry

Two personal stories illustrate cultural features taken up in this chapter. The first occurred in 2005. I was visiting my aunt who was a patient in a Catholic community hospital (not a fieldwork site). We heard a bar of a lullaby over the public address system. The physical therapist working with my aunt said delightedly, "That's the fourth one today!" She explained that the musical notes marked a baby's birth. This simple gesture alerted everyone reachable by the paging system that a new person had joined the human family and that someone in charge thought that notice should be paid. Although I did not ask, I suspect that no similar musical announcement occurred when someone died, to mark a diminishment in the human family.

The second story concerns a piece of medical equipment. While in the field I queried a member of the pain service in the teaching hospital for her opinion of a portable infusion pump she was working with on the table in the break room. My hospital also used this pump, and I disliked it. I found it unnecessarily troublesome to load, program, and maintain on patients' behalf, causing frequent beeping alarms and the need to consult with colleagues to troubleshoot. For years I had wondered why the hospital continued to supply such an unsatisfactory device despite complaints about it, especially when the type I had used in hospice home care for the same purpose was so much simpler. This pain service clinician at my research site stated that she handled the offensive machine perhaps "fifty times a day," and this familiarity did not lessen her own distaste for it. She said, "The hinges are cheap and break with big bags. The lock gets stuck. The upstream occlusion alarm is a software problem that they promised to fix while providing loaners, more than a year ago, but nothing has been done."

It was gratifying but still puzzling to hear her response. Much later, I had a similar conversation with pain service clinician in the hospital where I worked about the same type of pump. She had this to say:

> Other pumps I've used before that worked better were made by a company whose only business was to meet the needs of the customer using the pump. These pumps are made by a drug company. I feel sure that the hospital must get a discount on the drugs if they agree to use their pumps. So we have them. But because the profit on the drugs is so high, they don't have to pay attention to whether the pumps are particularly useful or not.

Her speculation was an example of the complex financial arrangements that enable hospitals to survive in the competitive marketplace of U.S. health-care. This manifestation of raw pharmaceutical power (Angell 2000, 2009; Callahan 2003) stands in contrast with the lullaby, which exemplifies the supposed purity of medicine and its goals. In fact, both are examples of mystification of the business of health-care, which directs attention to medicine's beneficence and maintains silence about its marketplace practices. "Every medical action is a transaction" (Middleton 2004).

In the United States, anxiety over the death of a particular group member has largely disappeared. To be preoccupied by the causes of death rather than the fact of death itself is a profound shift in social consciousness (Bauman 1992; Seale 1998). Focusing resources to eliminate death's immediate antecedents both discharges and exhausts public responsibility. It appears that the social contract is fulfilled by the maintaining of vital signs. More time alive stands out as the hospital's most culturally salient commodity, even as racial and socioeconomic disparities persist in health-care outcomes.

Specifically and most immediately in the hospital, this social mandate means rescue from crisis, instability, and the increased risk of death. These priorities express themselves not only through the infrastructure of acute care and its development, discussed in Chapter 2, but also through three major features of the hospital that interlock rescue with the burgeoning health-care industry: (1) technology and its resonating cultural features; (2) the connection of speed with productivity; and (3) the evolving structures that now determine how the care delivered in the hospital is officially recorded and paid for. Mystifying financial arrangements between and among the stakeholders of power and money in health-care, including some physicians and hospitals, insurance, government, pharmaceuticals, device manufacturers and distributors,[1] link these features and obscure them.

These veiled connections mean that bedside clinicians need never be aware of the fact that their actions on patients' behalf support industrial and ideological agendas (Taussig 1980). Tension exists between the business of medicine, which profits from social imperatives to diminish the disorder of disease, and the altruism of medicine, which demonstrates communal concern for its vulnerable members. The hospital houses this tension and exerts its own: it measures its own survival by its capacity to produce more time alive for patients while reducing their length of stay. All this pressure comes to the bedside of each patient in the ritual of intensification, especially if ambiguity about his condition is prolonged. It is evident in the Catholic community hospital in "Code 100," a frequently broadcasted warning that hospital capacity is overstretched and that clinicians should take appropriate actions to move or discharge patients. In the teaching hospital, the pressure manifests itself in clinicians' voiced discomfort and bedside actions when life continues overlong after supporting technology has been withdrawn. Chapter 6 depicts these manifestations of rescue as industry.

Why is this tension in the hospital significant? Sharon Kaufman (2005) has argued correctly that the procession of events and end-of-life decision-making are not actually autonomous activities, but are unswervingly shaped by specific hospital patterns. The overriding imperative within its walls is to "move things along" specific pathways. Kaufman does not address the invisible forces operating behind the patterns that make them so compelling, however. Ideological and cultural priorities motivate these arrangements while making them inscrutable to the actors involved. Patients, families, clinicians, and hospital administrators must grapple repeatedly with divergent cultural agendas that urge adherence to the social contract even as no curative stone is left unturned. At the same time, "futile" care should be avoided and the dying patients given comfort. Meanwhile, the hospital must continue to compete successfully among its peers for patients and qualified staff. Little guidance is available from ethical precepts, which fail to acknowledge the complex forces at work. The charge regarding each seriously ill patient is to construct a customized framework so that medicine and the family are innocent of wrongdoing, the hospital survives economically intact, and all do the "right thing" by the patient, whatever that may be. Because of the levels of mystification, none of the actors can be aware of, much less decode, the preset agendas operating in the background of this formidable task.

Rescue as Industry

A web of cultural values and financial connections links rescue and industry. As discussed in Chapter 2, the project of rescue engages the national interest in drama, heroism, individualism, and technology and makes them more compelling than a focus on public health, planning, or prevention. Rescue is last-minute and time-intensive, the challenge of meeting the impossible deadline. Stabilizing emergencies is individualized care that rights the wrongs of fate, demonstrates public compassion, and deploys a significant amount of equal opportunity. Focusing on more time alive on a one-by-one basis is an elaborate cultural representation, a fire-fighting strategy that consumes energy and finances in heroic display, capitalizing the markets that supply the necessary equipment and pharmaceuticals.

Unfortunately, the imperative to rescue adds cost, making trauma readiness a loss-leader for hospitals that commit to delivering this care (Taheri 2004). Intricate layers of transformation separate the bench (or the factory) from the bedside, obscuring the webs of connection. The hospital emerges as the liaison among all interested parties, stretched to serve opposing criteria of valuation. The hospital must emblazon the "purity" of compassionate medical care as it absorbs the stigma (along with the legitimacy) conferred by the expense of that care.

The obscurity of these connections not only complicates clinicians' attempts to care for seriously ill and dying patients (discussed in subsequent chapters), it also prevents the public from realizing how a focus on rescue eviscerates health-care's broader reach. The dual meaning of "bottom line" in terms of both life and solvency enables rescue and industry to be mutually reinforcing.

Industrialized countries meet the health-care needs of their populations by defining those needs in one of two ways: (1) by covering most kinds of care for everyone, with a provision for exceptional, more expensive care if certain conditions are met (System B below); or (2) by defining basic care very narrowly and paying for additional care a la carte (System A), a far more expensive approach (Engelhard 2005) (see Figure 5.1). Of industrialized countries, the United States spent 16 percent of GDP on health-care in 2005 (twice as much as Switzerland, the next highest), and bought much less quality in terms of whole population health (e.g., life expectancy and infant mortality) (California HealthCare Foundation 2006; Reinhardt, Hussey, and Anderson 2004). By 2009 estimates, the United States ranked 50th in life expectancy at birth among all the world's nations. Its death rate placement was 101st and its infant mortality rate was 180th of the 224 nations ranked (Central Intelligence Agency 2009).

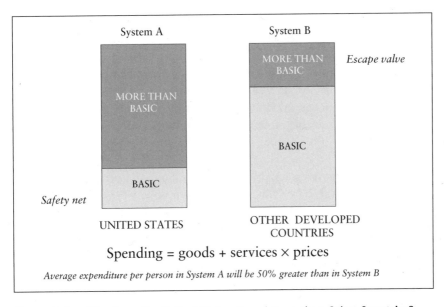

Figure 5.1. Why Does the United States Spend More than Other Countries? Source: Engelhard 2005.

Although health-care costs are not the main focus of this argument, it is instructive to notice what such high expenditures are *not* delivering in terms of longevity: infant survival or consistency from region to region (Wennberg 2006). Even these unarguable findings fail to grip the heart, however, in the same way that the promise of one's technological escape from death can. Permitting drug companies to advertise the benefits of unpriced prescription medications on the same newscasts that celebrate medical breakthroughs makes it difficult to assess the value of a health-care delivery system skewed toward emergency response.[2] How does one tell the puppets from the puppeteers or unravel the strings, when it all looks so life-like?

Mystifying Value

Michael Taussig notices that the business of medicine must convert intangible and unmeasurable features of the human relationship such as suffering, hope, compassion for the vulnerable, education, and experience into measurables—things that acquire a decontextualized life and power of their own. Objectification has unintended consequences. "Medical practice

inevitably produces grotesque mystifications in which we all flounder, grasp-
ing ever more pitifully for security in a man-made world which we see not
as asocial, not as human, not as historical, but as a world of *a priori* objects
beholden only to their own force and laws" (Taussig 1980: 5).

The preeminence of the measurable in the hospital seems to box up and
deliver what Americans value. At the same time, it transforms that thing of
value into unrecognizable pieces, so that it is almost impossible to interpret,
and it makes any other values that might fit into the box disappear from
view.

A physician in a group private practice housed next to the Catholic
community hospital shared this perception with me: "This is a good hospital. But people go where I tell them. If I said, 'I'm moving all my patients to
the hospital down the street,' all my patients would go there. Hospitals can
market all they want, but patients go where their doctors tell them to go."

This powerful statement intrigued me when I transcribed it, so I called
him back to ask a follow-up question: "If this is a good hospital, what
would cause you to change your mind and refer your patients somewhere
else?" He paused for a very long time. At last he said, "If they gave me a better deal on the rent. Well, and I suppose if there was better parking for the
patients. The deciding factor would be the financial arrangement between
the [group] practice and the hospital. I'm not sure it should be otherwise.
They get so much from physicians. Without us they wouldn't survive."

Here was a network of financial connections between physicians and
hospitals previously invisible to me. I knew that as a bedside nurse, my
labor was part of the hospital's overhead expense. In this role, I was naive
regarding the massive infrastructure of the health industry that culminated
in my bedside care. I remember being flabbergasted at the monstrous exhi-
bition of equipment at the first critical-care nursing conference I attended,
realizing for the first time that everything I placed in my hands and anything
that touched my patients was made by firms competing for (my) business,
and that perhaps the exhibitors were not delusional in thinking that nurses
could have some influence over purchasing decisions at their hospitals. But
in my day-to-day practice, the mechanism of those decisions continued to
escape me.

The mysterious connection between business and medicine in rescue
and the resulting quandary of ascribing value manifests itself on three levels: medical purity versus monetary legitimacy; technology as bearer and
expression of values; and how value in hospital care is codified for billing.
The overarching assumption is that more time alive is the unquestioned
priority, and the public expects the hospital to produce this commodity.

If death is the ultimate human problem and if individual rescue represents the promise of overcoming, it is not surprising that escaping crisis is prized in the economics of U.S. health-care. Technology is both the main engine of escape and also the main driver of health-care costs (Bodenheimer 2005 Part 2). What is surprising is how well Americans hide this fact and its implications from themselves.

Pure Medicine and "Filthy Lucre"

Myriad financial arrangements exist between physicians and hospitals. The Catholic community hospital contracted with an outside company to supply hospitalists because, they said, "Hospitals cannot employ physicians." Yet residents I worked with were being recruited by hospitals directly. These young physicians told me that their cohorts emerging from residency or fellowship programs will choose private practice if money is more important to them than time, or they will follow a research path into a teaching hospital if time is more important than money. A new medical office building with an ambulatory surgery facility and pain center was due to be completed in January next to the Catholic community hospital. In a managers' meeting that I attended, it was announced that shares in this facility would be sold to physicians. This was yet another complex financial arrangement invisible and removed from the drama of the bedside, cementing the importance of the medical marketplace to vested interests of hospital and physician alike.

On-the-job physicians not only write orders resulting in work for nurses, but their orders generate "stuff": drugs, lab tests, procedures, each with a financial ripple effect beyond calculation. Atul Gawande describes his understanding of this phenomenon:

> Physicians' after-expense incomes are a fairly small percentage of medical costs. But we're responsible for most of the spending. For the patients I see in the office in a single day, I prescribe somewhere around thirty thousand dollars' worth of medical care—in the form of specialist consultations, surgical procedures, hospital stays, X-ray imaging, and medicines. (2005: 53)

Hospitals and physicians are mutually dependent, especially in the business of rescue. Physicians need hospitals for supplies, equipment, drugs, OR space, and tools of the acute-care trade. Yet there is little if any overt reference or acknowledgment of these "actions as transactions" at the bedside. Why are they so hidden?

Without a broad system to ensure universal access to health-care, many rationing decisions must be made close to the bedside (Daniels 1986). Such a phenomenon implies one possible answer to the question: obscurity would help maintain innocence for everyone involved in care. Speaking from a background in anthropology and psychology, Howard Stein indicates the motivation behind this innocence: an association between time, money, and death.

> Thus, not only is money an embarrassing subject for physicians (wherein a sense of shame and humility can partly mollify patients' envy), and one that arouses guilt (for fear that one is exploiting the vulnerable); at a deeper level, conscious consideration of money issues threatens to undermine the physician's use of medical practice as a massive defense against biological time. Anthropomorphized, time is a formidable adversary, a menace who lurks behind every symptom, diagnosis, and treatment plan. If souls cannot be saved, perhaps at least bodies might be salvageable from death. (1990: 174)

Time to care for patients and more time in the patients' lives is the physician's goal, but time is also an intruder. To the extent that time and money are connected, money is a reminder of the physician's lack of control of death.

There is evidence that interactions perceived as communal, meaning outside of the realm of money, elicit more altruistic behavior than those connected to financial exchange (Hartzband and Groopman 2009; Vohs, Mead, and Goode 2006). Here we see the root of the separation of the idealism and purity of the medical project from the filthy lucre of what is economic. As the site of acute-care practice and the purchaser of its tools, hospitals became a major facilitator in hiding the connections between money and medicine, an arbiter between the pure and the tainted, housing both. It is a role that works as well for society as it does for physicians, keeping the bedside relationship free of contamination. Skill in coordinating the two is key to hospital survival. Although producing the commodity of more time alive, hospitals obscure the connection between what happens at the bedside and the medical industry that profits by it (drug companies, device manufacturers, research connections, equipment distributors, government, and private payers, to name a few). And although the insurance and payment structure, the pricing of medications, and other factors also conceal the movements of money throughout the health-care complex, hospitals are unique among them. Nowhere else are the moral drama and the high costs of the social commitment to care situated in such close proximity to market demands. It is no wonder that the association must be concealed.

Development of Cloaking

Jeanne Guillemin (1998) refers to the "cloaked economics" in the financing of U.S. health-care after World War II. Medical work of diagnosis and treatment seemed to be a "priestly art," somehow sacrosanct, so that the physician-patient relationship operated in a realm set apart from bills and reimbursement. In taking over the latter, hospital administration maintained that illusion. Guillemin also complains that bioethics helped muddy the waters by framing its areas of concern too narrowly, as if economics played no role.[3] In her view (1998), bioethics all along should have been scrutinizing physician relationships with the medical industry as closely as it studied their relationships with patients. Without the light of moral criticism, business relationships between physicians and hospitals remain opaque.

Stein and Guillemin focus on individual physicians, but it is important to note that resuscitation and its technological elaborations have been beyond the reach and the control of single practitioners since the American Heart Association declared speed to be more important than skill in the practice of CPR in the 1960s. This decision meant that first responders to the newly collapsed did not have to be physicians, which diminished their control over this practice (Timmermans 1999: 58–62). Nevertheless, physicians have been on the forefront of developing, elaborating, and deploying rescue interventions. The sophisticated techniques of advanced life support require the equipment and intensity of focused labor that only a hospital with skilled clinicians can provide. The infrastructure of medicine and hospitals, already favoring specialty care, was perfectly positioned to capitalize on the introduction of rescue and its related innovations (Grumbach and Bodenheimer 1995).

With the introduction of Medicare and Medicaid in 1973, fee-for-service (retrospective) payment systems gave way to prospective payment methods. Hospitals have had to deploy various strategies to compete, and many have not survived (Grumbach and Bodenheimer 1995; Stevens 1999). Before 1980, after the introduction of successful CPR in 1968 had shifted the focus to rescue, hospitals used technology to compete for physicians. During the 1980s, hospitals improved their market position by contracting with insurance plans and competing for patients rather than physicians. Their next strategy was to consolidate. This move reduced competition but increased their market power with insurance, enabling them to raise rates without losing insurance contracts, thus increasing the cost of hospital care.[4]

Interestingly, the actual charges for components of hospital care have been almost impossible to fathom, even as pressure mounts for greater openness. Hospitals have considered pricing structures and formulas to be proprietary information, and they vary greatly (Lagnado 2004). Behind the opacity of hospital pricing is a chaotic payment system. No one but the uninsured American is billed at full price, because all others have insurance companies or government entities such as Medicare negotiating a discount from list. "Only a handful of Americans truly comprehend the complex payment system for U.S. hospitals—mostly those whose job it is to set, negotiate, and study hospital prices. Self-paying, uninsured patients certainly do not understand these practices" (Reinhardt 2006: 57–58).

What *is* visible to the consumer and to the culture at large is the technology; the promise of medical breakthrough; the body-trauma shows; the purity of medicine and the progress of science. The hospital is the place where real drama unfolds, and true belief is still possible among the noninitiated. Guillemin ties the triumph of the ICU to its ability to grant maximum access to those in crisis, conforming to U.S. interests in nondiscrimination and even making up in some way for the impact of poverty on health (Guillemin 1998: 71). The display, along with the intensity of time and attention, confers legitimacy (as discussed below) and matches the priceless value of the loved one. Technology becomes the currency of justice, entitlement, and hope. For physicians, managing the technology demonstrates their fidelity to the fiduciary relationship both to the patient and to the social contract. The higher intensity and expense of ICU stays in the United States versus other industrialized nations therefore symbolizes social bonds, while appearing to be simply useful instrumentation, value free, neutral, and objective (Bodenheimer 2005 Part 3: 997; Osherson and Amara-Singham 1981). Technology transforms the taint of economics in medicine into a blaze of emancipatory and cultural power deployed for social good.

Technology as a Mystifier

It is a national custom to celebrate U.S. ingenuity by making technology a status symbol and a mainstay of biomedical care. Despite the supposed simplicity of Basic Life Support training in the American Heart Association's "chain of survival," rescue requires instrumentation as its tangible manifestation. The Pew Research Center's findings at the end of the twentieth century link technology inextricably with national achievement.

> When Americans today think about the nation's accomplishments during the twentieth century, about how life has improved, and even about the government's successes, technology is the answer. Nothing else is close—not winning the conflicts that defined America in this

century (the World Wars or the Cold War), not the civil rights movement that recast society, not the Social Security program that lifted so many seniors out of poverty. (Pew Research Center 1999: 3)

No more powerful economic engine exists in the United States than the human drama of medical rescue from death through technology (Bodenheimer 2005 Part 2). Its display transforms the taint of its expense (see below) into a mark of distinction, as its promise, partial success, and unending elaboration beguile its consumers and dampen skepticism.[5]

Technology defined broadly includes the pharmaceuticals, medical devices, and procedures used in diagnosis and treatment that represent manifestations of biomedicine—all that is coded as "skilled" rather than "custodial" care. It also stands apart from other kinds of patient care such as personal maintenance activities for patients (toileting, turning, mobility, nutrition), patient education, and psychosocial care. These are roughly the same distinctions used to differentiate hospital facility charges, counted as overhead, from ancillary charges, broken out and billed separately (see codifying value, below). Typically, technological care is bounded, easily differentiated and countable. It is ordered by physicians or licensed individual practitioners[6] and under their purview.

In 2003, one of the clearest forms of rescue, trauma care, became the costliest medical problem in the United States, surpassing heart disease and cancer (AHRQ 2005). Technological "bridges to transplant" such as dialysis machines and ventricular assist devices lengthen waiting lists for whole organ transplantation, a more problematic form of (as yet temporary) salvation from finitude. Since the advent of successful resuscitation, technology has proliferated and acquired the power to legitimize the value of both patients and hospitals while hiding patient selves and such social values that cannot be tallied. This ever-expanding materiality fills the eyes of clinicians and the public as it obscures their view of wider health-care needs and drives the costs of health-care delivery upward without limit (Bodenheimer 2005 Part 2). The quest to obliterate death's causes coupled with the fascination of puzzle-solving drives the research for innovative medical interventions. Competition and entitlement define the moral imperative of their diffusion through the health-care system. We explore these ideas in the next two sections.

Rescue's Salvational Connection with Technology

Resuscitation is a newly elaborated and highly charged moral duty in the continuum of social obligation to care for the sick and the dying. Building on both the ethical and hygienic understandings of the relationship between medicine and money, rescue gains moral sanction from controlling time through the intensity it brings and from its (sporadic) overcoming of death. Because it interrupts the specific body processes that immediately precede death, the obligation to resuscitate may be neatly isolated from both the illness itself and the particular meaning of individual death. The potential for deliverance and the requirement for speed sweep aside most competing moral claims in the quest "to err on the side of life," at least as far as hospital policy is concerned. Reclamation efforts cascade outward to mechanical ventilation, the placement of large intravenous lines, and intensive care, each intervention claiming "more time alive" as justification.

Rescue therefore exerts dominance in several moral domains:

(1) The potential to rescue from death and a universal mandate to do so increases the power differential between the well and the sick, obscuring the human vulnerability they share. Technology increases the power of the well who deploy it, obscuring this connection further.
(2) The duty to care for the vulnerable has been reformatted into the duty to stabilize the unstable, placing "more time alive" in a separate category of unquestioned (and presumably unquestionable) promise.
(3) "Rescuable" people therefore acquire greater moral legitimacy than those deemed "unrescuable."
(4) Economic outlay for medical crisis intervention is more easily justified than spending in other areas because it "errs on the side of life."

The veneer of potential salvation extends throughout the hospital in the form of response readiness. Hope, technology, and rescue reinforce each other, evading moral criticism in the ideology of the United States.

Byron Good's fieldwork among medical students indicates the strength of the salvational underpinnings of medicine, a finding that moves idealism into the realm of ideology. Biomedicine's practitioners and true believers look beyond medical instrumentation and its human and financial costs to the link it provides with hope and compassion. They intend that the suffering imposed by the human condition need not define it. "What I am suggesting is that medicine is deeply implicated in our contemporary image of what constitutes the suffering from which we and others hope to be delivered and our culture's vision of the means of redemption. . . . Health replaces salvation" (Good 1994: 86). This message of hope makes Paul Ramsey's injunction toward "solidarity in mortality" thirty-five years earlier sound fatalistic and almost like a betrayal of the cause (1970: 129). It is technology that arms this hope for health and salvation, as it did for the resident caring for Mrs. Turner. She detailed all the diagnostic tests and interventions she ordered as the uncertainty of Mrs. Turner's condition persisted, until her chief advised, "Don't keep giving this family hope." The resident's behavior of "very close regulation" impressed the family more than her words that Mrs. Turner's condition "went back and forth, with no headway." Her management of her patient exemplified Good's characterization of medicine by medical students: "From early on, many medical students speak of a kind of 'passion' required for doctoring. Not only do they seek a specialty that will maintain their intellectual excitement, but many describe their desire for a passionate engagement with the primal forces of sickness and suffering, a passionate struggle on behalf of their patients" (1994: 85).

Technology was the instrument of the resident's passionate struggle for Mrs. Turner as well as the vehicle of hope for the family. Many critics (Barger-Lux and Heaney 1986; Eisenberg 1996; Illich 1995b [1976]; Ramsey 1970; Taussig 1980) have expressed skepticism and disenchantment with medical progress over the years, but such unbelief has little meaning to vulnerable patients and families in the foxholes of serious illness.

Because the economics of this hope are hidden and often paid by others, in the eyes of the rescued, its cost is irrelevant:

> I remember, nine years ago, getting the bill for the heart surgery that saved my son's life. . . . I did not care how much was spent or charged to save my child. To me, all the members of the team deserved a million dollars for what they did. Others were footing the bill—so it's left to them to question the price. (Gawande 2005)

Even Good briefly decries the cost in dollars in placing hope of salvation in the "technical efficacy of medicine" (1994: 86). The revival of death movement through hospice and palliative care articulates what may be gained in terms of improved quality of life if seriously ill individuals renounce technology. But because rescue and industry are linked in a way that dying and industry cannot be gives untold cultural weight to the former. In contrast to critical-care nursing conferences, the organizers of palliative care conferences need not rent an adjoining exhibit hall to accommodate their industrial sponsors.

The extent to which hospital physicians rely on technology to shape their relationships with patients was illustrated when I asked a national expert in palliative care why the transition to palliative care was so difficult. He replied,

> If people just wouldn't have those hopes and dreams. It's difficult to say "How are you?" and really listen to the answer. It's much easier to close yourself off from the humanness and keep going. As

I get older I find it harder and harder to have those conversations with people younger than me or people my own age. And I'm reasonably well defended against burnout. I have great colleagues, I'm a rabid exerciser, I'm reasonably well put together psychologically, although others might have a comment, and, while it waxes and wanes, I have faith, and I have a very supportive family. So if *I* find these conversations difficult, then. . . . My colleagues in neuroscience and rehab say the same thing. What makes sense is to go in and say, "You'll never walk again. Just stop thinking it. Get over it. You can have hope, but it's false hope." That would be a hard-nosed way of going at it. It's much harder to say, "What are the three things you need today?"

These remarks candidly indicate the complexity of negotiating relationships with patients planted in landscapes devoid of rescue. His examples point to the barrenness of resources at the very time that they are needed most: when ordering more stuff can rescue neither the patient nor the physician from facing their humanness.

This difficulty points to a phenomenon underestimated by the critics of high-tech medical care: technology has become the essence of patient management, especially in acute care. To practice in a hospital setting requires that physicians must deploy the technology they have available to demonstrate their allegiance to their patients. To find that there is "nothing more to do" leaves them with unused fidelity on their hands. If no hope exists for producing more time alive, then the customary tools for relating to the patient are lost to the physician. It is no wonder that she is reluctant to give them up.

Routinization and Deployment

Procedures and interventions then are not neutral alternatives, an array of choices, but critical to the structure of the relationship between physicians and patients in the hospital. Several interlocking phenomena are at work here. The interest in salvation from death makes technology the lynchpin of patient management because it is proof of the social contract and the commitment to saving vulnerable lives, or at least to stabilizing them. Trying to solve the problem of more time alive fuels research, as does the intellectual satisfaction of tackling a fascinating puzzle (Kuhn 1996: 36; Nader 1996: 264). With capitalism, successful treatments such as cholesterol-lowering medicines not only make money for the investor, but also spur further research by revealing more puzzles, such as troublesome side-effects to minimize. Research and technology become circular, self-perpetuating phenomena. Once a treatment is routine, it becomes the paradigm, a require-ment rather than a choice (Koenig 1988). Such a "standard of care" ensures wide deployment through local competition (Grumbach and Bodenheimer 1995: 162). The fact that these treatments are available in many locations suits Americans' sense of entitlement. "More is better" is the view of tech-nology in health-care, but it does not translate into better health outcomes for Americans regionally or internationally.[7]

One administrator in the Catholic community hospital told me that phy-sicians use the phrase "standard of care," which to him really meant "physi-cian convenience standard." By this he indicated that hospital administrators feel the pinch when physicians use the phrase as a pretext to lobby for equip-ment acquisition. If technology is central to the physician-patient relation-ship, it is hospital purchasing departments that distill its expression.

The structure and hierarchy of economic outlay is hospital-specific, and sales representatives from drug and device manufacturers must become detectives to uncover its unique intricacies at each hospital in their terri-tory. One representative for bacteriostatic tubing for urinary catheters in the teaching hospital research site described it this way.

> It's a battle between infection control and the materials commit-tee. The two meet in the products committee. But you have to meet with them individually before you go to the products committee meeting. It's all more political than Washington. It depends on how much power each committee member has, because materials doesn't want to spend money, and infection control wants what's best for the patient. They always butt heads. If the infections control person doesn't have enough power, he has to rally support from other peo-ple on the committee. Every hospital is different in how this works.

For its part, the Catholic community hospital had five products com-mittees, according to a nurse educator. Office products could then be dealt with separately from surgical services. Equipment used by nurses obtained nursing input in the Nursing Utilization Committee, such as product testing of sequential compression devices placed on bedbound patients to prevent blood clots. This nursing authority was very circum-scribed, however. According to the nurse educator, "We are going to get new chest tubes now. Why? Because the new thoracic surgeon wants them. Physicians rule!"

Product introduction, purchase, advocacy, use, distribution, and dis-continuation practices are complex, under individual hospital purview, and not visible to outsiders. It is as impenetrable as the financial arrangements between hospitals and physicians and as critical to the production of more time alive.

Technology in the hospital acquires its own life, one that commands attention and propels its users forward. Its display and its redemptive ends distract attention from social values neither similarly adorned nor so vital to the economic engine. It is also a prime magnet for hospital charges, as we shall see in the next section, enabling the transformation of cultural priorities into dollars that contribute or detract from the hospital's financial health.

In her work in reproductive technology, Margarete Sandelowski sees both a coercive peer pressure to use technology and a pull from the technology itself in couples' reluctance to stop treatment in face of repeated failures to conceive:

> Like the gun, conceptive technology requires human beings to determine and achieve its purposes, but it also has an inherent quality of never being enough. In treating fertility, this "never-enough" property contributes to the problematic conflation of good treatment for infertility with quantity of treatment. I suggest that this confusion of the good with the sufficient is at the heart of issues of persistence in treatment that confront both couples and their caregivers. (1991: 31)

If these pressures are enigmatic to couples attempting to create life, "choices" between what is good and what is sufficient are even less clear for patients and families in hospitals facing prolonged, life-threatening illness. Here, institutional pressures overlay and complicate technology's promise, because time is money. The power to control the length of stay influences the assessment of value. To whom does this time belong?

The next section addresses this question. Conflicting social values are both expressed and concealed by hospital practice. The purity of medicine and the business of hospitals build on technology and its promise to maintain both life and the status quo. But all of these practices must be codified and transmitted to obtain cash from payers. In the next section, we see how these conflicting social values become billable events, and how the systems that do this reflect cultural priorities.

Codifying Value

A national health-care system in the United States might motivate some decisions regarding allocation of health-care resources to be made on the grounds of presumed greater good of the community. Hospitals and physicians now operate without such a framework. They themselves become the ultimate arbiters of both social ethics and social economics. Because of the emphasis on individualism, this role must be negotiated at the bedside of every patient, an unavoidable conflict of interests (Barger-Lux and Heaney 1986). It is here that the social contract, soaring costs, and the competitive marketplace must be balanced against each patient's clinical needs (Daniels 1986). To address but not solve this difficulty, a system has evolved that transforms competing social values into numerical expressions for mathematical manipulation for the purposes of tracking and billing. The term of art for this system ironically deploys the same word that clinicians use for resuscitation: *coding*. Even more so in the patient record (as opposed to the bedside), coding becomes the instrumental and rationalist means to achieve individualistic ends, also serving the health-care industry. Numerical coding translates the medical and procedural aspects (rather than the nursing care) of each "patient encounter" into minute descriptive categories. Coding makes it ever more possible to name and count the angels balancing on the head of each different pin (or patient), and nothing less than the hospital's survival depends on it. General illness tends to drain the hospital coffers; elective procedures (usually surgical) fill it up (Toner et al. 2006).

The patient's experience (or some representation of it) and the hospital's economic survival are intimately entwined through coding. But coding does even more than this; it supports the entire health-care enterprise. Coding is the foundation of other quantification efforts that use its categories in demographic research. According to the American Hospital Association (AHA) (2008: 1), ". . . the classification system is at the core of the information infrastructure," a powerful statement indeed. Coding serves as the language of tracking, of outcomes, and of "outcomes management." It is used for classifying hospital care, for health-care finance, and for grading the "Top 100" hospitals. It is the language of medical capital, both monetary and social.

Hospital care's essential value can be inversely related to the perceived cultural threat of the patient's condition, so that the weights and measures of coding reflect social priorities. But before conditions can be transformed into numbers, they must be recorded in text. Documentation of patient care in the medical record is the first step of mystification, one that is somewhat separated and hidden from the immediacy of attending to bedside needs. What is required is not just to save the life, but to write down or type in what happened, making a permanent record of the event. This nonheroic act is seen as a sidebar to the main action. A nursing colleague of mine once wore a T shirt with this message: "And on the eighth day, God charted." This phrase at once expressed the marginality of the act while associating it with creation itself, and both characterizations are apt.[8] The text, now torn from the life events that spawned it, undergoes further transformation in the basement of the hospital where weighty paper documents must reside. Here coders knead the text into numerical descriptors, exact to the fifth decimal point. Coding is the glue that fastens the rescue imperative to industry through the creation of a bill. As a seminar presenter described it, "Coding is the process of utilizing nationally recognized tools to assign a primary diagnosis, secondary diagnosis (if applicable) and procedures/services provided to a patient during the course of a hospitalization based on physician documentation in the medical record" (Lang 2004).

"Patient encounters," the units of exchange in billing for health-care, are not only the stuff of extreme vulnerability, compassion, and moral obligation, but through coding, they also become the fuel powering a health-care system that consumes far more of the gross domestic product in the United States than in any other industrialized country. To represent the care delivered, coders use preset formulas that mix tangibles and intangibles of the patient's primary and secondary illnesses, level of crisis, the medical equipment used, and clinician actions so that each variable carries a preset numerical value and weight. The codes representing any given encounter may or may not garner adequate reimbursement for the hospital when all is said and done, and this creates another level of mystification (see below).

The arcane nature of coding requires an ever more complex infrastructure that is ever less accessible to consumers and ever more invested in its own perpetuation and that of the structure it serves. Professional associations of coders claim 75,000 members, and they advocate that their members strive toward multiple levels of certification in the field. A medical records manager told me, "Coders are quirky—they have to have their desk and keyboard at the right height. They're very introverted. They just sit there and code, and like it. They're a hard group to manage. Now it's going on line and they can work from home. So much depends on coders, and they are paid $32,000 per year [2004]."

Coders use three major "vocabularies" for expressing different aspects of the patient encounter. Each lexicon has a separate history, purpose, and set of stakeholders governing its turf. Each is designed to render combinations of concrete and abstract concepts such as diseases, severity, risk of death, clinician expertise and position in the hierarchy, standards of practice, and time into numerical descriptors. These can then be manipulated and weighted to ascribe importance and garner reimbursement.

Coding, a hidden practice of "facticity" with its own hierarchies, reifies and obscures certain kinds of patients and practices. It naturally both reflects and reinforces cultural priorities while calling little attention to itself. For these reasons it merits consideration in more depth.

Coding Vocabularies that Name, Classify, and Weigh Value

If the survival of the hospital depends on its management of capital, both social and economic, then it must attend to cultural representations of value. In the United States, a collection of diverse, powerful entities (medical manufacturers and distributors, insurance companies, government entities, pharmaceuticals, research interests, some physician groups) vie for their share of the health-care market. Besides diverting time and energy away from social justice or ethical practice issues, the imperative to compete with each other forces hospitals to invest disproportionate resources to maintain a place at the table in the mystification of valuation in health-care. "Relative to hospitals paid under the much simpler national health insurance schemes in other countries, the contracting and billing departments of U.S. hospitals therefore are huge enterprises, often requiring large cadres of highly skilled workers backed up by sophisticated computer systems . . . strictly monitored and supervised by sizable internal control operations" (Reinhardt 2006: 59).

Hospital care is filtered through several national systems of coding to describe and establish its value for the various vested interests. Three of these major systems designate the significance of stabilization and rescue through naming, classifying, and assigning relative weight. Although the practice of coding enmeshes these systems, each coding strategy has its own role in privileging rescue and in marginalizing dying patients from valuation in the hospital infrastructure. Together they ensure that when compassion is tied to measurable, time-sensitive interventions, it can be institutionally supported. Open-ended waiting for death and therapeutic presence at the bedside, not yet codable, are far more difficult to justify.

Naming: Current Procedural Terminology (CPT-4)

To name something is to engage in the act of creation.[9] The Current Procedural Terminology (CPT), a mechanism for naming, was first invented in 1966, coinciding with the birth of successful CPR and the explosion of medical technology. Its basic purpose was to facilitate billing by assigning standardized numbers to correspond on a one-to-one basis with medical procedures provided by physicians.[10] Vested interests, principally the AMA, guard the creation of new CPT codes carefully, through a "transparent" process involving a seventeen-member editorial panel, a larger advisory panel, and 3,000 votes per year (AMA 2009).

Because it does not usually involve an intervention supplied by a physician, dying has no reality in this naming system. It cannot benefit from the validation CPT receives through billing and payment. Intervals of care that are not part of the calculus of reimbursement are accorded less stature. Without a name, dying is similarly beyond the physician's business domain, invisible and without reality. By reducing physician business to procedures, interpersonal aspects are similarly devalued.[11] Efforts to account for greater complexity in interventions have been addressed in the attempts to assign relative weights to physician work (see DRG below).

Classifying: ICD-9-CM

Naming, a CPT function, is a way of conferring social reality. This aspect of reality does not exist in isolation, however. To label a particular phenomenon is also to assign it a place in the social framework. If alcoholism is named as a disease, for example, is it more appropriate to classify this disease as an addiction, an enzyme disturbance, or as social maladjustment (Rosenberg 1992: xiii)? Classification is a more complex problem than naming, it would seem, and categories a more nuanced expression of values.[12]

As CPT is a system of nomenclature for reimbursement, *classification* forms the basis of the oldest coding vocabulary, now called ICD-9-CM. Its capacity for endless elaboration has made it useful for itemizing the details of illness and treatment. Based on the seventeenth-century London Bills of Mortality, it emerged in 1900 as the International Statistical Classification of Diseases, Injuries and Causes of Death. Its original purpose of tracking deaths and their causes enabled populations and countries to be compared. Its categories were updated every ten years. In 1949, the World Health Organization (WHO) adopted it and incorporated morbidity classifications with the mortality categories for the first time. With this greater elaboration, its uses for documentation expanded, even as society was becoming more engaged in pinpointing the causes of death as a way to combat death itself. In 1978, the United States published a new version of WHO's 1977 ICD-9 including more detail and procedures. With this update it was possible to examine the clinical data for individual patients for the first time, rather than large groups. This development provided more information than statistical tracking required, and it presaged the deployment of ICD-9 for individual billing when Medicare introduced the DRG system (see below) in 1983. Classification became ever more refined, capable of even more specificity than simple naming. ICD-9-CM (International Classification of Diseases, 9th revision,

Clinical Modification) is now owned (in the United States) by the Department of Health and Human Services and the Centers for Medicare and Medicaid Services, which maintain an "open process" for updating the system every six months (Centers for Medicare and Medicaid Services 2005).

From its origin as a system for tracking the causes of death, ICD-9-CM has evolved into the principal means of documenting all the barrages made by the medical system on the causes of death. This now-antique patched tracking tool has thus morphed into infinite numerical descriptors that "capture" diagnostic and treatment charges, and the burden of thoroughness falls on hospitals. Through ICD-9-CM, every admission is substantiated by a diagnosis; overhead expenses (facility charges) such as nursing can be claimed; and diagnostic and therapeutic procedures (ancillary charges) are enumerated (Stace-Naughton 1999: 2). Its required terminology has become so complex and divorced from common referents at the bedside that hospitals often employ specialized nurses to roam the units and place coding prompts in patient charts for physicians, so that money is not left on the table. One of these nurses in the teaching hospital explained the significance of her role: "Charges matter. Capturing charges matters. The hospital wants and needs more fee-for-service patients [privately insured versus Medicare or Medicaid]. We need more carve-out charges such as chemotherapy drugs. But systems and software for carve-outs and perfect capture are not in place to do this fully."

Where does dying fit into ICD-9-CM? Because it is more complete than CPT, we might expect dying to appear as a category or a diagnosis. But such is not the case. In the hospital milieu where almost every aspect of care has its slot, dying patients are uncategorized. They have no codable name or category (Buntin and Huskamp 2002). To say that a patient is a "no code" (equivalent to DNR) is, in fact, a double-entendre. Even if palliative care claims patients who are dying, they have no value in the hospital's "information infrastructure" simply because they do not appear in it. Dying patients in or out of palliative care have no official, classifiable reality.[13]

Therefore, patients who are "officially" dying in the hospital are unusual. They have undergone a change in status that has removed the privilege of categorization from them. The ritual of intensification culminates in identifying an empty, "unbillable" basket (Kaufman 2005: 91), an invisible category, and places the dying person in it. Medical jargon for this condition reflects its vacuum: "comfort care only," "withdrawal of care," or "withdrawal of support." It is not necessary to notice that often no one "owns dying patients," as a data analyst for palliative care pointed out to me, because their economic substance is nonexistent. Dying literally has no social or economic capital attached to it in the U.S. hospital. The next section explains by contrast how full every other category in the hospital must be.

DRGs: Adding Weight and Including Intangibles
For all their complexity, naming (CPT) and classification (ICD-9-CM) do not address the increasingly important issues of intensity, risk, and speed, however. This lapse was corrected in 1983 when Medicare introduced 300 (expanded to 541 in 2005) Diagnostically Related Groups (DRGs) to hospital coding. The requirement for speed both in patient rescue and in the hospital's productivity were now united and could be articulated ("captured") through the numerical descriptors of the patient encounter. The value of time and the power to control it could now be quantified.

DRGs revolutionized hospital billing procedures by introducing a prospective payment system to correct the overcharging that had been rampant in the retrospective (fee-for-service) arrangements of Medicare's first twenty years. By organizing patients into diagnostically related groups and defining payment schemes accordingly, Medicare loaded its reimbursement into the front end of the patient's hospital stay, making time (or "throughput") a critical factor for hospitals (see Chapter 6). It also enabled severity and the risk of mortality to be codified and added to the existing mix of ICD-9-CM and CPT through "added-value" formulas.

At the same time that Medicare and other payers were dissatisfied with charges coming from physicians and hospitals, they instituted changes to bring reimbursement for diagnostics and the higher payments for procedures more in line with each other. Atul Gawande describes William Hsaio's efforts to assign relative numbers to diverse medical work:

> Estimates and extrapolations were made . . . for thousands of services. (Cataract surgery was estimated to involve slightly less work than a hysterectomy.) Overhead and training costs were factored in. Eventually, Hsaio and his team arrived at a relative value for every single thing doctors do. Some specialists were outraged by particular estimates. But Congress *set a multiplier to convert the relative values into dollars*, the new fee schedule was signed into law, and in 1992 Medicare started paying doctors accordingly. (2005: 45, emphasis added)

Over the objections of many subspecialists, this multiplier method became the Resource Based Relative Value Scale (Riddick 1989). Along with physician expertise and experience, now payments could reflect such further intangibles as the degree of invasiveness of a procedure and its inherent risk of mortality.

DRGs did more than name and classify diagnoses and treatments; they weighted them and linked them to "appropriate" numbers of days in the hospital for particular maladies. The formulas and weights brought power and pressure along with new levels of complexity. Surgical work continued to carry consistently higher numbers and weights than medical work because of its invasiveness and risk, and the formulas did not improve the visibility or reimburseability of intangibles such as physician/patient interaction.

Hospitals could stand or fold depending on whether patients' lengths of stay matched their assigned DRGs as they compressed hospital time. Upcoding with comorbidities to make patients look more unstable or at increased risk of death became necessary to justify each day beyond the DRG norm. Collecting the necessary information for this practice costs hospitals time and energy that they can ill afford (Taheri et al. 2001). Hospitals face penalties and fines for upcoding, but insurance companies respond by downcoding and denying claims. The documentation nurse had these comments:

> Often palliative care patients come out "major" risk of mortality, not "extreme," even though they died. I don't know why cancer patients don't always come out "extreme" when they do die. It's an [inscrutable] program. You put in all the comorbidities you can, and it sometimes comes out "extreme" and sometimes "major." Respiratory arrest or code would always seem to be "extreme," but isn't always. Even the coders don't know. They put it all in, and can't tell how it will come out. If you could figure it out, maybe you'd be tempted to game the system and upcode too much. Young people who die—it's very serious and tragic, but because of their age, there are very few comorbidities, usually, so they don't get the highest ranking. Take Stevens Johnson disease. It's an autoimmune disorder that causes skin sloughing and the internal organs shut down. It's very serious. But the system calls it a skin disorder.

The unreadable enigmas she describes make billing submissions to payers resemble a form of supplication before the gods of reimbursement. The mystification is complete.

What are the implications of such a system? Using codes to paint the picture of the clinical journey reinforces limitless elaboration, detail and fragmentation. Alternative billing design could charge facilities by use; physicians could bill by the hour; hospitals days could be charged at different rates, based on length of stay (Taheri et al. 2001). The present arrangements privilege discrete events such as surgery rather than processes or repetitive actions such as education, rounds, hands-on care, turning patients, or simply being with patients. Nor does it adequately recompense medical practices such as preventative or primary care. Conditions and treatments with clear boundaries in time and space attract legitimacy in this system: time in the OR rather than postsurgical follow-up care. Patients cannot be admitted to the hospital without a clear diagnosis, which discriminates against patients in severe pain from an unidentifiable cause. Rather than encouraging continuity of care for patients moving between facilities that would lower overall costs, most hospitals and hospital systems are self-protective silo operations that reify the cultural emphasis on individualism and self-reliance on an institutional level. Sharon Kaufman is correct in her conclusion: "Simply put, at this point in history, dying people are not wanted in medical institutions, and it shows" (2005: 29).

Rescue and Industry Enmeshed

Current iterations of efficacious rescue emphasize speed and intensity of the response. Basic life support for circulation and breathing must be administered immediately and continuously until the Automatic External Defibrillator can be applied to the pulseless victim. The pungency of life-saving permeates the hospital, so clinicians always work against time, against deadlines, without questioning this inescapable pressure. Inside the hospital, the site of medicine and business, these axioms of medical rescue dovetail easily with those of productivity and profitability in the marketplace: speed, labor, and throughput. Because rescue is a universal offering, undeniable to most patients, all hospital areas must be aware of the potential need for speed and be ready to ratchet up the level of intensity in the blink of an eye. Thus, the medical atmosphere of rescue underlines the hospital's business interest in productivity and patient turnover—getting it done and getting them out, opening beds for new admissions.

If time is the enemy in medicine, the intruder that reminds the physician of finitude and powerlessness, it is not surprising that time is also the measure of productivity, speeding up the line, and in the hospital, of diminishing lengths of stay. Here the enemy is fought on both fronts in a joint assault. Mystification ensures that in the fight for more and better time alive, no one need notice the power of the partnership between rescue and productivity in maintaining the status quo.

The major role of mystification is to manage the preservation of innocence. So far the focus on more time alive as an ultimate value and the intensity of efforts that accompany its production have benefited capitalism extraordinarily well. The U.S. appetite for both rescue and the industry to support it seems insatiable. Mystification allows hospital inhabitants to celebrate the value of new life and the hope it promises with a lullaby without having to notice or attend to systemized gaps in care.

Notes

1. See Geyman (2003) for a status report on the medical-industrial complex.
2. See Batt (2007) for an overview of the ethics of health media reporting.
3. This is also the thrust of Daniel Chambliss's argument (1996).
4. See Bodenheimer (2005). Health-care costs have risen for other reasons as well, such as the consolidation of health plans.
5. Compare the effects of color, glass and light on creating consumer desire in early twentieth-century U.S. department stores (Leach 1993: 40).
6. This is a catchall term covering anyone who can authorize billable medical care, including nurse practitioners, interns, and residents.
7. Recent research findings (Wennberg 2006) indicate that increased use of technology in some areas of the United States does not correlate with improved patient outcomes. See Jost 2004 for an international perspective.
8. Michael Taussig comments on the act of objectification and of making permanent something that is transient; giving it life beyond its life. He says: "[M]edical practice is a singularly important way of maintaining the denial as to the social facticity of facts. Things thereby take on a life of their own, sundered from the social nexus that really gives them life, and remain locked in their own self-constitution" (1980: 5). Bruno Latour and Steve Woolgar (1979, 1986) have offered a fascinating study of how complex social processes are reduced to isolated, powerful items, malleable and useful to technicians. The fact's meaningfulness then pertains only to its usefulness.
9. Nancy Munn (1970) indicated that naming is an act of creation for the women of the Wawilak myth who created Murngin ritual. "With naming power they can 'create' the world though imposing upon it a social identity, by socially objectifying it and giving it a power of its own" (1970: 180). This phenomenon recalls Taussig's observation of the power of objectified reality that codes exemplify (AMA 2009; Munn 1970).
10. Now hospital coders connect CPTs with the hospital's ancillary charges (ICD-9-CM) and also to the weighted values of DRGs.
11. However, the ambiguity of assigning monetary value to communal actions is explored in Vohs, Mead, and Goode (2006).
12. Bowker and Starr (2000: 143) note the international tensions in the ICD system.
13. The cynical adage "'No code' means 'no care'" is true, in a sense. Such care is difficult to code, to charge for; it's a facility charge, not an ancillary charge. In a publication guiding hospitals regarding mortality figures, the Institute for Healthcare Improvement (2003a) conflates "no code" and "comfort care" into one category, an indication that they are the same from the standpoint of finance.

CHAPTER 6

How Rescue as Industry Minimizes Dying

The connections between rescue and industry are mystified in the hospital through technology and opaque approaches to valuation, as we saw in the previous chapter. Using a ritual of intensification to deliver on a promise of universal rescue keeps heroism, altruism, and the appearance of equity in the foreground, but it is an expensive endeavor indeed. Making the true monetary costs of this endeavor appear as an ancillary concern for hospitals, that is to say, hidden from view, is aided by the very elaboration and diffusion of those costs through the U.S. economy. At the same time, the dying patient has no vocabulary in the languages used and understood by acute-care reimbursement mechanisms. How do these conditions manifest themselves in the fieldwork sites and how do they influence clinician behavior to minimize the exposure to dying? Standards of care commonplace elsewhere in the hospital are not relevant as a mechanism for evaluating dying situations, as discussed in Chapter 1. The answer can be found by considering the phenomenon of time.

In hospitals, clock time is the enemy to be conquered in a dual mandate to save lives and maximize patient flow through the hospital. But more time alive is also the commodity that hospitals and clinicians produce through rescue, so it is something both precious (scarce, sought after, difficult to produce) and something to subdue—one produces time by working against time. Illness and injury interrupt the normal flow of time and life for the patient. The mission of rescue presumably spares no expense in channeling resources that will bring the illness or injury under control in an attempt to return time back to the patient. A dying person finds time hard to come by in this framework, because even when this precious commodity of time cannot be produced or overcome, it is still "owned" by the hospital and its clinicians in terms of their control over the tangible elements of care.

Cultural constraints dictate that time in the hospital may be claimed or granted by the viable only, those eligible to participate in social and economic exchange. The claim of dying patients to such wherewithal (outside of palliative care) is severely limited.

Clock time itself is a reminder of scarcity, but time in other contexts can carry far different meanings. Within time are changes and processes that clock time does not register.

> While birth-death and the rhythmic boundaries of the environment fundamentally entail becoming, clock time's invariable repetitions confront us with that which is irrevocably gone, with the relentless entropy of physical processes and with absolute finitude. Thus if we conceive of death in terms of clock time, we deprive ourselves of an essentially human understanding of that event: we dehumanize death. (Adam 1995: 54)

By changing "death" to "dying" in the last sentence, Barbara Adam could be describing dying in the hospital, a place that must run efficiently despite the chaotic illnesses within it. Hospital care reflects the priorities of the society. The understanding that rescue efforts were more effective, if applied immediately, harmonized happily with the efficiency and productivity that hospitals require. The ingenious, successful gadgetry invented to stabilize vital signs has not only saved countless lives but also ensures that the health-care production lines remain stocked and efficient. Marketplace competition guarantees that these priorities of speed dominate hospital activities. Divorced as resuscitation is from what Adam calls the "rhythmic boundaries of the environment," and tied instead to rescue and throughput, it is not surprising that dying, a process that is not (supposed to be) ruled by clock time, is a poor fit, especially when it occurs in the hospital's rescue beds (1995: 95).

The hospital's need to control the length of stay can color its view of the patient's social worth as diverse economic pressures limit the hospital's welcome. Efforts exist to find consensus so that death occurs with as little dying as possible, as discussed in Chapter 4. Each hospital in which I did fieldwork has a formula, so to speak, or a mechanism for decreasing the distraction that dying might present to the broader work of the hospital. The Catholic community hospital moves patients from one location to another and muddies distinctions among patients at times. Clinicians in hurrying environments that are more numerous in the teaching hospital unconsciously equate dying with suffering, thereby rationalizing actions to limit their perception of it and sometimes hastening death in the process. When a patient is deemed unrescuable or the ritual of intensification is closed down in the respective hospitals, these institutional mechanisms can take over, making families' and patients' needs subject to the hospital's own momentum.

This chapter explores how these phenomena play out for dying patients in the Catholic community hospital through its propensity to transfer unrescuable patients when beds are short, and in the teaching hospital through clinicians' associating time with suffering and wanting to limit both. These are different institutional manifestations of the same problem: the pressure to keep things moving and maximize "throughput" paired with the cultural mandate to minimize dying. How did it affect patients who died and their dying situations?

Issues of Throughput

Individual vulnerability, the pressure of time, and the social contract intersect most pointedly in the American hospital's ED. EMTALA in 1986 dictated that all comers to the ED must receive evaluation and needed treatment, whether or not they require admission to the hospital, and regardless of their ability to pay. But even as the ED has become the health-care resource of last resort, it is also expected to be a magnet for insured persons looking for correction of their acute illness or injury (O'Malley et al. 2005: 1). As the most accessible gateway to the hospital system's display of altruism and competitive innovation, the ED holds community service, technology, and market savvy in an uneasy tension. It continuously tests the hospital's financial ability to maintain these American ideals without discrimination, while attempting to attract customers covered by insurance. Because of this tension, EDs have become a benchmark indicator of the economic well-being of the hospital overall. As EDs increasingly substitute for primary care, traffic increases and costs mount for physician on-call availability, altruism comes under greater pressure. In 2005, the AHA reported that most hospital EDs go "on diversion" for intervals because staffed critical-care beds are unavailable. In the paradigm of stability and instability, bed turnover is no longer a function of patients' recovery. Now it reflects the hospital's bed management skills. An ED too full to accept another ambulance means a direct hit to the hospital's bottom line, because that ambulance often carries an insured patient (McConnell et al. 2005).

The "nerve center" of bed allocation and capacity in the Catholic community hospital is one person in an office located at the very back of the admissions department. I sought her out in my quest for the hospital's mechanisms of death tracking. A large flat-screen monitor on the wall dominates her small space. Displayed there is a grid with the location of every bed in the hospital along with its status: occupied, clean, or dirty. It reminded me of an air traffic controller. A nurse educator had told me earlier about the nightmarish task of assigning beds when the hospital was running at 112 percent of capacity: "I wouldn't want her job for anything. We're an old hospital with no private rooms. One patient on isolation blocks both beds. It's a daily problem. Constant complaints and no solutions."

Bed management (input, throughput, and output) is a continuous challenge. Hospital administrators are pushed not only by the economic pressure of the Diagnostic Related Group (DRG) payment system (see Chapter 5), but also by the shame and opportunity costs of periods when ambulances must be sent elsewhere. Diversion is seen as a black mark against the management. But diversion is a fact of life, especially for urban hospitals in the United States. Bed capacity is less meaningful than bed turnover, so identifying bottlenecks to patient flow is critical (Brewster and Felland 2004; Committee on the Future of Emergency Care in the United States Health System, Committee Board on Health Care Services, & Institute of Medicine 2006; Wilson and Nguyen 2004).

Diversion on the Ground

Coping strategies for continuous bed shortages vary between the two hospitals. In the teaching hospital (a very busy urban trauma center) one nurse manager explained: "The hospital is often on divert—patients can wait in the ED for forty-eight hours before being admitted. Part of this is the new rule that medicine [physicians] can only admit so many patients in a twenty-four-hour period, and patients are made to wait until midnight when the clock resets itself." So the capacity problem can be either too few beds or a shortage of human resources. The "new rule" manipulated time to keep the residents from being overwhelmed, regardless of beds, and ambulances were still forced to divert.

A Fall house newsletter was on display behind a glass case outside the administrative offices of the teaching hospital. One article described its strategy to handle the problem of diversion. The chief medical officer commented on an eight-point plan to reduce time spent on diversion, devised with input from employee groups. The new strategy would

> improve patient flow, decrease length of stay, and ultimately improve bed availability and patient volumes. Dr. __(CMO) said "Average length of stay and potentially avoidable days, two key measures of efficiency and throughput, have both improved significantly since

last fall. In addition, the most important measure of capacity, the number of discharges per month, increased 5 percent after our action plan was implemented. And while I think this is a significant improvement, I think we can do better."

Recognizing that capacity improvement is a system-wide result of cross-sectional barriers, additional tactics are underway to improve patient capacity. The result is that the ED has had 30 percent fewer diversion hours for July and August compared to prior months. A total of twenty-six adult diversion incidents in July and August. The CMO added: "We'll continue our efforts because ultimately this is about meeting the needs of patients who need our care."

This announcement came at about the same time as the Catholic community hospital implemented its own strategy. On the recommendation of outside consultants there, hospital management sought to eliminate diversion altogether by fiat. As described below, its methods differed from the collaborative approach of the teaching hospital, but its intention to prioritize service to the community exactly matched the message given by its competitor across town.

I first learned of the Catholic community hospital's Diversion Committee early in my fieldwork from an administrative nurse, who told me: "There is a Diversion Committee. It is very high-powered. They drive the bus. And that has a trickle-down effect. Today on the radio it said that [another area hospital] was having a big diversion. They had forty patients in trailers because of the flu."

I never encountered the Diversion Committee as such, but its "trickle-down effect" manifested itself in one of my first cases. Mr. Nguyen had been transferred from an ICU to a floor unit after life support had been withdrawn. My informants in the two locations disagreed: either he died in the elevator, or he took his last breath the moment he arrived in his new room. Regardless, his transfer was clearly untimely. The event upset the family, the staff on both units, and the manager of the receiving unit, who commented: "I'm not sure why he had to come here. They probably needed that bed. We get antsy when we don't have a code bed."

The floor nurse receiving Mr. Nguyen at shift change was overwhelmed with her other four patients. She later expressed her outrage that she could not give the situation more attention at the time. Still, she told me that the sending nurse had no choice: "The CCU manager was making the nurse bring him. They needed the bed. I think because we were on diversion or something. We didn't have to drag those people down here. In CCU they

needed to have a bed available, but they were not waiting to use it." The
anxiety motivating the transfer was the need to open the bed, even though
no taker for that bed was yet known. Both the nurse manager and the nurse
receiving the tenuous Mr. Nguyen understood and articulated this priority.

In the CCU I interviewed the sending staff to learn more about the
circumstances and the pressure for maintaining a "code bed," a designated
empty bed, clean and ready to receive any patient who may arrest on the
floor and require a quick transfer for intensive management after resuscitation. It seemed odd to me that administrators of a Catholic hospital would
prefer to take a chance on someone dying in the elevator than risk not having a bed for the merely hypothetical patient. When I questioned this priority, staff responses indicated their awareness of the economic and rescue
issues at stake.

> HC: Was it the pressure to have a code bed [that caused him to be
> moved]?
>
> RN: It used to be we didn't have to have one. They said for a while
> it was too expensive; we need to rent out every bed. It made the
> supervisors crazy not to have one. To wait until a code happens to
> move things around then. So it's gone both ways: code bed/no code
> bed—now we try to keep a code bed on the 5th floor.
>
> PCT (Patient Care Technician): I think they need to keep a code bed
> open all the time. Because one's crashing on the floor, and usually
> it's the same bed [on the floor you need to send the patient to]. You
> end up [almost] switching in the hallway.

Beds sitting idle create no revenue for the hospital, especially if they
are the "high-rent" ICU beds. Yet to hold and care for a fragile, newly
resuscitated patient on the floor while an ICU bed is cleared and cleaned is
awkward for staff who need to be getting back to their floor patients after
the code. Codes are unpredictable, and in a small hospital with limited ICU
beds, the quandary of the code bed is more immediate than in a teaching
hospital with options for greater flexibility.[1]

In their account of Mr. Nguyen's situation, the CCU staff mentioned
that the attending physician was someone less familiar to them. After discussions with the family the day before regarding his poor prognosis, the
doctor had written an order only to transfer Mr. Nguyen to the floor. This
was puzzling to them because there was no accompanying DNR order. On
the morning of the transfer, the physician came in and added the DNR to

the chart. But Mr. Nguyen was still receiving a high dose of IV medication to maintain his blood pressure, which the floor unit could not manage. The drip would have to be stopped before moving him, amounting to a withdrawal of life support that would surely precipitate his death. It was not clear that the physician addressed this important detail with the staff or the family. Even more significantly, the staff gave no indication that they found this omission to be an obstacle to the transfer. Expecting that Mr. Nguyen would indeed succumb without this medication, the nurse delayed turning off the drip until all the family members had gathered, only two of whom could speak English, a further obstacle to clarity about the plan.

> RN: By the time it finally happened the change of shift was coming. The daughter was okay. I turned it off. A half hour passed. They had a bed for him on the 6th floor. They wanted an open bed. There was not someone waiting. The next shift came. I gave report. I'm thinking, "Maybe he won't make it up there." That's what I feel bad about. The family wouldn't ride up with the patient. They all could have fit, but they wouldn't.

> PCT: They got him packed. We got the bed from upstairs. We tried to get the family in with us [in the elevator.] In the process we had to go downstairs twice. Half way up he stopped breathing. I bumped the bed. He started again. He stopped again. I bumped it again. He was breathing when we went through the door. They [the family] saw him take his last breath. I tried to get a blood pressure. We put oxygen on him. The family knew he was gone. I was pissed because it took so long to get him out. The elevator stopped on every floor.

The physician's order created the window for the transfer, but the "when" of the actual move was affected by various factors: the perceived priority of an open code bed, the receiving bed on the 6th floor, the arrival of the family, and the change of shift. The nurse delayed discontinuing the drip as long as possible because she was aware of the risk. Once she did so, the disorder that can be a part of the territory of dying erupted—in terms of the family's choices, the recalcitrant elevator, and death's premature arrival. After they declined to accompany Mr. Nguyen in the elevator, the family was waiting in his new room when he was rolled in, not breathing.

Mr. Nguyen suffered from being officially unrescuable and therefore no longer eligible for a bed in the ICU. In a climate of perceived shortage, this understanding of his status dominated the events that followed for him, preempting his unclear DNR status, his dependence on blood pressure medication, the missing order to withdraw life support, the language barriers, and the floor unit's overwhelmed nurses. The need to free Mr. Nguyen's bed in the unit for a patient in need of rescue took clear precedence in the minds of the clinicians in a similar way that it galvanized the resident in Ms. Hunter's case (Chapter 1). Mr. Nguyen's imminent death could not divert them from the execution of the mission.

Code 100

How did the pressure to "move things along" convert bed space into such a precious commodity in the Catholic community hospital? In most hospitals transferring a patient from one bed to another (even when in crisis) requires coordination and staging. As in other aspects of individual bedside care, the invisible hand that caters to hospital survival interests can be discerned. Such a transfer requires authorization from two quarters, physician and nursing. The physician owns the "whether" and often the "where" segments. After these aspects are known, nursing owns the "when" of actual patient flow. Physically moving the patient depends on discharges from the destination unit, bed cleaning, and staff availability for the tasks involved. Nurses often have some amount of autonomy in determining the timing. It is here that the administrative interests of the Catholic community hospital operated very clearly, as nurses sought to comply with their understandings of current priorities. The CCU nurse had the physician's order to move Mr. Nguyen, and she had already delayed turning off the drip during her shift in hopes that the family would arrive. What made further delay impossible?

Directives to move patients out of the ICU and maintain a code bed are part of administrative attempts to maintain throughput. The code bed issue intersected with "Code 100" in the minds of clinicians. It is common to hear the hospital operator announce over the paging system, "Code 100 is now in effect." Later staff hear "Code 100 is no longer in effect." The hospital enters in and out of this "capacity code" several times each day (Wilson and Nguyen 2004). To make sure all managers are aware of what is happening, their pagers beep with each change in Code 100 status. During my interviews I asked several clinicians to explain Code 100.

Nurse A, Neuro stepdown unit:

RN: But like today, it's a Code 100. That means we have to move patients out. If an ICU bed has a palliative care patient, they HAVE to move the patient. They have no choice.

Nurse B, Neuro stepdown unit:

RN: It took a while for other family to come. She died at 12:30. At 3:30 I said, "I can't keep her here." We were on Code 100. That means they were waiting for a bed for another patient.

Nurse, three East:

HC: Is it a problem to have patients transferred from ICU when they are about to die?

RN: Yes. It's a problem. It's a problem. It happens a lot. When they can't do anything. They make them DNR. As soon as they get that order, they transfer 'em out because they need the beds.

Nurse, ICU:

HC: What is the deal with the Code 100?

ICU RN: Code 100 means that we always have a code bed available. The supervisor knows at all times. A plan already in action. We always try and have one available.

HC: Has it impacted you, when you've had to get folks out?

ICU RN: Oh yeah. It's part of the deal. We can go pretty quick. Maybe it takes ten minutes to get the person down there.

Clearly, Code 100 mandates a special level of operation in which the rules and the hospital well-being can trump individual clinician judgments. This is significant because clinician understanding and actions illuminate "on the ground" practices that may or may not relate closely to institutional policy or intent. Clinicians expressed empowerment ("we can go pretty quick") or victimization ("no choice," "it's a problem") depending on their position as senders or receivers in the queue of patient movement.

These comments also indicate a routine conflation of categories (DNR, can't do anything, palliative care) corresponding to Mr. Nguyen's difficulties. For him, a transfer order and an order to forgo resuscitation became an indication to withdraw life support so that he could be moved. This coalescence of designations, each meaning unrescuable to the staff in the Catholic community hospital, differed from situations in teaching hospitals where painstaking lines are drawn around segments of nonrescue. The teaching hospital's infrastructure, its more elaborate rituals of intensification, and the numbers of people involved mean that distinctions relating to the presence or absence of rescue can be fudged less easily. But in this hospital for Mr. Nguyen, they all came together, inviting a just-in-time decision to create a rescue bed to which he had no claim. When the pressure to accept patients intensified in the summer of my research, this conflation became a particular problem for an entire unit of the Catholic community hospital (see below).

Strategies for efficient bed management in the literature suggest accelerating discharges from the hospital as a response to "capacity codes" such as Code 100 to maximize patient throughput (Brewster and Felland 2004; Institute for Healthcare Improvement 2003b; Wilson and Nguyen 2004). While acknowledging the relationship between ICU capacity and ER diversion, the literature does not indicate that capacity codes should exert pressure to move individual patients from the ICU to the floor (Angus et al. 2003: 641). The understanding on the ground can differ from recommendations in the literature, however. It was clear from the comments of the clinicians in the Catholic community hospital that diversion, Code 100, and having a code bed are issues cut from the same cloth. If beds are tight, patients must be moved as soon as possible, and it is everyone's responsibility to make this happen, seemingly without regard for the consequences.

This special duty to cooperate is remarkable in itself. It grows out of a merging of the hospital's Catholic and corporate identities. Messages from administration flow from either side, but the mixture in the messages is not always received without chafing. Chaplains are particularly sensitive to this phenomenon, exacerbated by the fact that their office is located next door to administration. The local diocese supplies a priest on staff for sacramental duties, but all the chaplains employed by the hospital are Protestant. Administrators frequently press them into service for projects serving a combination of corporate and Catholic priorities. Founders' Day was an example. For this event chaplains designed the program, which resembled a church bulletin, and administrators took leading roles in the program. The celebration, a call and response format with all the earmarks of a worship service, would have been held in the hospital chapel, if weather conditions had not intervened that day.

In this corporate atmosphere it is accepted that higher management will present administrative issues such as bed shortages and throughput as communal problems that require a spirit of cooperation from staff to solve. Employees, as part of the "family," become caught in dilemmas of administrative loyalty and patient advocacy. They misrecognized the true difficulty in the case of Mr. Nguyen, however: that they had been compelled by the system to withdraw the medication supporting his blood pressure so that a bed might be opened for no one. The hospital exerted this pressure on the staff without enabling them to put the situation in a context that would help them serve their patient as well as the hospital. In an atmosphere that actively supported Mr. Nguyen while he was dying, several things might have happened differently. The inadequacy of the physician's orders might have been more apparent to the staff; opportunities for abundant communication with the family might have been provided; the staff might have received permission to stop the drip after the transfer rather than before; and a key to control the elevator might have been available. Because an open bed was more important than Mr. Nguyen's dying situation, and everyone knew it, the staff would comply with the expectation to move him. Institutional support was withdrawn from Mr. Nguyen and from everyone involved in his care well before the nurse turned off his life-sustaining medication.

Three East: On the Brink of Comfort Care

The Catholic community hospital (340 beds) averages thirty-nine deaths per month. One acute-care (medical-surgical) floor, three East, is the "death and dying floor." Four of its twenty-five beds at the back of the unit were remodeled as hospice beds (so-called although no hospice or palliative care program was involved), and these rooms surround a homey sitting area. The other twenty-one beds remain regular general purpose acute-care beds. Several three East nurses pride themselves on their ability to work with dying patients. The unit's murky identity (is it med-surg or hospice?) serves the hospital in several ways. Here is just the place for patients whose legitimacy to consume valuable resources is likewise unclear. On three East they can at least be closer to "hospice," should they need it. The unit's reputation and seeming attraction for nurses (the nurse manager had no openings and a waiting list of applicants) comforts the hospital that it is caring well for its dying patients, even though formalized expertise in palliative care is not available. One of the chaplains observed: "When DNR is proposed, families don't want their loved ones put in a broom closet. They get sent to a less important bed. And everyone knows it is a less important bed. It doesn't matter where they go [after life support is withdrawn]. It's nice if they can go to three East with the pretty beds."

Once patients are no longer eligible for rescue, it truly "doesn't matter" where they go—they can be transferred anywhere, as long as the code bed is available. "It's nice" if they can go to a place that is pretty, but it does not matter. By the same token, unrescuable patients like Mr. Nguyen need not have a clearly defined care plan, once their disqualification for rescue is established. three East can therefore receive med surg patients, "hospice" patients, and patients whose status was unclear, perhaps "on the brink of comfort care" (see below), but who certainly are no longer rescuable.

Not surprisingly, three East averaged 28 percent of the total deaths for the hospital over the ten months for which I could obtain data, equal to all the intensive care settings in the hospital combined.[2] A three East nurse talked about the pattern of transfers she observed.

> In the ICU they send them automatically to us. When the ER's hoppin' they'll send 'em to us as soon as they extubate.[3] Sometimes they die in five minutes. Sometimes it can be a little stressful. The ICU is famous for sending us patients. We have four hospice beds. And the telemetry unit is famous for it. They give this grandiose report and then when they get here, they're like at death's door. "This patient's been made a 'no code'" and they call and ask, "Can we send him to your floor?" This is supposed to be a place that's good at it but the nursing supervisor and the docs—it's like we're a dumping ground. When they're actively dying they'll send them to us, and they'll die in transport.

The nurse's description of the unit as a "dumping ground" for dying patients echoes the administrator in Chapter 3 who referred to the dead as waste. The dumping phenomenon indicates the strong perception that as soon as patients anywhere else in the hospital are categorized as Dying (by extubation, by being made a no-code, or by being in the throes of death itself), hospital units want to get them off their hands. The nurse suspects that "the nursing supervisor and the docs" (who oversee transfers) are using three East's reputation for being "good at it" as an excuse, because the patients arrived too late to derive benefit from their skills.

In June, three East's share of the hospital's total deaths jumped to 39 percent and to 36 percent again in July. One chaplain attributed the increase of traffic on three East to the hospitalists, a new set of hospital specialists who contracted with private-practice physicians. Because hospitalist physicians work exclusively inside the hospital, they are often a boon to the institution in expediting patient throughput. Nurses could respond more promptly to changes in a patient's condition with access to on-site physicians. The contract began in April, and gradually more private practices were signing over their clientele to be cared for by hospitalists, should they go into the hospital. This change relieved private physicians from having to make hospital visits and enabled more continuous, focused care. The chaplain shared her impressions with me the first part of August about the impact they were having on three East:

> three East is a crossroads area. Patients are always on the brink of comfort care. When Dr. B was the admitting doc, patients would stay longer [on three East]. They didn't move. But with hospitalists, they're Johnny on the spot, and things happen. Patients are moved out. And now, the rest of the hospital is poised to send their patients to three East to die. They all want to send their dying to three East. Before, when they called at 2 in the afternoon for a bed, there wasn't one. Now there are beds. So that three East is having many more deaths than before.

During the day, private-practice physicians are busy with their office patients, and it is difficult to change their patterns of inpatient management. But with hospitalists always on site to expedite discharges, beds can open up earlier in the day. An unforeseen consequence was that other units could find space for their dying patients on three East and get them over there. The chaplain continued. "I've had two or three [deaths] a day there. The nurses don't like it. They say, 'This is a med-surg floor like any other. Put the dying in the four hospice beds and then put the other dying patients anywhere else in the hospital.' But even floor units are sending their dying there, and the ICU units are too. Because they do it so well."

The chaplain was reporting the nurses' distinct unease with this spike in dying patients to care for, and their wish that three East's alternate identity as "a med-surg floor like any other" could regain the foreground. The area's association with dying was too enticing and useful for that to happen, however.

Code 100, three East, and No Diversion

At about this time in early September, a new hospital administrator was hired to deliver a unilateral message of "no diversion" and to implement it. To be open to every ambulance at all times would have an impact on the entire hospital, starting in the ED. At a meeting for hospital managers in late September he explained the new initiative.

> We were on diversion an average of 200 hours in a month to 700 hours a month. If we are closed, and we're the flagship of the system, how do we make people want to come here? We will do everything we can to stay open. This commitment has made a difference

already. I heard a comment, "This hospital doesn't go on divert any more." This is the rumor now in less than a week.

(Just then beepers went off all over the room. The paging operator announced: "Code 100 is no longer in effect." People chuckled. He continued his remarks.)

We're off Code 100. In every area there is a spirit of support for not going on diversion, following the recommendations of our consulting firm. PACU (post anesthesia care unit, the recovery room) is willing to accept patients, and also the cath lab. August 13 to September 13 there were 150–200 hours of diversion. Then we were down to 1 hour and 46 minutes of diversion. The ER was packed last night. I heard a person in the ER say, "I heard this hospital doesn't go on diversion." All the staff are cooperating. We have the docs helping to get patients out so they are not waiting to be picked up. It is part of the admission packet here. A lot of things happen when the beepers go off [for Code 100]—it is a commitment to serve the community. Other people need to come here. You can be proud of [this hospital's] service.

He characterized the no diversion decision, born from consultation with an outside company, as "openness" and as a service to the community, just as the chief medical officer of the teaching hospital had described it in their hospital newsletter. Both hospitals framed the issue of being "closed" to ambulances as failing to live up to the expectations of the community, their constituency. If accommodating the "other people" who "need to come here" seems more important than attending to the (less cost effective) patients already in house, such a policy contrasts with the primary responsibility clinicians feel not to abandon the patients already under their care. Economics is at work here. The DRG framework front-loads the rewards to hospitals for admissions and discourages extended stays.

The "spirit of support" from staff that the new administrator cited for the moratorium on diversion could not resolve safety concerns I heard voiced for patients admitted to units not prepared to care for their particular problems. The chaplain stated:

No diversion means that there are patients everywhere. It feels like someone has (gesture of shaking a box hard or someone's shoulders, mixing things up). It means three East is dumped on even more with every Code 100. They talk about the hospice beds on three East, but there aren't any. It's a regular med surg floor where all the patients who are dying a bad death go—like they're dying but there's no DNR.

The policy of no diversion had changed the chaplain's characterization of three East. Its romantic hospice aura was gone, overwhelmed by patients simply dying bad deaths and filling up a med-surg floor. Her reference to "dying but there's no DNR" indicated patients in the fuzzy "not to be rescued" category. On three East, they were "on the brink of comfort care," but with the increased numbers, no comfort could be had.

Over the next few months, the hubbub and the complaints died down. The new administrator was less visible or less noticed. But Code 100 continued. In mid-October, three East's Care Manager reflected,

> It was a really rough summer. Really. I was worried about them [the nurses]. Three bad cases at once that went on too long. Also, we were getting so many dying patients. They see the word "hospice" on the door when they come in and they think the whole unit is hospice. But that's been addressed.

HC: How?

> I wrote a memo to [the Vice President for nursing]. And the Nurse Manager is very good about jumping on these things. The "no diversion" policy has led to many admissions and rapid turnover. Monday they admitted eleven patients. It takes forty-five minutes to enter all the stuff in the computer for each admission. Wednesday and Thursday they are usually very busy with discharges. But these guys really pull together to get it done. The no diversion was bad when it first hit.

The chaplain also told me, "Three East is in better shape." This was borne out by November data that showed locations of deaths more widely spread across the hospital. When I pointed this out to my chaplain informant, she said that "a decision had been made" so that all the dying patients were no longer going to three East.

When three East finally said no, the problem improved for them. But clinician propensity to transfer patients from ICU to floor units in Code 100 did not change. Patients who might be dying but were not now on life support could be moved, their place usurped by the potentiality of need. Clinicians physically moved patients to less premium places where meeting the societal obligation of hospital care was less burdensome for the institution, whether they were aware of this or not.

In the Catholic community hospital, then, the problem of time and its influence on dying patients relates to patient flow: moving patients who might be dying swiftly and efficiently to their appropriate locations according to capacity constraints. In the teaching hospital also time is too valuable a commodity to waste on dying. If a patient is officially Dying, then death is the goal, to be pursued in the name of limiting the suffering of everyone involved.

Throughput in Intensive Care; "How Much Longer?"

One way to minimize exposure to dying is to move unrescuable patients to the "less important" beds. Once that happens, the pressure seems to lessen, but the care plan needs be sorted out. In Chapter 1, Mr. Diangelo's DNR order did not clarify the interpretation or the appropriate response to his shortness of breath. Was he dying or not? Issues such as this concerned the staff of the Catholic community hospital much more than how long the patient spent in the new location, once he arrived as unrescuable. Unlike the situation with Mrs. Harper and her morphine drip in Chapter 1, clinicians in the Catholic community hospital rarely commented on the length of time it took for a patient to die nor did they find it an item of concern. One three East nurse described the attitude of a family member that she found puzzling as she cared for a man who was dying:

> The wife was asking "How many more hours? Minutes?" She wanted me to tell her exactly how long. I try not to make predictions. It's come back to bite me in the butt.

> From her asking me "how long?" I wondered, "Is there a plane that needs to be caught?" There was this sense of urgency. I was surprised with their aggressiveness.

Her perplexity regarding the family's impatience expressed a sentiment similar to what I heard from a new palliative care nurse while doing preliminary research. He had been giving comfort to a patient at the moment the patient stopped breathing. I commented:

> HC: That was pretty amazing to have two such deaths in one week.

> RN: Yeah! They happened in the same bed, too. They tell me to hold on to those. It's rare to be present when a patient dies.

The instruction to "hold on to those" indicated a shared recognition among his colleagues that to witness the moment of death, like the moment of birth, is a time of unusual privilege and portent. For these two nurses, the fact that dying has an unpredictable duration was a given. As one worked on three East and the other in a palliative care unit, both were far from the atmosphere of intense rescue.

By contrast, in the teaching hospital environment, time itself is a clearer preoccupation. In an institution that prizes the intensity of its rescue efforts, forsaking that approach is more dramatic and visible as an interval of acknowledged Dying is ushered in. In this period, all the participants (except perhaps the now-insensible patient) share open awareness of the patient's dying (Glaser and Strauss 1965). If life-supportive measures are being withdrawn, the interval of Dying may contain individual clinician practices operating below the radar of professional or institutional sanction. Clinicians in rescue environments rationalize their efforts to hasten death in the name of limiting suffering. They rarely connect this compassion directly with the mandate for hospital throughput, a link that is more than coincidence.

Clinicians in acute-care settings commonly express their desires for patients not to die alone, for families to be prepared, for goodbyes to be said, for the patient to be comfortable and for the dying to be peaceful. These wishes for control, orderliness, and lack of suffering on anyone's part are practically universal. Often clinicians' gratification with such circumstances is offered in contrast to dying situations they remember that were clearly not that way. One NICU nurse in the Catholic community hospital summed up her narrative about a dying situation that satisfied her by describing what it was not: "It wasn't messy, it wasn't ugly, it wasn't bloody, no tons of people in the room, it wasn't sudden. He was dying, and we let him." Her contrasting positive statement indicated how gratified she was with the opportunity to forgo the drama and potential chaos of an attempt at resuscitation.

What was notable in the teaching hospital environment especially was that along with these objectives of peacefulness and control, clinicians felt that the dying interval should also be both predictable and brief. Dying intervals ranging from ten minutes to two hours evoked an expression of surprise "that it took so long." Other clinicians articulated a similar partiality:

ICU RN: How lucky can you be to be extubated and die in an hour and a half?

Floor RN: It was perfect, routine, like the deaths I see every day.

ICU RN: She only lasted eight minutes. You can't complain about that.

ICU RN: The longer it is, the worse it is. Not that I'm trying to speed anything up.

Floor RN, after a code: In the long run, she was better off going quickly, the way she did. Otherwise (it would have been) slow with cancer.

ICU RN: Are we withdrawing [life support], or is it some slow, tortuous course?

To these nurses, good dying is dying that does not last long. Their reflections about these particular patients point to significant experience with other dying situations, enabling them to compare and create a personal standard for assessing how dying should be, and how this particular patient's dying measures up.

By contrast, when an informant from a setting more distant from intensive care mentioned the length of the patient's dying, usually no statement of judgment accompanied it. In one interview in the Catholic community hospital, I tried to prompt for such a statement:

HC: Was it a good death? Bad? Or was it sort of routine?

RN: I guess it was. It's hard to say a death is routine. It's hard to classify it. Sometimes we get 'em from ICU to die in a few hours. For some of us who have been doing it for a while. We go with the flow. It's part of life.

This nurse accepted that dying would take as long as it takes, and its duration and character were difficult to quantify. But clinician statements about the length of the dying process in the teaching hospital were often accompanied by the clinician's perception of its appropriateness, as in the comments above.

When the interval is "too long," clinicians in the teaching hospital often expressed their own discomfort in terms of what they thought the families were feeling. One major concern is that families might second guess the decision to withdraw life support if death does not come soon enough after the interval of Dying officially begins. Whether families actually articulate this anxiety or not (and some do), clinicians fear it, as Ms. Hunter's nurse did in Chapter 1. Certainly clinicians feel that a long interval can increase families' suffering.

ICU RN: The worst thing to do is—put them on a drip (to relieve pain or induce sedation) and it's agonizing the longer it goes, 'cause then you start second guessing.

ICU RN: We didn't want her family to be there a long time wondering "when is she going to go?" We were not wanting to lengthen the experience for them.

ICU RN: His family was very satisfied because it went quick. He didn't look like he was in distress.

Senior MD: I don't think we should delay. There was a patient in my [ICU] unit. Four hours went by. They had only weaned the vent settings [decreased support] maybe one level. I think we're doing a disservice to the family who's been told he's going to die, and they're waiting. And they think he's dead, or as good as dead. And he's just there, not dying.

This last statement frames death as a goal, a responsibility that clinicians have control over and "should not delay." If the patient is "just there, not dying," then time and everyone in it is frozen, stuck, unable to move ahead. This physician assigns greater weight to the waiting than to the patient's continued presence among them.

A prompt death likewise confirms death's inevitability. If the patient expires fairly soon after the withdrawal of life support, it establishes the "rightness" of the decision to withdraw. One nurse stated, "The comment we heard from the family was, 'I guess he really was sick if he died in thirteen minutes. It proved to us he was really not in there.'" In this case, the short duration of Dying "proved" not only the inevitability of death, but also that the patient's self had already departed. If he was not "in there," he was certainly not fighting to stay alive. Brevity provided reassurance that all contingencies and rescue efforts were fully exhausted.

Another concern was proprietary. Clinicians indicated that presiding over a dying interval that was completed within their shift was part of what was owed the patient in terms of good care.

RN: I feel like I'm not doing my job when I have to kick 'em out of here [transfer to palliative care]. If I do, I try to visit so I can close with them and for me.

HC: Would you turn up the drips (for pain control and/or sedation)?

RN: Oh, I'm not afraid to turn up the drips. In ICU beds, four hours is a long time to be hanging out.

Here the nurse indicated her view that part of shepherding the process appropriately for the patient and the family would be assisting death's prompt arrival with generous amounts of medications for pain and sedation. Her observation also indicates that dying "in ICU beds" should conform to a shorter time frame than dying elsewhere in the hospital. Another report of this proprietary stance came in a meeting about palliative care guidelines:

> In the meeting the ICU nurse reported that her colleagues were unhappy with the guideline to call palliative care if the patient survives for an hour after withdrawal. "They said that to transfer the patient [to the floor or to palliative care] 'looks like we're throwing him away.' They said, 'No, no, we'll take care of this.'" It was a matter of the nurses wanting the satisfaction of closure. (Excerpt from field notes)

Both of these reports reflect a sense of ownership of the process and investment in the outcome. To fear the appearance of having "discarded" implies that with a new lower status the patient needs their protection.

These comments receive corroboration from the relatively brief intervals between withdrawal of life support and the death of the patient in the ICUs of the teaching hospital, none longer than five hours during my research. Intervals in the Catholic community hospital are less clear, but range from a few minutes to a week. Often nurses in the teaching hospital describe dramatic increases they made in the pain and sedative medications at the time of withdrawal, which could imply the intent to limit suffering by hastening death. There were times that clinicians took actions that made it quite clear that death for the patient was the goal, as did Mrs. Harper's physician in Chapter 1. The chaplain's distress over this incident indicated its departure from the norm in the Catholic community hospital. Nurses and physicians in the teaching hospital related the removal of a tracheostomy tubes from comatose patients or the presence of paralytic agents when ventilator support was withdrawn. These were rare, but evident in several narratives. Certainly patients do live longer than five hours after withdrawal, because the palliative care unit regularly receives such patients, but the study design could not capture these data.

Short dying intervals in this teaching hospital are not an anomaly, according to literature that reports research on dying intervals in similar settings.[4] It may be true that dying intervals are relatively short in high intensity hospitals because the patients are sicker and treated longer, and therefore closer to death when treatment is withdrawn.[5] The use of large doses of medication for pain and sedation is also commonly reported in the literature, even though it is controversial because of the prevailing belief that these actions may hasten death (supposedly permitted under the Rule of Double Effect;

see discussion of bioethics in Chapter 2).[6] Still, clinicians believe that large doses of opiates are an antidote to suffering, and they administer them when withdrawing life support. Occasionally, they will admit that they do so to hasten death (Puntillo et al. 2001). According to David Asch's controversial study of clinicians, 20 percent of critical-care nurses self-reported that they practiced assisted suicide or euthanasia using lethal doses of an opiate. Even more revealing of prevailing attitudes is this observation:

> For example, nine nurses reported administering large doses of sedatives or opiates to patients while withdrawing them from mechanical ventilation. Although these activities may have been performed in part to hasten death, the central purpose was to relieve suffering for patients or their families *when death was already an explicitly accepted goal*. Such practices are standard in many critical care settings. (Asch 1996: 1376, emphasis added)

Asch's explanation of nursing actions indicates a belief that death is not just the passive endpoint of a dying interval but its objective as well. This understanding has two implications. First, it differs from a constructed narrative that supports merely the removal of the "unnatural" obstacles to death (Johnson et al. 2000; see Chapter 7). Second, Asch's reference to this behavior as "standard" indicates an unquestioned linkage among the concepts of suffering, dying, clock time, and the measurement of achievement. In this framework, when clinicians take steps to halt the rescue, a very broad permission "to limit suffering" appears to go with the territory, regardless of the definition, the method, or the means, and no matter who is in pain: the patient, the clinicians, the family, or the hospital. The torment of waiting is one that they have in common.

Certainly clinicians may often be correct when they suppose that families are really the ones who are anxious for death to arrive promptly after withdrawal of life support. But this argument does not address the power and motivation that clinicians have to control the interval of Dying, both in its framing and in the orchestration of its events. Whether large doses of opiates truly hasten death or not, clinicians in high intensity rescue environments believe that: (1) just to be dying involves suffering; (2) they have at least some power to shorten the interval of dying; and (3) that it is "better" when it is short. What is striking is that these actions and attitudes are prominent only in settings that specialize in rescue and virtually missing from settings more removed from this environment, including floor units in both hospitals and in palliative care in the teaching hospital. These findings suggest two questions: what makes attitudes about dying different for clinicians in rescue environments? What commonly held beliefs might these differences suggest? We consider these questions in the following sections.

Attitudes in Rescue Environments

The reader should not infer that community hospitals are not involved in rescue and stabilization. To stay on a par with other hospitals in the city, the Catholic community hospital offers a variety of intensive care settings with dedicated, experienced clinicians. Community hospitals must include a full spectrum of care to attract the staff the hospital needs to stay in business, and to ensure that paying patients will not feel compelled to shop around. By contrast, the teaching hospital is seen as both a research center and the care of last resort. As the only Level One Trauma Center, it is the core of the city's safety net rescue efforts. Its clinicians pride themselves on their ability to care for the "down and dirty," to be "in the trenches" caring for "the sickest of the sick." Here the mission of rescue is highly elaborated, specialized, central, and deliberate. Compared to the Catholic community hospital, the teaching hospital's management is more distant, and its layers and channels of hierarchy are less transparent. Rescue appears more pure without the distraction of hospital politics or overt coercion from administration. Intense industry in the form of machines, devices, procedures, research, and rapidly moving clinicians dominate the imagination in such a place. But the hospital agenda of throughput operates in both settings, nonetheless.

To understand clinician attitudes that accompany the decision to withdraw life support in an intensive care situation, it is helpful consider the scenario that precedes it. Opportunities exist in the teaching hospital environment to diagnose and treat more permutations of clinical problems, drawing out the ritual of intensification and its ambiguity. Experienced clinicians, burdened by 20/20 foresight revealing the ultimate sad outcome, may be anxious to foreshorten the ritual of intensification rather than watch it play itself out completely. Why delay when to do so only inflicts needless suffering on patients and families? Clinicians describe their attribution of vicarious suffering in feelings of increasing pressure and helplessness when they perceive procrastination in making the dying status official. They complain that to continue aggressive care is to flog the patient, or subject him or her to torture. The question taken up below and again in Chapter 7 is to tease apart the suffering of the caregiver from that of one receiving the care.

In their study using interviews with nurses and physicians, Oberle and Hughes found that the most commonly reported source of distress for clinicians was to witness the suffering of patients and families, which the researchers attributed to their "ontological commitment to the other" (2001: 713). Clinicians do indeed witness and often inflict patient suffering as a part of their practices.

> RN: That's what wakes me up in the middle of the night, is remembering putting them in the bag, or I think we're beating the crap out of them. It's inhumane stuff you're doing, even though it's not. Blood is everywhere. It doesn't look like you're trying to save their life, really. I don't tend to get upset until bagging [the patient after death]. I robot it, during [the time I am giving care]. It's a critical-care nurse type thing. Doing the tasks.

This description is chilling. To be engaged in resuscitation is a gory job of "beating the crap" out of a patient to save her life. The appearance of cruelty is so close to the real thing that it requires the nurse to turn herself into an automaton, something inhuman, until it is over and she zips the body into the plastic bag for its trip to the morgue. Then her humanity and full realization can be allowed to return. Being a critical-care nurse is less a matter of heroics than it is a deliberate dulling of feelings to cope with its contradictions.

During the ritual of intensification that may precede the code, patients often suffer as well. Clinicians attest to this, especially when the opportunities to deliver relief are inadequate, as Mr. Gomez's nurse did in Chapter 1. Families and clinicians expend a great deal of energy in bringing the ritual of intensification to an orderly close. The finish is clear. The air is let out of the balloon. With "everyone on the same page," synchrony is restored and loose ends can be tied up. Perhaps prolonged helplessness and postponing the demonstration of compassion for the duration of the ritual bring redoubled attempts at control at the end. What can clinicians do with their participation in "torture," exposure to grotesque appearances or procedures, angst over futility, families in chaos, helplessness over the ambiguity, and the lack of realism/realistic goals that they witness and describe (see Chapter 7)? Bring it rapidly to a peaceful, orderly finish. At last.

When it comes, the decision to withdraw life support is a manifestation of careful consensus that relieves the chaos preceding it (see Chapter 4). It indicates that the ritual of intensification and its implied gift of unlimited time are at an end. Clinicians have reason to believe that the interventions about to be discontinued have been supporting the patient's vital signs, and that these indicators will cave in when life support is removed. But patients do not always react to the withdrawal of interventions in the ways that clinicians expect. The withdrawal of life support appears to impose order on the dying situation by dictating an "official" Beginning of the End.

But the interval can bring its own unpredictability, ambiguity, and powerlessness. *All of these feel like suffering* to those dominated by clock time. Tolerance is low for patients in a rescue environment, teaching hospital or not, who are dying *for very long in what amounts to a public space*. In the Catholic community hospital, patients are moved when they are unrescuable. In the more intense rescue environment of the teaching hospital, prevailing ideals of peacefulness and confirmation of the rightness of the decision are attractive antidotes that may allow the Dying patient to remain briefly in a rescue environment. If the decision to withdraw life support is the keystone for wrapping things up for this patient, then the guiding principle about its aftermath may be "no regrets." If the patient dies swiftly, it "proves" she was clearly all but dead anyway. (If not, the patient can be transferred to a nonrescue environment such as palliative care.) The agonized decision-makers can be gratified, and more important, exonerated in their actions. If the dying and death are peaceful as well, then one need not carry the memory of suffering at the end. No one is overexposed to dying, and control is maximized (Kastenbaum 1978).

In this environment, it is interesting to note that by the time life support is withdrawn, the patients themselves may not be demonstrating signs and symptoms of suffering. Clinicians often administer medicines for pain control and sedation aggressively at this point, possibly in an attempt to give patients the benefit of the doubt; it is not always easy to assess distress in persons who are dying. Cause and effect may be difficult to track, because documentation is often less than complete regarding the details of withdrawal and medications given (Kirchhoff et al. 2004; see Chapter 7). Nonetheless, many patients are neurologically devastated at this point, which in itself is a common rationale given for closing down the ritual of intensification.[7] The question of consciousness is relevant to the assessment of suffering not only because it interferes with assessing pain accurately, but also because the self-aware clinician may see unconsciousness as a form of suffering in itself. To conflate suffering and lack of consciousness is problematic, however, as Kaufman points out:

> Of course there is no way that the nature and extent of such a patient's suffering—as both a state of being and an act involving reflexivity and engagement with the world—can be assessed. *Suffering* is often ascribed to comatose patients, yet subjectivity and agency are not. It is as though the person is perceived to be suffering because she can no longer consciously feel or experience. Yet suffering is a feeling itself, and conscious experience is intrinsic to

many ideas of what suffering requires. (2005: 303–304, emphasis in the original)

The question of whether patients who have lost the capacity to feel pain or be aware of it retain the capacity to suffer does not usually distract clinicians in rescue settings during a dying situation. Dying itself is perceived to be a form of suffering, even when the patient is unconscious. Concurrently, a lack of consciousness makes it easier for clinicians at the bedside to advocate for an end to rescue efforts, as essential personhood seems to have vanished already, presumably forever. These complementary impressions urge clinicians on. They need not ask themselves whether patients who are "not dead yet" are indeed "as good as dead." A shortened time in dying limits suffering for everyone, and this seems to be a worthy goal. It is rarely mentioned that minimal dying opens a bed sooner for the hospital and the needy public, but its presence in the background is undeniable. In Ms. Hunter's case, competition for her ICU bed boiled up into the foreground, overpowering the method of withdrawing ventilatory support. In Mrs. Harper's case, the new physician's decision to start the morphine drip occurred after laborious discussions with her husband regarding the need for transfer. In these cases, as Asch described, death was the "explicitly accepted goal."

Clinicians express more discomfort with patients who seem to linger and associate time with suffering more frequently in the settings where rescue is most fully elaborated. One chaplain perceived the connection: "It's like we code them quick, and then when it's over, we want it to be over quick." The pain of "when will it be over?" is related to the momentum, the technological "stuff," and the need for speed that typically dominate rescue environments. It infiltrates dying situations palpably, even after the drips are off and the machines have left the room. Settings farther removed from rescue were more impervious to this pressure.

Cultural Attitudes Displayed

The fact that clinicians in rescue environments can be dominated by clock time when their patients are finally officially Dying indicates how devoid of value the society around them finds dying to be. Dying's ostensible emptiness makes it offensive, and the time and space it takes up in the rescue environment is begrudged. The "revival of death" movement in general, and hospice and palliative care in particular, influence this arena very little because they are prescriptions for private behavior, not for patients in public view, occupying the important rescue and acute-care beds. Even in the protected spaces of hospice, families and patients often defer to the expertise of the professionals for guidance in how to act, as the popular culture offers few resources (Walter 1994). The terms "death bed" or "death watch" no longer carry social currency (Harmon 1998). Persons in the United States rarely have access to a set of norms that would suggest appropriate behavior or rituals to undertake at the bedside of a dying loved one such as getting them dressed for the occasion (see below). For most people, if dying is anything it is an aberration, a blankness of waiting and dependence, set apart from social or capital exchange. How does one buy a card or a gift for a person or a patient who is "officially" Dying? "'The Dying' are expected to wrap life up and go" (Lynn 2005: S1).

Few clinicians in acute-care environments indicate openness to the possibility of working creatively within a given dying situation. Some embrace the new initiatives in training in end-of-life care that assuage the moral distress of rescue, but the scenarios in many end-of-life training programs[8] envision conscious patients with orderly, predictable trajectories in their dying processes (such as Mrs. Morgan in Chapter 1) rather than the wide range of dying situations that typically occur in the hospital. More commonly, clinicians fill the dying interval with medications, compassion, and prayer, and often wish it to be short, as though it had little or nothing to offer its participants. Framing the time for families as an opportunity for retelling stories and for honoring the dying patient, and marking the significance of the moment can open up the dynamic (Chapple 1999). Such an approach recasts the time in the dying situation as "an open-ended generative time of caring" rather than simply an uncomfortable reminder and confirmation of the finitude of clock time (Adam 1995: 101).

But in the rescue environment generated by a nation accustomed to movement and progress, such orchestration can go only so far. In a recent dying situation, we were withdrawing life support for my patient, and I was able to do several things "right": I explained to his family that he had never died before, he had this one chance to define it his way, and I told them, "He gets to take as long as he wants." I worked with them through the day to help them come to terms with the combined dread and wonder of being with someone who is dying. They seemed satisfied. But the next morning they arrived with a new question: "Why aren't we taking him back to surgery?" His continued lack of death seemed to indicate that he still had "fight" in him, and that the decision to discontinue curative treatment had been in error. The waiting that his dying entailed was simply too difficult to endure and understand.

Waiting itself, a major activity for families in the hospital, garners little nurturing from clinicians or hospital administrators, nor from society generally.[9] How can clinicians or hospitals afford to inhabit any space of waiting, when the "greater good" of still-viable patients compete for their attention? They must submit to the pressure to move patients who might be dying as far as possible from the sacred space of rescue, and do it quickly. While one inhabits a space that affords the gratifying display of technological power that clinicians apply to correct their patients' vulnerable states, it is difficult to remember the value of dependency as teacher and convener (Hauerwas 1986; Vanstone 2004: 54–57). If the mission of the hospital could be reframed as caring for the sick rather than as housing procedures and stabilizing the unstable, it is an open question whether the humanity of helpless and dying people would command more social and economic investment from the population at large (see Chapter 9).

Nurses in the Catholic community hospital understand that their roles include getting patients who are not rescuable to someplace else in the hospital and worrying about the details of the care plan later. Clinicians in the teaching hospital's rescue environments minimize dying by equating it to suffering and limiting everyone's exposure to it in the name of compassion, which also coincides with the need for throughput. Each formula for minimizing contamination by the dying intertwines with economic pressures and hospital well-being. Clinicians conform to the prevailing ideals, either not realizing how the impetus for movement influences the overall treatment of dying patients or else helpless to turn the tide. At the core of the diminishing is not so much the economic pressure, however, but the seeming absurdity of making the care of the dying a widely public concern. In an acute-care environment built around episodic and goal driven patient encounters, states of continuous being that are impervious to improvement (wellness, chronic illness, and dying) are unwelcome. Informed by social values that make it critical to get the better of dependence and adversity, Americans cannot embrace dying that happens in the public square.

Exceptions to these general rules do occur. In one particular case, the clinicians in the Catholic community hospital were able to reach beyond this void to honor another tradition. A nurse, a chaplain, and the physician in the ICU cooperated in a daughter's wish to dress her Chinese mother, Mrs. Lee, for death according to Buddhist custom.

RN: She had to be pretty when she died. She had beads and belts on already. She had lipstick. The daughter wanted to know, "Could she be dressed in these?" Before she was extubated. It was important to this lady. It took her two hours to come back here with the clothes. It had to be three layers of black clothing, socks and shoes. On top of the swan and the foley.[10] She was to go to the morgue in what she had on. We put her in the body bag. I wrote a note in the chart telling them please to leave these on her.

This simple act of agency blended public and private priorities. It brought tradition, community, faith, subjecthood, and the ministrations of Mrs. Lee's family into a public space of rescue. The acknowledgment of a state of Dying brought responsibilities and expectations forward. For clinicians to comply with the request, they had to adjust the sequence and timing of withdrawal accordingly. To dress Mrs. Lee for death reversed her unmaking as she had entered the hospital with her flu and pneumonia.[11] When they were finished, the decorations for Mrs. Lee's journey to death enshrouded the devices of failed rescue.

Notes

1. By the 2008 direction from The Joint Commission regarding patient safety (Goal 16), many hospitals are trying to reduce the unpredictability factor of codes by deploying rapid response teams. These clinicians are trained in critical care to help manage floor patients whose potential for instability has increased (The Joint Commission 2009; Scott 2009).
2. The percentage of deaths occurring in the ICUs of the teaching hospital was 57 percent.
3. Remove the breathing tube, indicating the withdrawal of life support.
4. Here the dying intervals for children and adults were comparable to my own findings. Kirchhoff et al. (2004) reported a dying interval for adults in the ICU ranging from 3 minutes to 17 hours, with a mean of 133 minutes. Burns et al. (2000) reported that death after withdrawal of life support from children occurred in less than four hours in 85 percent of cases. Zawistowski and DeVita (2004) described a range of 30 to 270 minutes in their pediatric study.
5. In one of the few studies to compare community hospitals to teaching hospitals, Keenan et al. (1998) reported less time after death in the ICUs of teaching hospitals than in community hospitals. They explained it as sicker patients in the former or slower methods of withdrawal in the latter.
6. Wilson et al. (1992) reported that low doses of such medications tripled during and after the withdrawal of life support for adults, and the dying interval averaged 3.5 hours. In a study that contradicts the widespread understanding that large doses of opiates hasten death, Chan et al. (2004: 286) "found no evidence that the use of narcotics or benzodiazepines to treat discomfort after the withdrawal of life support hastens death in critically ill patients," reporting

    dying intervals ranging from 1 to 890 minutes (14.9 hours) after withdrawal of ventilator support in seventy-five adults.

7. Prendergast and Luce (1997) noted that of 179 patients for whom withdrawal of life support was recommended, only six were able to participate in the decision.

8. These include End of Life Education Nursing Consortium (ELNEC) for nurses and Education on Palliative and End of Life Care (EPEC) for physicians.

9. See Vanstone (2004) for a thoughtful treatment of this problem.

10. A "swan" is a major intravenous line placed to measure heart pressures, nicknamed for one of its inventors. A "foley" is a catheter inserted through the urethra into the bladder that drains urine, also named for its inventor.

11. For compelling descriptions of how persons are unmade by medicine and by pain, see Katharine Young (1997) and Elaine Scarry (1985) respectively.

CHAPTER 7

Order out of Chaos: The Ritual of Intensification

To do what can be done until the outcome is repeatedly negative drives the default approach to care of every patient. There is no clear conception of how to balance goals of treatment and goals of comfort or the demarcation of where the limits of doing everything meet those of doing what can be done. A clear articulation of goals is almost impossible.

—Drought and Koenig (2002: 120)

In the previous chapter, we considered rescue and industry on the ground, time, and the impacts of these factors on dying patients. In this chapter, I return to a closer look at the ritual of intensification that precedes dying. Every hospital admission without a positive trajectory involves uncertainty. This uncertainty must ultimately be resolved in a way that removes the patient's immediate entitlement to acute care. Either the patient's restored stability moves her out of the hospital or a decision is taken that the goal of stability is no longer worth pursuing. The chaos of illness and the inconsistent control of it can make such a determination difficult. If the patient does not clearly get better or worse, the ritual of intensification imposes a structure designed to resolve the uncertainty. It suspends the hospital's concentration on clock time to apply rescue technology, hopefully to enact improvement, but at least to get to the bottom of the problem. Patient complications require time "off the clock" to resolve. The clock time of production and shift work involves predictable, repeatable patterns. It does not account for bodily rhythms, change, or creativity (Adam 1995: 52). With ritual procedures and a suspension of clock time, everyone feels that things can be sorted out. This allowance for variability serves the ideals of individualism, equality, and technological rescue as it also generates a rationale to start the clock once again. The interval cannot last too long before the pressure for movement reasserts itself.

Without characterizing it as ritual, Sharon Kaufman makes this interval the subject of her excellent book . . . And a Time to Die (2005). In ethnographies of twenty-seven patients, she foregrounds the issues for clinical staff, families, and patients around resolving uncertainty, pointing to the invisible force of hospital imperatives, especially "moving things along." Problems arise when patients become "stuck" in a "zone of indistinction" without movement. She very skillfully draws attention away from bedside dilemmas to these much broader systems issues. In concentrating on the complex ways in which patients become "unstuck," however, she omits the broader contexts of ideology, power and economics influencing the configurations of clinical uncertainty in the hospital. She also sidesteps clinicians' internal conflicts about how patients should be classified, concentrating on the unified face shown to the families and patients. What happens to the patient after all the struggle with decision-making to certify him or her as officially Dying likewise merits little attention. My own experience at the bedside as well as my research indicates that multilevel conflict within acute care is in part a reflection of the burden clinicians carry to enact these life-death transitions on behalf of the larger culture (Gerardi 2007).

Bioethics literature has given exhaustive treatment to the problem of end-of-life decision-making, but bioethics also does not frame it in terms of ritual.[1] The act of relieving a social entity of its obligation to rescue one of its members requires ritualization to enable its misrecognition, however. Seeing this process in the context of ritual puts clinicians in the role of ritualizing agents (Bell 1992). They enact a social transformation of the patient when technology dissembles rather than saves and a new story of individualism and suffering must be constructed. The inexorable demands of ritual operations victimize not only the patient but also the clinicians, families, and the hospital itself.

If death can be permitted only after all the contingencies have been explored, the ritual of intensification supplies a framework for their pursuit. The ritual provides a cultural rite of passage à la van Gennep (1960) in that it isolates and transforms patients, but this ritual does not provide a mechanism for reincorporating the dying patient into society. In fact, it justifies the removal of the patient from public purview or obligation. This transformation is essential to society's interests, and it is beyond the control of any one person. Using Catherine Bell's definition, the ritual of intensification carries the necessary four earmarks making it a ritual (1992: 81): Each patient's clinical course is unique, so that the ritual of intensification can be tailored to particular situations. It is strategic, in that clinicians clearly use it to work toward system interests along with patient goals. The ritual of intensification enables "misrecognition," a critical component. That is, ritual agents see themselves as responding appropriately to a set of circumstances. They do not see how their actions enable them to reshape their understanding of the circumstances before them, creating a comforting congruence among what Bell calls the "main spheres of experience—body, community, and cosmos" (1992: 109). Finally, in its search for incontrovertibility and consensus, the ritual of intensification provides redemption. At a critical social juncture the ritual reproduces and reinforces the existing power relations while minimizing moral misgivings.

A national ideology of rescue that stood unchallenged in the acute-care system would not allow resuscitation and stabilization efforts to cease until death or rescuer exhaustion set in. Here, bioethics and the revival of death movement step in to make alternatives and ritual transformation possible. Permission to close down the ritual prior to death draws from the rubric of autonomous choice and consent, allowing clinicians to withdraw or withhold life-supportive measures under particular circumstances. The revival of death movement supplies the consolation prize in the form of the "comfort care" alternative, offered when hope for recovery is to be officially abandoned. With these ideas in mind, clinicians and families use the ritual unconsciously to transform the patient from Living and a Part of Society *to* Dying and Removed from Official Public Concern. It allows them to do this while divesting themselves of responsibility, a feature of the ritual's redemptive power. This is a delicate and painful negotiation, critically important to a society that lionizes egalitarian rescue. It requires overt evidence of having grappled resolutely with death's ultimate undoing on the patient's behalf, along with a mechanism for making the humiliation of defeat orderly and explainable. The ritual of intensification allows those in power eventually to reformulate the goal of their beneficence away from continued life and toward the priority of limiting the suffering of this particular patient, and to do it at a time that serves the interests of the system and the society at large. Meanwhile, the ritual and its technology stand as proof of their good-faith efforts.

The ritual of intensification interrupts throughput, but it cannot do so forever. The urge toward the resolution of uncertainty metamorphoses into generalized suffering and pressure to close down the ritual. Clock time is an anathema to ritual, and it reasserts its power (Myerhoff 1996: 149). We look first at the economic origin and impact of this pressure. Then we examine the chaos of illness addressed by the ritual and the interpretations of suffering it generates in each hospital as time passes. What is the ritual's agenda? What features belong to it? Building on the conjunction between time as *costly* and time as *suffering*, we consider the tipping point that reclassifies the patient and closes the ritual. Its operational efficacy is tested and proven with successful negotiation of the family hurdle. Finally, the issue of suffering returns through the consequences of disorder, when the ritual of intensification fails to control the chaos of illness and death, fails to transform the patient, deepens his liminal status, and exacts a toll on clinicians.

Time as Costly; Moving toward the Goal of Resolution

Since DRGs were implemented in 1983, Medicare and Medicaid ensured that the U.S. hospital's commitment to delivering its gold standard of care for each patient must waiver. Time's passage imposes direct costs and opportunity costs. Rescuing and getting patients discharged as soon as possible adds up to a double imperative for hospitals. Extended care for any patient, whether or not her care is reimbursed at higher private pay rates, can "block" rescue beds for potential patients, resulting in opportunity costs for the hospital.[2] Medicare and Medicaid admissions will pile up direct costs as well as opportunity costs when they outstay their DRG allotments.

Because the rescue mandate cannot be separated from the economic calculus, Level One Trauma Centers (such as the teaching hospital research site) are especially hard hit financially. The front-end loaded reimbursement design of DRGs does not match the combined direct expense and opportunity cost of the most complicated rescues (Taheri et al. 2001). This shortfall jeopardizes the hospital's ability to fulfill its social contract. Just as unstable patients require intense interventions applied promptly for the best outcomes, hospitals likewise incur their greatest expenses early in the patient's stay. The survival of both the patient and the hospital becomes time-sensitive (see Chapter 5), supporting Kaufman's observation that the imperative to "move things along" is as "natural as air" in hospitals (2005: 98). But to what goal? What galvanizes all this movement?

Uncertainty compromises both the present and the future, as Eric Cassell reminds us. Present suffering (worse when unexplained) is exacerbated if it seems unending, if one cannot anticipate relief at some date certain to come (Cassell 1991: 36–37). This uncertainty is particularly difficult to bear because it represents the difference between the reassurance of ongoing life, the restoration of orderliness on the one hand and the yawning abyss of death, separation, and the unknown on the other. Clock time demands that every admission be brought to closure, since patients in the hospital are guests, not residents. Meeting these needs means different things depending on one's role in the drama. Patients and families seek resolution of the illness or injury itself as their priority. The hospital and its staff work toward "dischargeability" as their goal. As long as the patient is recovering, these objectives mesh nicely. But with the uncertainty of prolonged serious illness, they diverge. The ritual of intensification offers transformation by reworking the narrative of the patient's clinical course and allowing the two paths to rejoin. Should patient death be the ultimate outcome, the mechanism of discharge, an explanation for irreversible deterioration, must be constructed ahead of time. This elucidation must be very customized, so that it does not insinuate finitude for other existing lives or power structures. Armed with the new certainty constructed through the ritual of intensification, the clinicians, the family, and the hospital can bring resolution to the admission, survive, and move on.

Virtually every hospital clinician carries the burden of hospital survival unconsciously in her practice simply because the hospital provides the turf and the "stuff" for the mission of patient care. It *is* in the air, as Kaufman says—it pours from the oxygen flow meters on the walls; it powers the beds; it is folded and stacked in the linen carts, stuffed in the drawers of supplies; and it pops out of carefully opened sterile packages. It is impossible in this environment not to be working toward goals of completion. As a chaplain in the Catholic community hospital put it,

> CH: We set goals. The system is geared toward goals. We have to be *doing*. When we're not clear. . . . With the palliative care pathway, we have a name for doing nothing. There's all this pressure, as if, "I'm not doing good care until we determine the plan of care." When we can't determine it, we're uncomfortable. [It is as if they say] "I'm a bad nurse if I don't know what I'm [supposed to be] doing."

The "pathway" she mentioned was a method to justify palliative care, allowing waiting and watching (or "doing nothing") to appear more legitimate in a goal-driven atmosphere. Many clinicians refer to it as "comfort care *only*," indicating its limiting and limited status, even though skilled palliative measures can be very complex and aggressive. A nurse at the teaching hospital described the generalized discomfort of delivering care without a clear direction, the suffering of uncertainty: "We were in a difficult place for nursing. You don't know what your job is. I said to the docs, 'I'm uncomfortable; we're not doing some things. We need to declare a path instead of letting him linger.' *It was not fair to him*" (emphasis added).

"Not doing some things" meant deviating from the egalitarian demands of rescue and stabilization. Here, the nurse identified it as the team's responsibility to "declare a path," to exert control over whether the patient "lingered." As a part of the team, she shared a sense of guilt. She recast this distress in terms of the patient's interests. "Declaring a path" would not only clarify her position and her work, it would also benefit the patient. The attribution of fairness made "declaring a path," imposing orderliness, a moral obligation.

It is one thing for the patient to be "stuck," as Kaufman puts it, in a "zone of indistinction." Clinicians cannot allow *themselves* to be so. To be dependent on the team to "declare a path" is one way to feel stymied. To be at the behest of the time of others is troubling. Barbara Adam compares the "archetypal time" of the woman giving birth to the clock time of her hospital attendants: "It seems clear that a woman's entry into the time of her labouring body disrupts the attendants' sense of time, and that it raises for them the spectre of uncertainty, separation and death" (Adam 1995: 49).

It is comforting to channel those spectres toward the goal of resolution. Within the ritual of intensification clinicians know how to proceed, satisfying the demands of the hospital's ticking clock of opportunity costs. Moving toward the goal of certainty exerts mastery over clock time in its role as a reminder of time running down toward death.[3] In acute-care's efforts to win back time for the patient either by enhancing life or preventing a "premature" death, time is nearly always produced by the hospital in a satisfying way.

But uncertainty plus the march of time portends a bad outcome for the patient, as nurses recognize. They are flummoxed when their foresight about the ending does not enable them to close down the ritual of intensification. To stabilize vital signs without recovery on the horizon appears to them as a "bridge to nowhere," a black hole without redemption. Any hope for the future retreats into the distance, and the goal of "more time alive" turns sour. A nurse in the Catholic community hospital put it this way: "It was frustrating because we were full and we knew this man was going nowhere except to heaven. It was costing more money. He was on big drugs. Because our hands were tied. There was nothing we could do except continue."

The nurse voiced the team's helplessness in terms of the hospital's capacity and *its* well-being, now that the patient's ultimate fate was sealed. She wanted the ritual of intensification to close down, because "this man was going nowhere." Yet, because of forces beyond their control, clinicians' "hands were tied." Longing for an ending shows a desire for the restoration of predictability, a comfort that clock time provides. Drawn-out uncertainty is a form of suffering for hospital insiders who project it onto their patients rather than acknowledge it as their own. In doing so they perhaps underestimate the importance of critical care to patients and families (Matsuyama, Reddy, and Smith 2006). A dubious or clearly tragic patient outcome and the search for answers again bring clinicians closer to their own inability to control the forces of life, an uncomfortable place to be.

If physiologic uncertainty is truly at an end, why keep at it? What can possibly be the purpose of continuing this ritual in which clock time is suspended? With certainty's arrival, it seems to the nurse that normal life and routines can be restored at least to the clinicians, and limiting the suffering of the patient can and should become a paramount concern.

Suffering the Ritual of Intensification

The normal preeminence of clock time in the hospital must submit to the priorities of rescue at first, but it is restive. Technology's dazzle holds little charm for clinicians if it does not produce clear results. This is why the ritual of intensification can engender a sense of being "stuck" in Kaufman's "zone of indistinction," even as forces and movements swirl beyond individual control. Ritual is a practice that transcends time and allows meaningful operations to occur (Adam 1995: 38). It offers the constituents the time to wait: for healing, for responses to interventions, for strength and resilience that nutrition will surely provide. Meanwhile, they can also act: clinicians maintain their patient's stability, forestall and react to complications, tend the machines of life support, adjust the plan of care, and lend their support to patients and families. These, in turn, pray, rally their communities, interpret events, hold the rest of their lives together, and fight the illness.

Rescue delays the movement that clock time demands while it seeks resolution, but the discord of this interruption does not dissipate. It emerges in various characterizations of suffering which introduce tension into the ritualization. Before examining the content of the ritual of intensification, it is important to consider its context at the two hospitals and the pressure of time common to both.

The Chaos of Illness at the Two Hospitals

Illness creates its own particular indeterminacy, justifying the open-endedness of the ritual. Clinicians impose routines and habits of practice on illness's more familiar manifestations (Koenig 1988), constructing and interpreting milestones as they occur. It enables them to produce technical control and an orderly process. Although physicians in both hospitals routinely write orders for procedures, in the teaching hospital it is rare for one person or constituency (other than the family) to dominate the course of the ritual or its duration. In the Catholic community hospital, however, certainty seems to come more readily. A single test or a marked deterioration can precipitate closure there more often than in the teaching hospital, and one phone call can bring the ritual to a halt (see below).

The location of deaths in the two hospitals reflect differences in ritualization practices. In the teaching hospital, 654 deaths occurred in ten consecutive months. Of these, 57 percent ($n = 372$) occurred in ICU settings. In the Catholic community hospital the total number of deaths for the same ten months was 388. Of these, 28 percent ($n = 109$) occurred in ICU settings. This indicates that patients were *eliminated from rescue and transferred out of ICU more readily* at the Catholic community hospital, partly because its relative percentage of ICU beds to total beds in the hospital was smaller (9.7 percent versus 14.5 percent at the teaching hospital). Without interns and residents to serve as the labor force managing extensive stabilization 24/7, clinicians' expectations of controlling every elaboration of illness generally may be lower. Although the teaching hospital serves as a regional referral center, hospitals within the city almost never transfer their sickest adult patients there.[4] Thus, the very intensity of rescue available at the Catholic community hospital has a lower ceiling than in hospitals with more resources, whether city residents are in a position to recognize this limitation or not. Neither hospital can rely on resolving an admission by transferring that patient to a facility with more elaborate technology or expertise than it possesses on site. The buck (and the patient) stops here.

In the Catholic community hospital, then, stabilization *for its own sake* is less of a given, an expectation, meaning that the tipping point for the ritual (see below) can be more by fiat, be less complete, and come sooner in the patient's clinical course. The permutations of illness are accordingly less chaotic. The everyday operations of illness management are less predictable and patterned at the Catholic community hospital than in the teaching hospital. Patients can be tipped away from rescue more easily than in the teaching hospital, but perhaps not all the way to another definitive care plan. Compared to the teaching hospital, the care plans of the Catholic community hospital may be less specific, physician presence more sporadic, staffing less abundant, and individual clinical behavior more arbitrary. A nurse who had practiced at another teaching hospital where interns and residents were typically within shouting distance had changed jobs recently. Now she worked in the ICU of the Catholic community hospital.

She described her frustration with the new complexity she encountered in contacting private-practice physicians.

> ICU RN: We spend lots of time calling physicians. It's a nursing judgment who and when to call. You talk over the situation with other nurses. [Private practice] docs are very strong in various areas. You get to know who's strong and in what area. When they get paged, docs are being called out of appointments. They hate it. They (seem to) hate to come in. You have to figure out who to page. Cardiology? Pulmonology? The attending? The one on call for any of these? The house doc?

She told of an ICU patient who developed respiratory difficulty and a rapid heart rate. Her condition seemed to put in question the orders that were in place to transfer her to a stepdown unit. With the patient in this doubly tenuous situation, it was unclear which physician should be contacted. The nurse spent several hours calling different physicians and obtaining orders, but the patient was ultimately transferred without physician examination. The nurse's take on it was that besides trying to get the proper care for the patient, her calling around was an attempt to keep physicians out of trouble. But she wondered how much risk they perceived: "While I'm trying to save your ass, docs keep passing the buck. I'm trying to prevent the bounce back [from the floor to the ICU]. There's not enough accountability. No one is looking over the shoulder of the docs."[5]

Those with less formal power in the hierarchy, such as nurses, chaplains, and social workers, can combat physician inconsistency by taking matters into their own hands: contacting families on their own, calling in the physicians they like, and bypassing the ones they do not when this is possible. Nurses who fear that a patient will require an imminent code that will be detrimental can take matters into their own hands. They can prompt closure to the ritual of intensification by making a key phone call to a physician or family member. Problems might come afterward, when transfer to a nonrescue bed does not bring a new care plan with it, but this seems less troublesome.

In the teaching hospital, rescue is more elaborated and its closure is more carefully defined. More people are involved throughout, bringing a sense of predictability and a broadly perceived understanding of how stabilization and rescue should proceed. This understanding does not differ greatly from the Catholic community hospital, but the expectation of conformity both from patients' body systems and from coworkers is higher in the face of the greater chaos of illness in the teaching hospital. Even coming from a teaching hospital myself, I was struck by the enormity of sickness in the bloated, bleeding, leaking, discolored bodies clinicians described. Stabilizing them with so many interventions can feel overwhelming. Clinicians seem to have their fingers in the dike of cascading events, spinning plates, dancing as fast as they can. In the midst of this, they cry. They berate themselves for being too jaded or for engaging in self-protection. I witnessed tears from nurses in the Catholic community hospital as well, but their suffering seemed more straightforward and less existentially related. Mr. Wayne in Chapter 2 was one of those desperate cases, like a fire burning out of control. His nurse talked about how she had expected to cry, had waited to cry when he died: "The son just broke my heart in little pieces. When I got home I told my boyfriend, 'Maybe I'm just not caring.' I was feeling guilty, afraid I wasn't caring enough."

The family's grief had touched this nurse deeply, but she found she could not react. When the family sought her out after Mr. Wayne's death to thank her, she said, "I felt bad. I didn't do what I normally do with families. There was nothing I could have done for them." The nurse had not lived up to her own standards of caring. The enormous effort she and the staff had expended was clearly important to the family, but in her own eyes because Mr. Wayne had died, it became "nothing," and she had failed to empathize with them in their grief.

Clinicians in both facilities expressed guilt over their complicity in causing the suffering they witnessed and projected onto their patients. Mr. Gomez's nurse declared, "He was in [heart] failure! Why were we doing this? Making his last hours a living hell?" Clearly, she included herself among those tormenting Mr. Gomez; using the "we," she drew a clear separation between herself and "those" who fail to communicate about impending death: "They don't tell the families. They don't sit down. How can they not tell them?"

It is no wonder that clinicians take satisfaction in relating a "good death" and in the same breath differentiate it from their memories of horror. Having achieved some orderliness in a universe of general chaos, nurses in both hospitals frequently spoke in comparative terms,[6] as these examples illustrate.

Oncology nurse, Catholic community hospital:

RN: It's not always this smooth. I've had 'em worse, way worse.

ICU nurse, teaching hospital:

RN: It was hard on the staff. She'd been here a while. Three months. Four months. Everyone took care of her. I was happy to see her out of her misery. We didn't have to code her. It was more peaceful. The family had time to prepare. It was calmer than a code.

Clinicians in each hospital use their own strategies to control the chaos of illness, but the dissonance created by managing time and ritual are common to both sites. The narrative that must be constructed for families must not resound with this tension, however. If possible, it must be both logical and linear. If the appropriate content is missing, the tipping point can be delayed, causing frustration among the team. We explore this phenomenon in the next section.

Hope and Suffering in Time: Technical Dying, Bodily Dying, and Torque

Jane Seymour provides a useful differentiation between what she calls technical dying and bodily dying. Technical dying involves the content needed to explain the patient's deterioration and death, most important to families and physicians. Physicians need to articulate certainty, provide a defensible explication to the puzzle, powered by technologically produced objectivity: numerical measurements, lab values, and scans. This diagnostic information (technical dying) combined with visible bodily dying allows the team to "naturalize" the death in their narrative construction about events (Seymour 2000). If the bad outcome can be understood as an aberration, ascribable to the patient's uniquely intractable physiology, then the patient's dying and death can be seen as both inevitable and also neatly confined. Families need to hear an authoritative explanation of what went wrong, usually from the physician (Kirchhoff et al. 2002). To fix the blame for the outcome firmly on the patient's body exonerates medicine, the hospital, and the family. This (now understandable) death must leave everyone else safe from its contamination.[7] Clock time's pressure can be kept at bay while the ritual of intensification works toward this end.

Seymour recognizes the primacy that technical dying holds over bodily dying, but she does not point to the gap between them and the problems it can cause. Clinicians who are not physicians are often less interested in drilling down to what they see as superfluous details of certainty and order. For them the obvious changes in the patient's body (bodily dying) are completely compelling. In their view, this physical evidence alone provides all the certainty anyone could wish, decidedly sufficient to close down the ritual of intensification. To be convinced of this sad outcome reorients their priorities and brings forward a moral imperative to limit suffering. Accordingly, they declare to one another and often to the physicians that the care plan should target eliminating patient distress, changing the patient's code status, and preparing the family for the inevitable, regardless of the cause of the deterioration. Delaying closure of the ritual to pursue more definitive diagnosis would prolong the patient's suffering and subject him/her to the threat of resuscitation, an anathema in their view. Clinicians abhor both its brutality and its inefficacy in cases of serious illness. The survival rate for CPR is less than 20 percent overall.[8] "Holdouts" who continue to cling to rescue, whether doctors, family, or systems issues, can appear villainous. One of the nurses in the Catholic community hospital expressed her distaste for pointless aggressive treatment: "I'd like to have an ad, instead of the drug ads, showing patients contracted, intubated, people pushing on their chest, and have it say, 'This is your loved one after you've loved them to death.'"

This nurse, who would be standing in for society and the family to "push on the chest," despised the box they put her in: having to deliver bone-crushing compressions because of their "loving" directives. Another nurse objected to the ongoing suffering of a patient she considered to be unrescuable. She saw it as part of a pattern, a common delay in closing the ritual related to a lack of physician frankness.

> RN: It's just not fair. Treatment goes on too long. They're admitted from the nursing home with no quality of life there. They're DNR. But they're ordering all kinds of tests. They're end stage Alzheimer's and the first thing they do, the doctors throw a feeding tube in them, give them antibiotics, fluids. They go back [to the nursing home], and two weeks later they're worse, and they're back in. [The physicians are] not talking to the family, and not being honest about the fact that in six months they'll still be unresponsive and they'll still have bedsores.

This nurse was complaining that alongside the patient's misery limped the lack of resolution, a sense that the ordeal was not only endless but that, *because the outcome was certain*, the patient's suffering was now pointless and should trump all other considerations. Previously, when the outcome was not so clear, the patient's suffering was also less compelling, a part of the price to be paid for the chance at more time alive.

This association between clock time, certainty about the future, and intensity of suffering figured significantly in the course taken by the ritual of intensification. The difference between technical and bodily dying and the important meanings ascribed to them by different constituencies caused tension and conflict. Geoffrey Bowker and Susan Leigh Star describe the phenomenon of "torque," of disjointed time lines that creates consternation

(1999:27). This overarching disquietude is the stuff of moral distress, a salient concept in nursing literature (Hamric 2002; Jameton 1984; Nathaniel 2006; Oberle and Hughes 2001). The perception of bodily dying often precedes the orderliness of technical dying. Clinicians closer to the patient and lower in the hierarchy (nurses, chaplains, respiratory therapists, interns, residents) can find the gap between the two to be almost unbearable.

Clinicians' consistent compassion comes through in their narratives. Physicians' and nurses' understandings of the charge to care well for the patient brings different behaviors and prescriptions of fidelity, but everyone wants to do the "right thing."

Chaplain, Catholic community hospital:

No one could step in and say, "This is wrong." It was pain being inflicted on a dying patient. There was constant anxiety that was increasing. That room was sucking the life out of them. There was this bad energy that weighed down the whole unit. Nothing could be done to allow him to die with dignity.

ICU RN, Teaching hospital:

During that day, the day he died, everyone worked out their feelings except the daughter. They said they wanted to really look at him. But he was only perfusing [getting circulation to] certain organs. I tried to explain this. I showed them his feet. Not in a crude manner. I told them, "Yes, he's living if you look at the [his vital signs], but if you look at *this*." His feet were black. I wanted a peaceful end of life for this man. My goal was to keep him alive until the family reached closure. I cleaned him up. I lowered the lights. I wanted to make him look as normal to them as possible. . . . I prayed with them. They sang. This was throughout the entire day. He was my only patient. I was really busy, but I was able to be there with them. I offered them everything I could emotionally and spiritually.

ICU RN, Teaching hospital:

I called the mom again. I told her the day before not to be worried till I got worried. I told her, "I'm very worried about him. I'm worried now."

To discern bodily dying in a patient is to witness suffering without purpose; to imagine its future resolution through death (or through transfer to "comfort care") as a blessing. This diametric opposition exists without nuance for many clinicians. As long as uncertainty persists about the outcome, suffering can be subsumed as a means to an end, just as the ritual of intensification can suspend both the demands of clock time and the hospital's need for efficient discharges. Nurse perception of bodily dying strips the ritual of its usefulness for her, and she can imagine the suffering from illness and hospitalization only increasing as the ritual continues. Hope for improvement in the patient's condition can no longer be the workable avenue of redemption. This realization brings unavoidable tension and torque.

Feared suffering for the future piles onto present suffering (Cassell 1991: 36). Because past suffering has been squandered, gaining no chance at recovery for the patient, clinicians' fiduciary duty as compassionate moral beings requires intervention now to prevent future suffering. Although families continue to engage in making meaning around the illness and its treatment and physicians seek orderliness through the explanation of non-recovery, such priorities are opaque and inaccessible to many clinicians. To them, little else can be relevant when compared to the immediacy of their patient's suffering accumulating in clock time, *whether this suffering can be confirmed or not*. Now it is important to them to characterize the patient as suffering, not only to deflect the reality of their own suffering, but also so that nurses especially can see themselves as agents with the means and intention to relieve that suffering. For the ritual of intensification to continue under these circumstances simply twists the knife in the imagination of these clinicians. Once bodily dying is clear, the uncertainty of the timing of the tipping point to close the ritual (see below) causes distress. The chaplain in the Catholic community hospital said: "They are prolonging his death, prolonging his death, prolonging his death. No one has talked to the family and explained to them that he's dying. In an attempt to avoid the discussion, they will lab-rat him to death; the doctor says, 'We'll see if x y z works.' Knowing full well he is dying."

Resolution in terms of the patient's bodily dying was clear to this chaplain, but she was powerless to enact it. She felt as trapped in the ritual of intensification as the lab rat she invoked, blaming the physician for not opening the cage door that would free them all, especially when he seemed to know better. Any beneficence in his action was invisible to her.

Meanwhile, Kaufman indicates that families value the continued attention of technological intervention for their loved one and the hope it represents, even as they cannot "know what to want."[9] In my practice, I have observed that physicians demonstrate their fidelity to the patient by orchestrating the elements of instrumentation required to manage acute illness (adjusting vent settings and antibiotics, ordering tests, monitoring fluid balance), and they are loathe to dismantle this tangible stuff of relationship. Tending technology is a manifestation of commitment.[10] Each participant seeks a resolution to the situation that allows one to live with oneself, but mutual comprehension of varying perspectives across physician and nursing disciplines is rare (Oberle and Hughes 2001). The twisting time lines or torque regarding the primacy of bodily dying versus technical dying during the ritual of intensification troubles clinicians whose position in the hierarchy does not allow them to close the ritual. When it finally comes, resolution brings consensus, an end to ambiguity, the realignment of timelines, renewed direction and momentum, the opportunity to relieve suffering, and the relief of torque, as discussed in Chapter 4.

Nurses' moral distress over continuing to fight when the cause seems lost links resolution of the admission, suffering, and *time*. Even though they may act only as a kind of Greek chorus, commenting on the action to their colleagues without direct influence over the "plot," nurses give voice to the pressure of clock time through the temporal urgency of pointless suffering that they ascribe to the patient. The ritual of intensification and its machinations cannot suspend time indefinitely. Just as the speed of the rescue response maintains stability, and prompt bed turnover enhances the hospital's bottom line, closing down the ritual of intensification as soon as possible can be seen to restore dignity to the patient and limit the suffering of all concerned. Time that was formerly the commodity, the hope, and the prize is now transformed into time as suffering, especially in the teaching hospital where rescue is at its most intense.

Using the Ritual of Intensification to Shape the Chaos of Severe Illness

Recall Mrs. Homan, the 51-year-old patient described in Chapter 3. Her longstanding emphysema, steroid-compromised immune system, and continuing gastrointestinal complications were interfering with her recovery. Even with support for each compromised body system applied during the weeks she spent in the Catholic community hospital, she could not gain the strength she needed to breathe without the ventilator. The clinicians discussed transferring her to a nursing home, but their strong preference, motivating them to call an ethics consultation, was to discontinue their "torture" of Mrs. Homan by withdrawing life support and allowing her to die. Her brother disagreed with them, saying "I have more faith than they do."

Mrs. Homan's ritual of intensification had the power to interrupt the hospital imperative to "move things along" and command an open-ended interval, because the ability to stabilize the patient disrupts the proximate causes of death. Daniel Callahan comments on the cultural shift enacted by rescue and stabilization: "Just as fatalism, the resigned acceptance of destiny, was dismantled in favor of the medical management of death, so also were all those attendant rituals, habits, and practices that were able to give cultural and religious meaning to death, to give it familiar place in public and private life (1993: 33).

Callahan's view is that without the rituals that gave meaning to fatalism and made it bearable, the "medical management of death" stands naked. But, in fact, the ritual of intensification has become *the* ritual regarding death's approach. In the United States, it must display the twin values of equality and individualism as it reformulates the chaos of illness and uncertainty into an orderly narrative. By engaging fundamental societal values and asserting cultural control over dangerous life circumstances, Callahan's "medical management of death" through the ritual of intensification and its aftermath does the necessary work of the culture around death.[11] Or does it?[12] The governance is not perfect, of course. Even as machines and infusions support vital signs, bodily chaos erupts.

ICU Nurses, Teaching hospital, three separate cases

RN Case 1: The fact that we couldn't turn him with his [lung condition]—he had bloody plugs. It was horrible. He had a huge decube [bedsore] on his bottom. It was leaching out everywhere. His bed was saturated.

RN Case 2: We kept pumping blood into him, blood into him. . . . What we were dumping in, he was bleeding out. It was tons of stuff. . . . He just wouldn't stop. It was so bloody. Housekeeping cleaned the floor six times in an eight-hour period.

RN Case3: He looked terrible because of the subcutaneous [under the skin] air everywhere. His eyes were swollen. His skin was starting to tear.

Such situations cry out for interpretation, for context, and containment. Even if it does not win the day, the ritual of intensification orchestrates the situation by directing the narrative and making explanatory sense of the chaos. As it continues, the ritual of intensification allows ever more contingencies to be explored, bearing witness to its participants' heroic intent. If it does not ultimately bring recovery, the ritual serves the social order by tipping the balance away from further rescue efforts. Sufficient time, elaboration, and suffering accrue to make closure possible without censure[13] through shifting the narrative of the illness. The ritual enables an important legacy to be created as time and interventions mount. The clinicians could point to their extraordinary efforts on Mrs. Homan's behalf (multiple weaning attempts, extraordinary interventions to aid digestion, treatment of sepsis and GI bleed) *along with* the time that had passed. Eventually, they were certain that she was dying, and having drawn that conclusion, they regarded further treatment as prolonging her suffering.

Besides providing a framework and an explanation, the ritual alters the patient's status in society if the road to recovery is not available. The ritual serves as a classificatory tool, able to eject the patient from the socially favored public sphere of rescue to the dreaded and private status of dying, again with little or no recrimination for the participants or for society in general. Indeed, a successful ritual of intensification redeems them all. In this way, the ritual is critical to the "certification" of Dying and its accompanying reduction in social status (Rappaport 1971: 69–70). The ritual succeeded for Mrs. Turner and Mr. Mendez in Chapter 3, but Mrs. Homan's brother was not willing to accept the dire prognosis. He had seen her come through difficult times before. He dismissed the clinicians' assessment, saying they lacked faith. In doing so, he also rejected any alteration in Mrs. Homan's status. In her case, the ritual failed.

For Kaufman, the time the patient spends in the "zone of indistinction" is itself undefined and inchoate. Eventually, the "time is right" for the ritual to end (2005: 153). In fact, the sense of "rightness" occurs because clock time is pressing and relentless. Nurses often call attention to it by declaring that the duration of ambiguity itself "proves" a bad outcome. Uncertainty's hiatus is over. The ritual's interruption in clock time finally builds enough pressure that clinicians unconsciously search for a tipping point to close it down, shift the balance of power, and prioritize patient comfort. The process time already "spent" in operating the ritual becomes an ally when clock time reasserts its dominance.

Agenda of the Ritual of Intensification

The ritual begins when patients appear not to respond to initial interventions, or when complications set in (see Figure 7.1). It is helpful to consider what elements the ritual of intensification contains to understand its variation in the two hospitals and the obstacles to its closure should clear recovery be elusive, as happened for Mrs. Homan. Things cannot "move along" and the ritual cannot be closed down until all criteria are met. If destabilization and death occur before the agenda can be fulfilled, the order is disturbed.

(1)   *Clock time submits to process time to resolve uncertainty.*[14] Because allowing time to pass is a primary component in reducing uncertainty, an open-ended opportunity to produce answers is allowed (Buchman et al. 2002; Cassell 1991: 231). For the patient and family, this is a time of waiting, watching, and trying to understand. For staff, this time is filled with performance, work, and interacting with the patient and family about these actions and their interpretations of the patient's response.

(2a) Clinicians stabilize, watch, diagnose and treat patients through the hospital's in-place *technology and infrastructure.* They enact procedures, measurements, scans to generate seemingly objective data confirming a mixed response. The ambiguity persists along with continued stabilization efforts, if they become necessary. Where labor and technological resources are less plentiful, as in the Catholic community hospital, the ritual is more easily closed (see discussion of what factors shortened the ritual below). As long as the potential for crisis and rescue exists and both resources and management can be brought to bear, patient care strategies that would make this technology extraneous (such as palliative care) are almost unthinkable.[15]

(2b) As technology and infrastructure define the shape of the ritual of intensification according to each hospital setting, clinicians work to *discern the riddles* the patient presents and to plan the next steps of care. If cure is elusive, an explanation must be found, and reasons for the poor response ultimately pinned on the patient (Callahan 1993; Seymour 2000).

(3)   *Clock time intrudes.* Continuing interventions combined with a sense of mounting clock time make the goal of returning the patient to a preadmission "baseline" seem distant rather than just around the next corner. As the future retreats behind continued ambiguity, assumed and discernible suffering begins to chafe.

(4)   Eventually, a *tipping point* arrives to shift the momentum from a continued rescue stance to something else. Certainty's arrival or permission to end the quest can be based on a new piece of information, a new interpretation of existing information, or some other factor, such as the neuro consultation for Mrs. Turner. Clive Seale points out the key role that such proof of irreversibility plays in the moral and social order:

> The preservation of health is a form of bodily capital, and medicine is pledged to preserve it, and to help individual patients in its accumulation. The preservation of health and life as an ultimate

and sacred good is an underlying premise of medical ethics, together with an ethical commitment to ensuring that death only occurs as a result of *technically irreversible disease processes*. Together, the application of these principles enables the separation of adventitious or unnatural deaths from natural deaths, so constituting order from disorder. (1998:78, emphasis added)

With CPR as the egalitarian default, almost all deaths are considered to be adventitious and premature in the U.S. hospital. The ritual of intensification is the mechanism that sorts the technically irreversible processes from all the others.

Primary among the "irreversible disease processes" is severe neurological impairment (see discussion below regarding what could shorten the ritual), as it was for Mrs. Turner. Her family could recall that she had never wanted such an outcome for herself. In Mrs. Homan's case, the realization that she would never wean from the ventilator formed the tipping point. The time had come to get her into a long-term care facility able to handle ventilators, and this added pressure to the argument.

(5) *The narrative shifts.* As events unfold, the health-care team (larger in the teaching hospital, smaller in the Catholic community hospital) discuss the patient among themselves informally and use meetings with families and patients to interpret events more officially. In doing so, they construct internal and external narratives. The internal narrative may contain an assertion of bodily dying, and disagreement among the team may occur. While the search for an orderly explanation of technical dying continues and timelines are torqued, the external (and official) narrative will continue to portray a plan of aggressive care. With the tipping point comes the attempt to shift both narratives (Johnson et al. 2000; Norton and Bowers 2001; Seymour 2000). Technological interventions are recast from serving as supportive extensions of the body to being unnatural and prolonging patient suffering. Mrs. Homan's nurse declared, "this is not faith keeping her alive—this is machines doing it." This statement reflects the change in perception from hope in a transcendent technological power to seeing technology as the bridge to nowhere. Reconstructing the narrative is generally more problematic in the teaching hospital because of greater numbers of staff involved and longer, more elaborated rescue. In the Catholic community hospital, defining the post-ritual plan of care becomes the stumbling block.

(6) *The family hurdle.* If they have been fortified with a technical explanation for their loved one's sad state, families can often be persuaded to

"let go" (Swigart et al. 1996). In recounting the patient's clinical journey for families, clinicians cite the time already bought and "spent" during stabilization as partial justification for reclassifying the patient as unrescuable and closing down the ritual. But families often object, as did Mrs. Homan's brother. When the ritual fails to convince everyone of the "rightness" of its transformative effects, disorder, dissonance, and distress follow. The ethics consultation called by Mrs. Homan's clinicians was their attempt to reestablish control. If the family agrees, the patient becomes unrescuable (Dying) and may acquire one or another denotation of this new status, such as a DNR order and/or transfer orders. Life-supportive measures may be withdrawn. Or things may go on unchanged until the patient dwindles toward death.

The fact that an agenda seems to exist and that time pressure increases is not to suggest that participants are aware of it or that the ritual is necessarily a linear or orderly process. Informants combined internal and external narratives in their descriptions using the ritual of intensification to apply order to chaotic elements as they unfolded. Diagnosis and treatment were of a piece—they appeared to be chronological, when facets of either might have been simultaneous, reversed or missing altogether. The strategy of ritualization seeks resolution to the illness (and to the admission) by supporting the patient and "buying time" for recovery. Failing this, it can achieve resolution to the admission by making the patient's body responsible for removing the patient from public concern. The action of the ritual and the time spent on it proves to the participants that the public concern is *justifiably* exhausted. At the same time, it maintains the illusion that Dying is an aberration from which all may yet be safe, as the responsibility for this particular death lies with the patient's intractable body, not with the system.

Figure 7.1 places the ritual of intensification within the broad phases of the clinical course for the seriously ill patient in the hospital.

Not on the Agenda

Palliative care and symptom control are certainly not in this lineup, while the ritual of intensification is in force. Aggressive treatment does not rule out attention to symptom control, however. Intubation is frequently accompanied by continuous infusions of pain and sedative medication to ease its discomfort. Certainly clinicians attempt to relieve patient distress consistently, but attention paid to these issues is secondary compared to rescue concerns. This stance contrasts sharply with one of the examples of orderly dying, withdrawal of life support (see Chapter 3) when, as clinicians dismantle

TRAJECTORY ONE (Most Patients)	TRAJECTORY TWO Used when Trajectory One Fails; Patients Seriously Ill		
FIRST-CLASS STATUS	FIRST-CLASS STATUS, OUTCOME UNCLEAR		SECOND-CLASS STATUS
Rescue and potential for rescue	Ritual of intensification; Rescue and potential for rescue; Technological support for instability.		No rescue planned; Instability and deterioration expected; Perception of crisis unlikely.
Patient admitted and treated; Straightforward recovery; Clock time undisturbed; "Moving things along"; Little or no obstacle to normal throughput.	Recovery stalled; Ambiguity, "zone of indistinction" (Kaufman 2005); Complications, perhaps with stabilization modalities; Discharge postponed, open-ended; More complex technology and management applied; Clock time suspended in favor of elasticity of process for resolving uncertainty; Waiting for patient to "declare himself"; Patient's suffering often secondary to the demands of producing more time alive; Stability is achieved for some patients from this point.	Time passes, Pressure builds; More sensitivity to suffering as outcome appears more dire; Bodily dying may become obvious; Puzzle solving, technical explanations not yet complete; May be called "flogging" or "torture" by nurses.	Ritual closing down with tipping point, family hurdle; Institution of DNR and/or withdrawal of life support; Patient "certified" as Dying; Palliative care possible; Patient transferred to non-rescue bed; Redemption possible through relief of suffering.
TEAM SYNCHRONY	TEAM SYNCHRONY	TORQUE & TENSION	TEAM SYNCHRONY USUALLY RESTORED
Profitable	Profitable, but decreasing.	Opportunity costs exist at least, with possible direct costs.	No profit; may be undocumented, unreimbursed care.
TIME ⟶			

Figure 7.1. Trajectories.

technology and hopes for recovery, they meticulously replace them with "comfort care" and the relief of suffering. Only when clinicians perceive rescue as futile does patient suffering acquire iconic power to motivate a transformation in the plan of care.

Mrs. Oliver was a relatively rare exception to that rule. I describe her situation because even though it was uncommon, such cases leave a more powerful impression on clinicians than dozens of orderly, ventilated, and well-medicated patients. Mrs. Oliver, 66, had done poorly after heart surgery in the teaching hospital.

> RN: Then her kidneys failed and she needed continuous dialysis. Then from her [medications to keep up her blood pressure, the circulation to her extremities was compromised] and her skin was sloughing. She blistered and sloughed, blistered and sloughed. Her tongue was necrotic. I told the doc she was uncomfortable every time I touched her. He told me, "That's not pain." Those were his exact words. Then I excused myself to take a blood pressure pill.
>
> HC: How awake was she?
>
> RN: She was very aware—much of the time. [That's why it was so bad.] I advised for her to get more pain medication. The surgeon felt otherwise.
>
> HC: What was the surgeon's justification?
>
> RN: He said she was confused due to her liver failure. I said, "When I ask her if she has pain, she nods yes." The surgeon said, "She would say yes to anything." But she clearly had a grimace, she was clearly uncomfortable. She was really sick. [I wanted to] make her comfortable. She became a DNR, too. After that they might have been more liberal with the pain meds.

In the view of the surgeon, pain medication might have interfered with assessing Mrs. Oliver's liver function through her waxing and waning mental state. His assessment that her signs of discomfort were "not pain" frustrated the nurse enough to go in search of her own medication to calm her blood pressure. For Mrs. Oliver to "become a DNR" was an indication of the successful conclusion of the ritual of intensification when floodgates might be opened and symptom control could become primary rather than secondary.

Unanimity among clinicians who are certain about the patient's outcome does not always bring about the tipping point for the ritual of intensification. Various issues and system norms may intervene to postpone consensus, as we will explore now.

Factors that Prolong the Ritual

Within the ritual of intensification, a sense of urgency builds steadily toward a deliberate, intentional resolution of the ambiguity. The momentum behind this urgency is invisible to the participants involved, who must attribute the rationale for change to the patient's circumstances (Kaufman 2005:131). Even so, its culmination arises less from the patient's physiology than from sources unknown to the participants that are influencing the shape of the ritual of intensification, whether brought about by resuscitation or by less dramatic technology. Factors exist that shorten the ritual of intensification, discussed in the next section. For now it is useful to consider the markers of special legitimacy capable of diffusing this urgency and delaying the tipping point. Certain habits of practice and factors within the system stand against the resurgence of "moving things along," while they may have little to do with the individual patient's circumstances.

Habits of Practice: Assuming Personal Responsibility

When the perception of bodily dying alone is too weak to halt aggressive treatment, nurses and other clinicians become frustrated, unable to comprehend what hidden agenda the physicians might be following. Physicians themselves may be unaware both of nurses' frustration and nursing's social norms (Buchman et al. 2002; Oberle and Hughes 2001). Nurses often single out surgeons as particularly intractable. According to one: "Surgeons have a certain lack of—I'm generalizing now—empathy and connectedness to people. Maybe they have to do that to take parts out and mutilate them. They are not part of the gameset if there is nothing surgically to do. They don't follow [the patient] continuously. They don't see patients as human beings with feelings."

Some nonnursing observers attribute the callousness perceived by this nurse instead to be an *excess* of feeling, a high level of accountability and shame regarding patient death reinforced as a part of their socialization to the profession. Surgeon and anthropologist Joan Cassell and her colleagues call this proprietary feeling the "surgical covenant" (Buchman et al. 2002; Cassell et al. 2003). Such a sense of personal responsibility would mitigate against closing down the ritual of intensification, as one cardiology fellow (clearly not a surgeon) confirmed to me: "Yes that's true. [Surgeons think that] once they give them a sternal scar (through surgery), they get a God complex, and those patients are not allowed to die until after they leave the hospital."

Not only does the surgeon have the power to rearrange the patient's body, but also to interfere with time itself to prolong the ritual of intensification. Because surgical procedures provide the main contribution to the hospital's bottom line as they enact dramatic bodily changes so relevant to the rescue culture, it is not surprising that surgeons can delay the resurgence of clock time by refusing to declare "technical dying."

Certain other factors touch cords of personal responsibility for any physician, such as iatrogenesis (hospital-acquired illness) or physician error (Casarett, Stocking, and Siegler 1999). Yet another prolonging factor can be seen in the teaching hospital where residents move to a different service each month. Here, a patient who is far along in the ritual of intensification is often maintained during the transition. The new team needs time to get to know the patient, become acquainted with the family, and compare their own assessment with the information they received on sign-out, as they take the patient under their wing.

Habits of practice favor certain categories of patients for more extended treatment. The ritual of intensification carries more momentum for younger patients, those with few coexisting illnesses, and/or a high functional status prior to admission. Occasionally, a pediatric or neonatal patient merits transfer to the teaching hospital when clinical needs exceed the capacity of the Catholic community hospital. Jessica Muller and Barbara Koenig (1988) found that if the patient's demographics match those of the young physicians treating her, they are more reluctant to close down the ritual of intensification. A patient who is *"part of the hospital family"* (i.e., an employee or a member of an employee's family) motivates clinicians to extend the ritual of intensification.

Physician practice in most acute-care settings involves itself with the management of the patient's technological requirements, and no comparable channel to demonstrate her fidelity may present itself, as was the case for the physician caring for Mrs. Turner in Chapter 3. The prospect of dismantling the technology for any reason, even for imminent death, can look and feel too much like abandonment, a sin for any clinician. Even if technical and bodily dying are established, dogged fidelity to a particularly favored patient can delay closure.

Habits of practice among new interns and residents influence the ritual's duration in the teaching hospital. A principal clinician in the palliative care unit made this observation.

RN: During the first three months of the year (July–September), everything is more slow and inefficient. New interns have to check with others before writing orders or making decisions. The radiologists are reading a hundred x-rays that won't be ordered next May. Plans are slower. I suspect length of stay is at least a day longer on average. By May and June, palliative care consults are up and the unit is full of palliative care patients. By then, the interns get it. They realize they can't save the world. Right now (August), it's all about teaching.

Palliative care does not usually become a viable plan of care until after the ritual of intensification is complete. This palliative care clinician naturally saw a longer duration of the ritual as slow and inefficient. Clearly, the network of teaching hospitals supports the learning curve required for residents and interns to manage patient complications and become familiar with the ritual as a necessary part of graduate medical education, even though it extends the patient's length of stay. Getting to the bottom of the conundrum posed by the patient is key. A terminal diagnosis is insufficient to curb the ritual of intensification in a young, previously stable patient in either hospital. If the patient is deteriorating quickly without a technical explanation, rescue efforts are redoubled, as was the case for 32-year-old Mr. Jordan, a cancer patient of four years who was suspected of selling his prescribed pain medications on the street. A young hospitalist physician who worked shifts at the Catholic community hospital described Mr. Jordan's history.

> MD: He would lose prescriptions and run out of them five times too soon. Finally they kicked him out of the pain clinic at the teaching hospital. One doctor there would write him daily prescriptions, but he complained about having to come in for them when he was weak from chemo. He came to this hospital to escape [their discipline]. While he was in the ER here he was suddenly short of breath. They intubated him. They could find no reason for it. They could not ventilate him. It happened at the change of shift, and Dr. H and I stayed and worked on him till 1 AM. . . . We didn't do chest compressions, but we did the vent and pressors. With his metastatic disease. . . . The family asked for an autopsy, and I just got the preliminary results, which show ARDS [Acute Respiratory Distress Syndrome]. But we don't think it's that. It may have been a PE (pulmonary embolism, a clot in the lung).

A sudden, life-threatening, and mysterious complication required stabilization first of all. Stabilization allowed time to find the explanation. Mr. Jordan's youth and the disorder of his acute distress trumped the terminality of his underlying condition. The crisis caused clinicians to scramble and to keep struggling with the question even after the patient's death. Bodily dying and terminal illness were irrelevant.

Habits of Practice for Private Practice versus Teaching Physicians
Lacking plentiful ICU beds and physicians in training, the Catholic community hospital routinely has fewer resources to manage and prolong the ritual

of intensification, a factor in closing down the ritual (see above). Meanwhile, teams and the involvement of larger numbers can delay the closure of the ritual in the teaching hospital. An oncologist in the teaching hospital offered this comparison: the attending MD said, "It's the relationships. In an academic setting you have to explain it to so many more people. It's easier to keep going than to have those discussions. In a private hospital, it's just the attending, the nurse and a few family."

By "explain it," she meant any divergence away from the ritual of intensification. If the inertia she describes and the time of year can work to extend the ritual in the teaching hospital, fewer "relationships" in the Catholic community hospital may not grease the wheels of the process. Despite the lack of comparable resources, individual habits of private-practice physicians can still work to delay the ritual's closing.

Informants described wide variations in physician behavior that influence the closing of the ritual through communication issues, unilateral decision-making, and lack of physician accessibility. One of the few studies comparing community and teaching hospitals found that private-practice physicians in community hospitals may have less experience in dying, engaging in troublesome conversations, and in changing the care plan.[16] An RN at the Catholic community hospital put it this way: "The doctors, they hedge a lots of times. Sometimes they aren't good at getting the no code."

Her observation was borne out by instances in which a physician was notified that his patient was being resuscitated and yet refused to come in. Family wishes regarding patient code status were occasionally misunderstood. These negatives were balanced by reports of physicians who: (1) stepped into the breach left by their colleagues and apologized for their actions; (2) explained the dying situation to everyone's satisfaction; and (3) exhibited "pastoral" behavior with families. Individual physician behavior worthy of praise or blame was reported far less frequently at the teaching hospital, perhaps indicating fewer unilateral decisions of note.

Accessibility to physicians in private practice can be challenging, a difficulty somewhat alleviated when hospitalists were introduced into the Catholic community hospital. One nurse there blamed the demands of private practice for the obstacles preventing physicians from doing the difficult job of closing the ritual of intensification. She observed:

> RN: Our private-practice docs make very short visits. They're in and out. They come in after office hours. They're gonna see a whole lot of patients real fast, and then they're gonna be outta

here. I can't figure out how they cannot know they're dying. They lose it all in talk. They don't want to put the picture together. It never occurs to them to look for death as a possible alternative to what's going on here. It's what you've been trained to see. What you're looking for.

This description indicates several issues that would delay the closure of the ritual of intensification: office hours cause physician visits to inpatients to be too short and episodic to "put the picture together." Private-practice physicians typically see patients alone without the teaching hospital mechanisms that require peer discussion. These factors may reward preexisting ideas, or "what you're trained to see."

Receiving care from one's personal physician while in the hospital may be very satisfying. It may also be more idiosyncratic than that of a teaching hospital, where patterns generated by physicians practicing in hierarchical teams are the norm. Private-practice physicians have their own ideas about patient management. More important to this discussion, they may ignore a patient's wishes to have CPR withheld. A CCU nurse explained the rationale behind this unilateral decision:

RN: Everyone is a full code, coming through our doors. If they have a durable DNR[17] order, for twenty-four hours we can honor that. Then otherwise they become a full code. Because why come to the hospital? Because you want help. Sometimes the docs think "I can ride 'em through this." They can override the [patient's express desire for] DNR because he thinks he can get them through it.

Habits of physician practice in the teaching hospital may influence the duration of the ritual of intensification for different reasons and in different ways than hold true in the Catholic community hospital. In both settings, however, system norms rather than the patient's physiology account for these differences.

System factors dictate varying levels of "ownership" and authority in the patient relationship. The physician and/or team who admits the patient "owns" the responsibility for and the privilege of directing that patient's care. Cross-cover physicians, by definition, are not primary, and they often defer major patient management decisions (such as closing the ritual) until the return of the primary team or attending physician with the more "legitimate" physician/patient relationship, as in the cases of Mr. Diangelo and Mr. Gomez in Chapter 1. Such delays occurred in both hospitals.

Floor nurse, teaching hospital:

RN: With night float, it's usually "keep 'em alive till seven and five." But our docs know the patients.

Stepdown unit, Catholic community hospital:

RN: [She didn't go to hospice] because it was the weekend, and on call doctors don't make those decisions.

For Mrs. Homan in the ICU of the Catholic community hospital, the ritual of intensification extended for several days because the physician was going out of town. This occurred despite a family meeting earlier in the week that had resulted in an agreement to withdraw life support. The RN said: "[T]hen he went away for the weekend. He didn't tell his partners what to do. [Mrs. Homan's] respiratory rate was in the 50s, so the partners put her back on [full ventilatory support]. She sits like that all weekend."

In teaching hospitals, residents feel caught by their own untested judgment, patient suffering, and their low position in the hierarchy when they consider advocating for the closing down of the ritual of intensification. One intern in the pilot study expressed this difficulty, along with a clear understanding that "fighting to live" rules out comfort:

MD: Even though she looked like she was on death's door, the attending wanted to keep going. There was this disconnect between the attending and [lost articulation], but being an intern two weeks on the service, I didn't know if this woman could turn around or not. The nurses were upset. I was in the middle. . . . It's hard to balance between fighting to live, and therefore you can't give the morphine and the narcotics, versus we're going to call it a day and give you comfort care. The closer they get to death, the farther away the attendings get. It's not a criticism, it's just an observation.

Another intern in the pilot study expressed his sense of helplessness based on his position in the hierarchy. He said: "There's always a high degree of variability [in the dying situation] based on where the patient is and what service they're on and who the attending is—all things that are out of control of house staff."

Of all these system factors and habits of practice, perhaps only what is relevant to the technical dying explanation makes its way into the narrative of the illness' course constructed for the family. After all, few of these factors can be related directly to the physiology of the patient. But each can delay the arrival of the tipping point, the decision that moves the patient away from rescue.

Tipping Point and the Family Hurdle

The tipping point brings the ritual of intensification to an end and allows the normal hospital agenda of "moving things along" to resume. Assuming the patient does not die before this tipping point arrives for clinicians, it affords perfect hindsight to construe the present tragic situation as orderly and the patient's dying as inevitable.

Defining the Tipping Point

The tipping point is the official decision taken by clinicians *among themselves* that justifies a change in the patient's official status from living to Dying. Clinicians recognize it as the official backstage signal to redirect the narrative constructed for the family and patient, sometimes referred to as "hanging crepe." For insiders, the ritual has done its work successfully, allowing them to bring dying into open awareness with the benefit of the technical dying explanation (Glaser and Strauss 1965; Moore and Myerhoff 1977; Seymour 2000). Acknowledging the significance of putting disease in the appropriate frame, Kaufman states, "Dying does not become institutionally recognized or named, and thus is not really happening, until medical staff interpret discrete measurements as irreversible and fatal."[18] She refers to this as a "moment of new understanding" (2005: 205). The expressions for this moment in both hospitals indicate both exhaustion and helplessness regarding medical or social responsibility, and the shifting of the onus to the patient:

Teaching hospital:

"He was past the point of medical care."

"We can't help her."

Catholic community hospital:

"We've done all we can. The fight is done."

"We were prolonging the inevitable."

In these phrases and in the expression used for Mrs. Turner, "Don't keep giving this family hope," clinicians understood and agreed that the appropriate medical task now lay along some path other than aggressive care. The patient's clinical state may not have changed, but her time in the ritual of intensification has run out.

But Kaufman also acknowledges that it can be less of an epiphany than a negotiation, a "mutable phenomenon, always linked to the politics and rhetoric of the patient's condition" (2005: 237). Ivan Illich describes the physician as the representing society at large, especially important at this juncture.

> Like all other major rituals of industrialized society, medicine in practice takes the form of a game. The chief function of the physician becomes that of an umpire. He [sic] is the agent or representative of the social body, with the duty to make sure that everyone plays the game according to the rules. The rules, of course, forbid leaving the game and dying in any fashion that has not been specified by the umpire. (1995a: 205)

Illich's observation speaks to the assumption of order in the ritual and the anticipation of the control of death, as the illness and its instability have also been if not completely controlled, at least subject to explanation. The attending physician is held legally responsible for the patient's plan of care, so the search for order in the official narrative corresponds with accountability to the system at large for the patient's nonrecovery. The hierarchy dictates that it is the attending physician through her authority, then, who decides when technical explanations are adequate, whether the tipping point has indeed been reached, and how the new plan should be presented to the family.

Just as particular patient demographics may lengthen the ritual and beat back the pressures of clock time, antithetical circumstances have the opposite effect. Characteristics influencing clinicians to close down the ritual more swiftly include the patient's advanced age, admission from a nursing home, poor functional status, and/or multiple coexisting illnesses.[19] Family requests can also shorten the ritual, which happened a handful of times in both hospitals (Prendergast and Luce 1997). Clinicians are more likely to raise arguments among themselves that continuing the ritual is "futile" care and a waste of resources in such cases, a transparency that reveals the powerful forces seeking resolution of the admission. Finally, bodily dying itself can sometimes become a tipping point. If the patient is deteriorating, nurses often take steps on their own, especially if they wish to avoid having to inflict a code on a patient (see the section on suffering, below).

A major influence on clinicians for closing down the ritual is the patient's neurological status. Because it is so strongly connected with postmodern ideas of personhood (Kaufman 2005: 293–295) and perhaps because of the existence of the phenomenon of brain death as a legal rationale for the withdrawal of life support, clinicians make an argument for the tipping point using a quality-of-life argument and dignity, as they did both for Mr. Mendez and Mrs. Turner in Chapter 3. Clinicians considered both patients to be rescuable until a stroke or other consequence of the illness resulted in an inability to respond. The hastening of Mrs. Harper's death (Chapter 1) was certainly influenced by her neurological devastation. A nurse in the neuro ICU described her lobbying the resident for closing the ritual on a patient: "I talked to the resident, I said, 'He has no life. He is vegging. It would be cruel to trach and peg.' And we did decide to make him a DNR and withdraw care. I said, 'He's not here. His body is here, but he's not.' The resident talked to the attending. He talked to the family, and they did decide on withdrawal." Here, the nurse equated "no life" with the lack of conscious awareness ("he's" not here). His resulting nonhumanity ("vegging," like a vegetable) presumably should elicit a humane action from the staff, that is, the declaration of a tipping point.

If a patient with a devastating head injury survived the initial trauma, he would need a trach and peg (tracheostomy for better airway protection and surgical placement of a feeding tube, that is, "PEG" tube, percutaneous endogastric tube) for long-term stabilization. These procedures required consent from the family. Such a conversation could pave the way for nursing home placement or for withdrawal of life support, depending on its outcome. Either would close the ritual and resolve the admission. In the nurse's description, the decision about the trach and peg became a tipping point for clinicians, later accepted by the family. I commented to another neuro nurse in the teaching hospital that physicians often neglect to include the prospects for the patient's quality of life in consent discussions such as these. In particular I noted that saying "nursing home" could bring more reality into the family's understanding. She replied,

> RN: The word "diaper" works even better. That's universal. "Trach and peg" is medical and seems okay. But "diaper." You can see people cringe. Everybody knows what that means.

> HC: Because it's the word that means indignity.

> RN: I tell people to try to work the word "diaper" into their conversation. Because that's really how it is for them.

Her advising others of this strategy indicates the strength of the felt need to steer a course away from rescue to another plan. This exchange betrayed our shared bias that it would be "better" and "more dignified" for everyone if the "less-dignified" path to the nursing home were not chosen, and the patient were allowed to die.

The certainty of permanent unresponsiveness colors the U.S. clinical perspective more dramatically than most other kinds of physical devastation. But the agendas of some cultures may prevent it from being determinative. Withdrawal of life support may be less compelling for people from nonindustrialized settings and from certain religious traditions. In Anne Fadiman's account of Lia Lee (1997), her unresponsiveness made no difference to her Hmong family, who took her home and continued to care for her. Numerous institutions in the United States are designed especially to care for unresponsive patients (Kaufman 2000, 2005). Nonetheless, the confirmation of severe neurological injury often serves as an effective tipping point in the ritual, making it possible to close it down.

For a surgical ICU nurse in the teaching hospital, the very extremes of treatment needed to sustain her patient defined the tipping point by signaling his demise. She described the last hours of Joey, a teenager who had started out with an ulcer and was now in multisystem organ failure and supported by four machines.

> RN: [His blood pressure was marginally acceptable.] But we had him on such jet fuel to do it!
>
> HC: What do you mean by jet fuel?
>
> RN: (naming his IV meds): Epi, calcium, boluses and boluses of bicarb. To me that's like a continuous code. He declared himself. Point five of epi per minute.

Each one of these powerful medications has a role in the algorithm of Advanced Cardiac Life Support and may be given as a bolus[20] during resuscitation efforts. If one of them restores the patient's heart rate and rhythm, it may then be given as a continuous infusion in the postresuscitation period. Joey needed three of these to maintain even a very low blood pressure. Interpreting the patient's condition by way of the treatments he requires is a method of studying an ambiguous oracle, in this case the patient's body. The notion of the patient "declaring himself" involves making the patient responsible, thereby absolving the caregivers and the family from responsibility for deciding about death. This nurse was using both of these concepts as evidence in constructing the Joey's narrative, as researchers such as Johnson et al. (2000) have observed.

Significance of the Tipping Point

However consensus arrives, with the tipping point the clinicians managing the ritual of intensification now agree that the required transformation is (tragically) manifest. In applying technology without time restrictions, the ritual has done its work to "certify" the transformation as far as they are concerned. Competing interests that may have delayed the tipping point have retreated, so that the time is "right" (see Kaufman below). Clock time reasserts its primacy. Official certification of the dire outcome untwists the time lines, unites the staff, and holds out the promise of rapid resolution (assuming the family also acknowledges the transformation). This decision to openly *name* the dying means that sufficient quantities of social motivation exist to reclassify the patient, making his subsequent, expected deterioration explicitly not a crisis requiring public attention. Movement can resume. In Illich's words: "Technical death has won its victory over dying" (1995a: 207).

Assuming that the family agrees, this reclassification may come in the form of a "comfort care only" care plan, a DNR order, the physical transfer of the patient to another bed, a palliative care consultation, the withdrawal of life support, or some other named status that obviates full resuscitation, the expected obligation of the social contract. The tipping point also validates the patient's suffering, that it has been "enough," earning this change in status (Kaufman 2005: 75). The flaw is that the transformation lowers rather than raises the patient's status in society and privatizes rather than celebrates the fruits of that suffering.

Complete and Incomplete Tipping Points
Not surprisingly, the tipping point varied by hospital cultural practice, as certain other studies have indicated.[21] Greater elaborations of technology are available at teaching hospitals, enabling stabilization in the face of a greater variety and number of complications. Expanded layers of human hierarchy and power among physicians and administrators matches the higher pitch of chaos, rescue, and urgency for control found in these settings. Patterns of practice influence clinical norms, demanding conformity. In the Catholic community hospital, nurses, social workers, and chaplains jockey for position more freely, and the tipping point reveals these variations.

The tipping point is more sharply defined in the teaching hospital, just as rescue interventions there are more elaborated. The change it brings about in the plan of care is more complete. In the Catholic community hospital, it is easier to have a "no code" (more common parlance than DNR) written for a patient, but the plan for care afterward is harder to pin down. It is as if patients can be tipped away from rescue, but not all the way to comfort care. One example was Mr. Wallace, who was 49 years old and died on a floor unit. The nurse described his situation.

RN: He was critically ill, very critically ill. When we got out of report, the night nurse said he wasn't breathing, so we went in together. He'd had an elevated temp, he was tachy, he was on a lot of oxygen. The night nurse asked, "If he's comfort care, why am I giving meds every hour"? If there is no order for palliative care, we do every treatment that is ordered.

HC: You have a palliative care order?

RN: We have a palliative care pathway. The docs know about it. It's a six-day pathway.[22] No vital signs, meds for comfort only, nothing invasive. It's death with dignity, the way I see it. For a patient you know is terminal. Nothing but morphine and turning the patient. Had we had an opportunity to do this during the night—it happened so quickly. He was gone when we arrived this morning. It was hard.

HC: Was there a DNR order?

RN: He was a no code. . . .They wanted him to go to a hospice bed. We throw terminology around. I'm not sure physicians always know what they mean, hospice or palliative care. Medicine seems more in tune than surgery. There were many doctors to call on this patient: pulmonary, renal, neurosurgery, neurology—

HC: Were all these consulting physicians?

RN: All consulting on him. MJ was the attending.

This nurse described Mr. Wallace as "critically ill," a "no code," "comfort care," being cared for by many doctors, but without "the opportunity" for hospice or palliative care, because "physicians don't always know what they mean." Because of this, nurses "do every treatment that's ordered," even though the plan of care seems to contradict itself. Here the hard work of signification seemed to be complete simply with the designation of his unrescuable status. Imminent death and symptom control may not rise to the level of crisis, as they did not for Mr. Diangelo, and seemingly fail to command further attention or definition.

In the teaching hospital, clearer stipulations about the care plan are the norm, reflecting a higher expectation of control of the situation among the staff. Nurses can be more insistent in getting the interns and residents to clarify orders for patient management, but they are much less likely to violate the ownership of the tipping point itself than are the nurses in the Catholic hospital. Instead, they work inside the hierarchy to influence the decision, (as did the nurse who advocated using the word "diaper") and because of the numerous invasive procedures requiring consent, family meetings may be more frequent. These mandated discussions for consent can function as status reports and reviews of the patient's "big picture." At times, the procedures themselves provide new and definitive information, prompting a tipping point. Families may initiate changes on their own, as they did in three cases.

Suffering Related to Tipping Point

Because getting to the tipping point can resemble abandonment by the hospital and the clinicians in a society where the production of more time alive is a democratizing value, *it must be construed by everyone as the only decision available.* When nurses conclude that the patient is dying, they countenance changing the care plan on the basis of limiting suffering and promoting the patient's dignity as the only thing left to be done. Everyone needs to believe that they are backed into a corner. The influence of time, throughput, and the itch to resume control when illness has won must not appear to have an influence in closing down the ritual of intensification. Accordingly, all these forces are read and articulated as the importance of dignity and limiting suffering, as Kaufman describes:

> For its part, talk about dignity is often connected to ideas of *suffering*, especially in attempts to assess the role suffering plays in a patient's experience of critical illness and of hospitalization (whether or not the patient can articulate his or her suffering). Dignity is also invoked in the deliberations among staff and family about *whether there has been enough suffering.* (2005: 75, emphasis in the original)

Kaufman does not indicate that the accrual of suffering goes hand in hand with the consciousness of clock time. "Enough" suffering is clearly a construction that others can project on to the patient, if she or her body cannot communicate subjectively. But such a judgment can occur only after some interval of time's passage.

As the ritual proceeds and dying (bodily or technical) materializes, the pain of not moving things along for clinicians becomes indistinguishable from patient suffering. Everyone suffers as resolution is postponed. A chaplain at the teaching hospital reflected on a particularly troubling case regarding a patient with a devastating head injury.

> CH: *I* wanted it to be over. *Staff* wanted it to be over. When you've been through it hundreds of times, thousands of times—you know the outcome—we forget that families are seeing it for the first time.

HC: (revealing my own bias) We want to save them suffering, but it's our suffering we're saving.

CH: Yes, we want to limit the ambiguity of when it will be over. How long will we have to live with it? Our definitions of the end-point—endgame—are different than the family's definition.

Such different perspectives between the family and the clinicians bring their respective sufferings. Clinicians witness, inflict, and project suffering onto their patients. Their angst regarding bodily dying and a foreseen, preventable resuscitation attempt are greater motivations for them to close the ritual and limit everyone's suffering than such foreknowledge seems to be for physicians, as discussed above. One nurse working nights in the Catholic community hospital's ICU described a situation that compelled her to pick up the phone and convey the necessary information to the family herself. Then she called the physician to close the deal:

RN: I called them. I told them she would die. She had almost died the first night. Then she got better. And then got worse again. I told them we had nowhere else to go. "We've done everything. If we resuscitate her, she may come back, but she won't come back as good as she is now, and with the first compression we would break ribs. Or I will take the same care of her and keep her comfortable." I called the attending, actually the guy covering. "I can take a verbal DNR order from you. Are you comfortable signing it?" "I'm comfortable if you're comfortable."

In the case of Mr. Gomez in Chapter 1, even in her distress the nurse did not take a similar action. In only one case did a nurse in the teaching hospital report approaching a family on her own. Such independent action was more prevalent in the Catholic community hospital.

The tipping point is an acknowledgment of powerlessness *without humiliation*. It affirms that even as the illness has overmastered the patient and everyone interested in her welfare, her clinicians can appropriate the power of certainty and order, blandishing its reassurance. Comforted themselves by the social attention that the ritual of intensification has afforded the patient and relieved that official Dying now banishes him from the arena of public concern, clinicians hope that his own comfort care may now begin.

The Family Hurdle and Closing Down the Ritual
Once the tipping point is reached internally, the stress on clinicians relaxes somewhat as their timelines and understandings are reunited. Before the

ritual of intensification can be closed down, however, the family must be on board with the plan clinicians have formed. Broaching the unrescuable territory involves giving the bad news—e.g., naming what is abhorrent and proposing next steps, such as a DNR order or a withdrawal of life support. As Peter Metcalf reminds us, "Rituals may make a show of power, but they run the same risk as other shows: they may fail" (Metcalf and Huntington 1991: 6). The family's willingness to accept the new plan is the test of the ritual's operational efficacy in performing its transformation of the patient from living to dying (Moore and Myerhoff 1977: 12–13). Kaufman elaborates on the stumbling block this hurdle presents:

> Life-sustaining treatments are promoted until *it is time* to stop; then the pathways shift course and promote, or even dictate the acceptance and facilitation of death. Patients and families are expected to conform to both these directives and to switch in a smooth and timely way from making life-prolonging moves to making preparation-for-death moves. Unsurprisingly, patients and their families often balk at having to make the switch. (2005: 153, emphasis in the original)

Whether or not families get on board, for clinicians the momentum has shifted completely. They are now uniformly pessimistic and ready to move on. They see their further engagement with the patient as mopping up, as anticlimax. To continue aggressive care at the behest of the family feels disorderly and untidy to clinicians, who blame families for their lack of understanding and prolonging patient suffering.

ICU RN, Teaching hospital:

RN: People look down at families and think, "They're never going to [decide to] withdraw [life support]." I think sometimes they don't ever get it.

ICU RN, Teaching hospital:

RN: I would have let him go a while back. He'd been through so much. But the family, they make the decision. . . .We added more stuff, added more stuff. After he died, he didn't look peaceful. Some people look so peaceful. He didn't.

Mrs. Homan's nurse asserted that machines were more responsible for her continued time alive than her brother's faith. He wanted her to be kept alive until her daughter's birthday the next week, a wish that told the staff that he was not in touch with her reality. Only at the urging of other family members did he agree to the withdrawal of life support.

Successful negotiation of the family hurdle depends on clinicians' ability to change the narrative for families, a delicate process. Nancy Johnson and her colleagues have described its complexities after observing the internal discourse of ICU rounds and external meetings with families. By making the patient's body appear as the "author of the story," clinicians, especially physicians, must replace the present murky picture with certainty that recovery is impossible, proven over time by the patient's body's resistance to rescue interventions. Clinicians must reformulate the family's understandings of culture and nature. The ventilator, the dialysis machine, and the blood pressure infusions must shift from adjunctive and supportive to alien and unnatural. To offer to limit suffering is seen as the more important goal "now," as "treatment and technology become the villain." A "natural" death (without technology) allows "greater forces" to take over and helps to distance clinicians and families from culpability for the death (Johnson et al. 2000).

The presence of any form of an advance directive can strengthen the case to close down the ritual of intensification, because it allows clinicians to attach not only terminality to the patient's body, but also a formal statement of her own volition not to be "maintained." Even without an advance directive, it is important to characterize the (often unknowable) patient intent in a particular way. Johnson and her colleagues comment:

> Discussions about what the patient would have wanted, however, appear to be less about patient desires, goals, and motivations in the context of the dying experience—as proponents of advance directives and adherents to the dying with dignity movement would have it—and more about assigning moral agency for the decision to limit treatment to the patient. (2000: 287)

In this context, the documented reluctance of African Americans to use advance directives is justified (Crawley 2005; Dula and Williams 2005). Clinicians and families can use patient statements about limiting aggressive treatment to reinforce the "rightness" of their own conclusions, as happened with Mrs. Turner.: "The last thing she wanted was this." With or without an advance directive, U.S. ideological understandings of individualism and equality (articulated through bioethics) constrain clinicians. They may not use the tipping point unilaterally to close the ritual without outside consent from patient and/or family. How did they fare in the two hospitals in obtaining this endorsement?

More than half of the accounts of patient deaths at each site mentioned the family hurdle aspect of the patient's care: forty-seven of seventy-three cases in the teaching hospital and forty-nine of eighty-two cases at the

Catholic community hospital. Among these, it seemed that there was more resistance in the Catholic community hospital, where 33 percent of families resisted and 35 percent accepted clinicians' judgment. In the teaching hospital, 51 percent agreed with clinicians that the patient was dying, and 28 percent did not. In the remaining cases, the family hurdle itself evaporated, either because the patient or family initiated a halt to treatment, or the patient's death preempted the discussion. If this is an accurate representation, then one may speculate that the higher intensity of rescue in the teaching hospital was itself persuasive.

The study's retrospective view limits this interpretation of the data, however. It is impossible to know from the data whether some patients stabilized without dying after families insisted on continuing treatment. Further, categories of resistance to negotiating the hurdle are difficult to quantify because of factors such as timing. If a family resists and then agrees to a DNR order just as the patient is being overwhelmed by death, is this a "successful" negotiation just because chest compressions do not occur? How soon before death does family agreement to limit aggressive care need to occur to "count"? In some cases, physicians were at cross-purposes with the family, delaying agreement. It is difficult to separate these instances from those in which physicians withheld resuscitation, overriding family wishes. It appears that the success of changing the narrative and negotiating the family hurdle maintains the semblance of linear progression in the chaos of illness more than it presents an invitation for family input in the direction of care. By going through the motions of "respecting autonomy" in changing the narrative and presenting the new story to the family for their endorsement, the clinicians prove to themselves that they are not bulldozing the family, even as the illness is overpowering everyone.

Catherine Bell states that in ritualization, "the hegemonic order being experienced must be rendered socially redemptive in order to be personally redemptive" (1992: 116). This is a key component. Only after the patient's body is assigned full physiologic responsibility for its own dying, and the "hegemonic order" of the social body (rescue, equality, and individuality in terms of autonomy) triumphs through the ritual of intensification, can clinicians feel personally innocent of (redeemed in) demoting this patient to the category of "Dying." If families agree to this characterization in time, clinicians might be able to orchestrate a "good death," supplying an even greater dimension of orderliness. If not, the ritual of intensification fails, ushering in disorder and perhaps conflict, as occurred in Mrs. Homan's case.

Both the tipping point and the family hurdle are critical to closing down the ritual and achieving an orderly death. This action transforms relationships along with the patient's status. Physician fidelity, mediated and expressed almost entirely through management of the patient's technological "stuff," must find new avenues of expression; the level of official concern and display gives way to private dignity; the physical location of the patient and the plan of care may change. Physicians and family are exonerated, and the status of medicine and the position of the living vis-à-vis the Dying emerge intact.

Consequences of Disorder; Unsynchronized Dying

To be acceptable in the U.S. hospital, death should happen with as little dying as possible. Clinicians attempt to impose order on the chaos of illness through the ritual of intensification, and this process exacts some amount of suffering as the price of its transformation. Open awareness of Dying is the unsought reward, the nonprize called "dignity," earned for the suffering imposed by the ritual, bringing along a reduction in status, an outcome uncharacteristic of most rituals. A benefit it appears to bestow is the opportunity to apply a further rubric of order to this newly certified state through the withdrawal of life support and/or the transfer of the patient to palliative care.

But the torque of twisted time lines cannot always be neatly resolved. Lack of consensus and alignment leads to "bad" deaths: patients can deteriorate and palliative care not be applied "in time"; "unnecessary" codes are called; codes last "too long"; or compromises regarding resuscitation procedures occur, such as "chemical codes": medications only, without chest compressions to provide circulation of the medications through the patient's body. Clinician pain and powerlessness in these situations is palpable. A nurse had been in the room when the patient suddenly died. She reflected on the subsequent resuscitation attempt. She said: "When she stopped breathing it was so peaceful and calm; then there were all these people engaging her in a battle to make her come back. So different from dying in your sleep."

Unexpected codes could be orderly in the sense that to rally instantly to patient collapse is emblematic of the mission in acute care. Nurses are central to this rescue effort in their roles as first responders. Paradoxically an *expected* code brings profound disruption. Foreseeing the need for resuscitation means that the patient is already seriously ill, teetering on the brink of collapse. One nurse put it this way: "It was pretty ugly . . . we should tell families, 'This code will be barbaric.'"

Besides the brutality of chest compressions alone, success can be ephemeral. Said an oncology nurse at the teaching hospital: "I do not want to code this man. We'll bring him back just to make him suffer more." If such codes cannot be forestalled, they represent disorder in the extreme. Accordingly, nurses often take steps. They press physicians hard for a change in code status, as Mr. Gomez's nurse did, or they abandon protocol and approach the families directly.

Nature of Clinician Burden

Clinicians represent at least three disparate interests: the hospital in which they work, where the bottom lines of physical and economic survival coalesce; the society/culture they live in and bring with them to work that prizes more time alive, minimizing suffering, and dignity in death [van der Geest and Finkler 2004]); and their (suffering) patients, the focus of their practices, who want simply "to breathe, to escape the place, to get better, or to die" (Kaufman 2005: 28). In the role of ritualizing agent, the clinician

> already possesses schemes that he or she can deploy, more or less
> effectively, to produce actions that are more or less coherent with
> each other and with a larger view of the whole of life. . . . One
> appropriates and thereby constructs a version (usually neither very
> explicit nor coherent) of the hegemonic order that promises a path
> of personal redemption, that gives one some sense of relative domi-
> nance in the order of things, and thereby some ability to engage and
> affect that order. (Bell 1992: 208)

While participating in the ritual of intensification, then, the clinician chooses from among his varying interests to construct an understanding of the whole and his role in it. As individuals they may be helpless to control aspects of the procedures, the illness, the agenda, or the outcome. Nonetheless, clinicians can act to increase their own sense of agency. Taking action to limit suffering (by calling a family member, advocating with a physician, or "doing every treatment that's ordered") are strategies clinicians use to assert their own agency through endorsing or contesting the ritual.

To lobby for limiting the suffering of another deflects guilt from one's own complicity. Serious illness in the hospital brings moral situations fraught with uncertainty, which we have seen is a source of suffering in itself. Clinicians constantly make decisions and perform actions without complete knowledge of their meaning or their consequences, and often they cause pain. The entire experience of hospitalization is not one that most patients would choose for themselves; it is an experience they would prefer to forgo. Escalating skills in rescue and stabilization have unhinged the moral ground, creating a new form of life that does not include the subject's conscious participation.[23] Clinicians and families need places of unquestioned moral refuge, and limiting what appears to be the needless suffering of patients provides this sanctuary.

Suffering seems to earn interest and intensity over the course of the ritual of intensification, as discussed above. The imposition of clock time and suffering's accrual can consume clinicians who project and worry, imagining suffering in the future as added on to the suffering of today.

> [S]uffering has a temporal element. For a situation to be source of suffering, it must influence the person's perception of future events. . . . Note that at the moment the individual is saying "If the pain continues like this, I will be overwhelmed" he or she is *not* overwhelmed. At that moment the person is intact. Fear itself always involves the future. (Cassell 1991: 36)

By invoking the suffering of the patient, clinicians recast more time alive, moving it from an ambition to an abomination. But the fact or extent of actual suffering from the patient's point of view can be difficult to ascertain, masked by neurological compromise due to illness and/or medication to ease its burdens. Elaine Scarry (1985) has articulated a strong connection between discerning physical pain and political objectives. A similar unacknowledged linkage occurs here. As the redemptive understanding of generative time for ritual recedes and clock time resumes its former ascendancy, the suffering of clinicians and patients corresponds with hospital financial suffering, all of which accrue, building pressure for a denouement. To opt out of rescue, to violate the prevailing norm of seeking more time alive as the primary goal applied to every patient equally, this patient's individual autonomous interests for dignity and freedom from pain must be configured to outweigh that norm. As the ritual of intensification's prediction of certain death ushers the patient out of the realm of public concern, it opens the door to full pain relief. Relieving today's pain now can redeem both yesterday's and tomorrow's suffering for the patient and for the clinician as well.

And the clinician's suffering is not to be minimized. Kathleen Oberle and Dorothy Hughes call on "administrators to recognize the burden carried by practitioners who are required to witness suffering as part of their daily work" (2001: 713). Stanley Hauerwas goes further and says that clinicians are "tainted" by this exposure. "Through their willingness to be present to us in our most vulnerable moments they are forever scarred with our pain—a pain that we the healthy want to deny or at least keep at arm's length" (1986: 79).

This lived burden of witnessing suffering rests on the shoulders of clinicians because those who work with seriously ill patients may be the only ones who cannot escape its daily reality. Such witness compels acknowledgment even in the United States, where self-reliance rules the day. The accrued effects of carrying this burden with little apparent societal support or guidance are not known.[24] The ultimate problem is that clinicians are the ones who must assign the patient to second-class status and justify doing so on whatever basis is afforded by the ritual experience. Hospitalized patients cannot become residents of the facility. It would be less wrenching if, in the words of Peter Metcalf, "the gradual disentanglement of the living" (Metcalf and Huntington 1991: 84) from the dying did not also force this abandonment. Could the tipping point be reframed as a reward, an achievement, something that represents a public position of honor for patients and their families? If so, it could be a turning point that would secure some status with charisma or symbolic capital attached to it (Bourdieu 1998: 102). The next two chapters begin a consideration of such possibilities.

Notes

1. A few exceptions exist. See Myers (2003) and Mohammed and Peter (2009).
2. I am grateful to J. Brian Cassell who clarified this for me in a private communication.
3. This recalls Howard Stein's reference to medical practice as a "massive defense against biological time" (1990: 174).
4. Occasionally, a very sick child would be transferred from the Catholic community hospital to the teaching hospital.
5. As the hospitalists took over inpatient management for more private-practice physicians, this problem may have decreased. See Chapter 6.
6. Laubach, Brown, and Lenard (1996) attribute this offering of contrast in clinical narrative to cognitive dissonance.
7. See Callahan (1993: 65–67) for a discussion of the need to separate causality in death from culpability and its connection of the need to do this with the disappearance of nature.
8. See Jones, Brewer, and Garrison (2000). And see the discussion in Chapter 4.
9. See Kaufman (2005: 31). Kirchhoff et al. (2002) indicate that it is also a source of denial and magical thinking.
10. Muller and Koenig (1988) describe this phenomenon well, but they do not bring in the concept of fidelity. See Good's observations (1994: 85–87) on moral drama and the passion for medicine. Physicians can interpret having to manage the "stuff" of patient care as a way of suffering with their patients.
11. These criteria set forth by Moore and Myerhoff (1977: 17–18), T. Turner (1977: 61), and V. Turner (1967: 41–42).
12. In Chapter 9 we consider a modification.

13. Culpability, per Callahan (1993).
14. For a helpful discussion of the differences between clock time and process time, see K. Davies (1994).
15. "Because we can" was an excuse that nurses gave to each other when they felt that aggressive treatment was going on too long, rather than "because the patient needs it" or "because that's what the family wants." This reference to simple availability as a motivator is borne out by regional variation in patterns of care (Wennberg 2006). Availability obviates choice.
16. Keenan et al. (1998) speculate that greater experience and intensity in teaching hospitals may mean that physicians broach the topic of withdrawal of life support sooner in these sites than occurs in community hospitals.
17. A durable DNR is a Do Not Resuscitate order written by a physician for an outpatient, such as a hospice patient, and it travels with the patient from one facility to another.
18. Kaufman (2005: 93), echoing both Glaser and Strauss (1965) and Rosenberg (1992).
19. A unilateral decision to withhold treatment at the outset or along the way was unusual, but it happened in five cases, three in the Catholic community hospital and two in the teaching hospital. Keenan et al. (1998) note that this happens more often in community hospital settings.
20. A bolus is a single concentrated dose of medication pushed rapidly through an intravenous line rather than dripping it in over time.
21. In a survey of 386 hospitals in California, Zingmond and Wenger (2005) looked at early DNR orders (i.e, those written within the first twenty-four hours of admission). After correcting for patient characteristics, they found a higher use of early DNR orders in nonteaching hospitals, as well as those that were rural, smaller and for-profit (rather than nonprofit). They also found a tenfold variation across counties, noting that early DNR use was much lower in the urban Los Angeles area than in urban San Francisco. They attributed hospital variation to differences in hospital culture, and the regional variations to differences in physician practice and patient preference, a view supported by other studies (Dartmouth Atlas Project 1998; Prendergast, Claessens, and Luce 1998).
22. See Chapter 6.
23. Marilyn Strathern (1992: 174) and Kaufman (2005: 324–326) have noted this.
24. Moral distress takes a toll on the clinical workforce, however, according to Aiken et al. (2002).

CHAPTER 8

Ritual Display, Palliative Care, and Trust

The family hurdle, then, is a crossroads of trust. If the patient is dying, what needs to stay alive and be preserved for clinicians, the hospital, and the family at this moment? Does the prospect of palliative care measure up as a viable alternative to rescue? How will clinicians maintain the credibility of the salvational system they represent while conceding its failure to produce more time alive for this individual patient?

Rescue as Ritual Display

Joanne Lynn, architect and primary investigator of the influential SUPPORT study (1995), has reflected on the focus of American health-care delivery:

> The care system we now have reflects its origins—powerful men who were worried about heart attacks. That is an outrageous over-simplification, of course, but still fundamentally true. A citizen can get 911 services almost anywhere in the country; and surgeries, devices, drugs and hospitals have had ongoing investment and yield profits. But don't risk finding that you need a home health aide on the weekend or need help opening a jar on the day your arthritis acts up! (2004: 134)

Rescue from death or from a discrete, limited problem through hospital EDs seems more accessible to persons in the United States than meeting simple, ongoing health needs. How does such a narrow, expensive approach to health-care delivery survive? One answer is to consider the health-care focus on rescue and technology as a form of display put on by those who benefit from the present architecture of the health-care system to be appreciated and consumed by those who must live and die within it. Although it may seem altruistic to use heroic measures to save any individual from calamity, the centrality of such a focus in national health-care functions as a form of bargaining that maintains the status quo of social hierarchy. Its benevolent appearance contributes to its efficacy as a cultural representation. It attempts to make up in extravagance in rescue what it lacks in continuity in meeting other health-care needs. As such, its ability to engender trust at the bedside is equally spotty and unpredictable. Clinicians' success in negotiating the family hurdle depends not only on their personal sincerity, but also on the perceived quality of the display contained in the ritual of intensification. If palliative care functions often as an assuagement offered for the discontinuation of the ritual, how "choosable" does it appear? We explore how the palliative care movement works to insert itself into the hospital environment as well as into the ritual of intensification. Finally, we consider whether either approach is worthy of trust.

Because clinicians deploy technology in rescue as agents of a social contract, their actions appear to represent pure altruism, emblematic of the public's interest in extending itself and its resources for vulnerable individuals in its midst. Richard Titmuss recognizes the power of such an impression. He argues for the importance of maintaining volunteerism as the engine of blood donation, so that blood continues to be thought of as a "gift." He promotes this spirit of altruism as a crucial element in engendering trust in the quality of the blood supply (1997 [1970]).

Trust is also the currency at stake in the ritual of intensification, tested in the family hurdle. But several features of the ritual may play havoc with trust: the unequal positions of power among the participants in the ritual of intensification; the drama of serious illness; the dazzle of energy and manpower required by rescue and technology; and the high stakes of its promise of salvation from death. Society channels this form of social altruism through clinicians to patients and families. The ritual of intensification honors the patient and family by its elaboration, intensity, and display. These features at first seem limitless, deployed entirely for the benefit of the one person in trouble. The ritual destroys a wealth of disposable medical equipment on the patient's behalf.[1] The capacity and authority to mount such a display, while aimed at the patient, demonstrates the wealth and status of the society. Zygmunt Bauman calls this display the "stratifying magic," and he connects it to the important project of engendering trust. "The exorbitant price of the gadgets adds to the prestige and, indeed, to the perceived trustworthiness of those who operate it; it also gives a new lease of [sic] life to the hopes of those on whom the gadgets are to be tried, and protects those hopes from being disavowed by the lack of practical success" (1992: 143).

Not only is the display expended by society in the hope of saving this person's life, but also in the interests of engendering enough trust in the system's good intentions so that when the time comes to limit the gift, the family will acquiesce to the dishonor of its withdrawal. If families agree with clinicians that it is best to shut down the ritual of intensification and allow a natural death, their trust is a form of reciprocity, limiting the display and conforming to its unspoken authority (Adloff and Mau 2006). And what about reciprocity in kind, a traditional cultural expectation? How can such extravagance be repaid, and by whom? In its disguise as a benevolent gift at the bedside, the ritual display of rescue appears unconnected from economic exchange because of its universal application and the mystification of its reimbursement (see Chapter 5). The separation between bedside care and finances makes it possible for the relationship between the givers and receivers of care, even technological care, to appear to be free from the reciprocal obligations of material exchange. But the filthy lucre will not be denied. Every health-care cost decried as excessive is seen by someone else as appropriate payment for goods and services rendered. Because the display of technology in rescue is beyond the capacity of most individuals to afford, many of its recipients and their families are ruined. But this aspect, too, is mystified and unspoken.[2] The cost of care is not often raised at the bedside. In the United States, when individual collapse occurs and rescue is needed emergently, families and patients have little choice but to participate in receiving this gift. Indeed, almost no one would refuse it, even if capable of unfettered choice at the time. The capacity to begin this process for anyone in need is a source of national pride. It distracts Americans from focusing on the mediocre aggregate outcomes they purchase with their high-cost health-care (Jost 2004), as discussed in Chapter 5.

For clinicians and the hospital, the stakes in the family hurdle are high. If the ritual fails, clinicians will need to continue in what they consider to be futile treatment, even resuscitative measures, which will inflict meaningless suffering (in their view) on the patient and deprive him of a good death—that is, a Dying that is private, prepared, orderly, and calm. The stakes for the hospital are continuing direct and opportunity costs. If clinicians succeed in negotiating the family hurdle and changing the narrative, the family (and patient) accept the new order. It specifies that the patient is dying from the failure of certain body systems rather than from any shortage of efficacy in medicine, and it ensures that the family, the clinicians, and society itself can survive with minimal guilt. Steps can now be taken to free that bed for a rescuable patient.

But the stakes are even higher for the family. If they had been relying on the social contract to guarantee that every contingency would be explored to hold back death, a new narrative that seeks to close the ritual may appear as betrayal of that contract. The choice offered to families whether to keep going or stop is designed to honor the patient's autonomy.[3] But to discontinue the ritual of intensification devalues the patient. It serves as justification for putting him or her away from the mainstream concerns of the hospital and perhaps from these very clinicians as well. Under these circumstances, the choice may appear to the families as abandonment, discrimination, and/or murder, to which they would be accomplices (Kaufman 2005: 100, 175). If "erring on the side of life" has become the only legitimate way to say "I love you," any alternative course may be too self-incriminating for them to consider.

In the context of the family hurdle, trust depends partly on history of the patient and family's experiences with the health-care system. According to clinicians' understandings of bioethics in the United States, informed consent or refusal of treatment almost always allows individual autonomy to override clinical beneficence. Families can and do sometimes insist that aggressive treatments continue, ensuring that their loved one remains a focus of cultural attention. In only five cases did physicians flatly overrule such family requests for continued rescue and/or resuscitation. Such a low number convinces clinicians that ultimate treatment decisions really belong to the families.

And what do clinicians have to offer in place of rescue at the time of the family hurdle? Common parlance refers to aggressive treatment and rescue as "doing everything," while the tipping point and the family hurdle emphasize "nothing left to do." This refers to the extravagance of the ritual display compared to the void left by its discontinuation. But even with all its energy, intensity, and elaboration, the focus of rescue is exceedingly narrow: maintaining vital signs that are compatible with life through the support of organ systems. All other concerns virtually disappear in favor of ensuring hemodynamic stability for as long as necessary. Attention to other important aspects of the illness (pain, immobility, stress, nutrition, function, overstimulation, anxiety) remains secondary, limited, or rarely, even missing altogether. In this framework, the "official" status of Dying has much in common with states of disability, aging, and chronic illness. Each is a condition of unredeemable human frailty, lacking potential for amelioration in a rescue paradigm. Such states of being are marked as "other" and are feared in mainstream U.S. society, to be avoided or sublimated. It would seem that finding creativity and meaning in the human condition is more quixotic than the hope of rescuing humans from it altogether.

If accommodating the vicissitudes of existence is often beyond the capacity of the U.S. health-care system, it could widen its attention to the parts of being seriously ill that this tunnel vision leaves aside. Hospitals certainly employ pain specialists, occupational and physical therapists, nutrition consultants, and chaplains. But they usually remain secondary to the "real" work of rescue and stabilization.[4] Palliative care reverses this hierarchy and executes these tasks as its primary responsibilities, leaving rescue aside. Can this be an avenue for trust?

Once the ritual of intensification is exhausted, clinicians may improve their chances at the family hurdle by having something positive to offer as a replacement. Palliative care might provide a corrective in hospital settings where rescue is lionized and dying is invisible. It might at least help clinicians who need to show that they are not simply abandoning the patient when they propose closing down the ritual of intensification. In the next sections, we explore palliative care and its place in the framework of the ritual of intensification, its potential for modifying that position, and its capacity for engendering trust. How might patients, families, clinicians, and hospitals judge its strengths and weaknesses as an additive or an alternative to the ritual display of rescue?

Palliative Care as a Vehicle for Trust

In the teaching hospital, the palliative care unit staff provided guidance to ICU clinicians: If a patient lived for an hour after the withdrawal of life support and seemed stable enough to survive transport, she would be welcome in the palliative care unit.

Ms. Snyder's case represented an example of such a transfer. Opinions about appropriate clinical practice came into conflict in her case based on diverging opinions as to the proper interventions regarding patient suffering. An advanced practice nurse in the palliative care unit at the teaching hospital described what transpired when his team was called in to consult on Ms. Snyder, who been requiring mechanical ventilation in the medical ICU.

> RN: We got a palliative care consult last week. The ICU team thought she wouldn't survive extubation, and told us to come back in the morning. When we came back she was extubated and on 40 mg of morphine [per hour by IV infusion]. She looked comfortable! Our fellow's recommendation had been to put her on 2 to 4 mg per hour after extubation.

> I asked why she was on so high a dose. They went ballistic! They said, "Where is your compassion?" They said it was in the protocol [for withdrawal of life support], but I've never seen the protocol. I've asked before, and they say they can't find it.

I'm proactive, I just want to go with the science. I said, "Just give me an idea of where you're going [with this dose]." The chart said she was grimacing, and they went up to 4 to 6 mg. She looked uncomfortable, and they went to 6 to 8. I said, "I'm with you on all that." But after that, nothing! The chart is silent. They were beyond defensive. We brought her down here [to the palliative care unit] and shut off the morphine, and never turned it back on. She was comfortable and the family was happy. She died five days later. I haven't seen this [dosing level] in a long time. And I've never seen the defensiveness.

This nurse, an expert in pain control, and the palliative care fellow (a physician between the level of resident and attending) respond when units or physicians seek specific help with a dying patient or with symptom management. The nurse objected to Ms. Snyder's high morphine dose as incompatible with "the science," that is, with clear indication of patient discomfort that would support adjusting the dose to such a high level. The reaction of the ICU nurses was telling in its force and its content. For them, the time for science was done now that the ritual of intensification had closed down and synchrony had been restored. In their minds, the job of nursing allowed and perhaps dictated (per the unfindable protocol) the unmitigated relief of suffering. The high level of the morphine infusion expressed the genuineness of their compassion. If the consultation was supposed to assist them in caring for a Dying patient, why would the palliative care nurse, of all people, not understand their position?[5]

ICU nurses who had been following the science of rescue were now free at the withdrawal of life support to deliver their unlimited compassion to Ms. Snyder, demonstrating fidelity to their relationship with her and making it up to her for what she had suffered. The palliative care team, demonstrating its biomedical legitimacy by conforming to evidence-based practice, was in its turn expressing fidelity to standards that benefited Ms. Snyder and her family. Which view deserves trust, and in whose eyes? We address this question by considering palliative care's place in the revival of death movement, how it is understood and practiced in the two hospitals, and national strategies to promote palliative care.

Palliative Care and Hospice

In Chapter 3, we considered the revival of death movement as a subaltern voice speaking on behalf of dying patients and offering a nontechnological vision of privacy, order, and control. Hospice, the most visible iteration of the revival of death movement, is especially compatible with certain kinds of dying, specifically those with a trajectory of gradual decline typical of some cancers. It envisions dying as a particular interval at the officially declared end of a life. It contains an orderly process, predictable changes, and support that enables patients and families to adapt to inevitable, usually gradual physical decline. Because the Medicare hospice benefit was designed to reimburse providers using a daily rate rather than by piecework, referrals to hospice early in the trajectory carry maximized benefits for both the patient and the provider. This form of reimbursement is suitable for home care, with processes to bring symptoms under control, to teach patient care techniques to families, and to help them prepare for a proximate but unpredictable deadline.

Hospice has coexisted poorly with the thrust of acute care in hospitals, and not only because most hospice care is delivered in nonhospital settings. Even though many hospitals have hospice programs attached to them (including the Catholic community hospital where I did research), comparatively little cross-fertilization has occurred between the two (Last Acts 2002). Besides the stigma of death that hospice carries, reimbursement rules dictate that a patient must be discharged from the hospital and admitted into the hospice, even if he remains in the same bed, because the reimbursement mechanisms for the two are irreconcilable (Cassel, Ludden, and Moon 2000; Huskamp et al. 2001). The lack of a mechanism to reimburse hospitals for explicit care of the dying (see Chapter 5) is a major obstacle for institutions considering such programs. Insurance companies often deny payment even for complex care if the patient has a DNR order (Cassel, Ludden, and Moon 2000). Payment patterns thus underline a "forced choice" between "mutually exclusive goals" (Morrison 2005: S-81).

Despite this philosophical and financial incompatibility, a significant opening for ingratiating hospice principles into acute care to ameliorate the state of hospital dying came in the mid-1990s with the publication of the SUPPORT study. Not only did this investigation expose hospitals' poor performance regarding dying patients, it did so in a venue that the academic health-care community could not ignore: multi-sited research with a before and after intervention involving 9,000 patients. It showed that patients' pain was undertreated and their preferences were ignored by attending physicians, but this was not all. Phase II of the study indicated that even when physicians were aware of their shortcomings, wished to do better, and a mechanism for improving communication was provided, information sharing and pain control remained poor (SUPPORT 1995).

The study was galvanizing. Soon after its publication, funding from multiple sources appeared for studies and start-up programs designed to address the issues it raised. The American Academy of Hospice and Palliative Medicine took shape at the same time, and the *Oxford Textbook of Palliative Medicine*, the first of its kind, was published. With this convergence of events came the opening for hard science and hard research dollars to move into the hospital under the nondeath, medical-sounding rubric of palliation. Surrounded and cloaked in the legitimacy of medical education, research, and clinical intervention, "soft" hospice principles had a chance.

But even as palliative care may insist on its distinct territory from hospice and on its expertise in alleviating the complex side effects that accompany intricate treatment regimens, palliation is still neither rescue nor is it often technological. The problems it addresses are life changing, but not life-saving and not lucrative. Rarely can it tap into pharmaceutical or other corporate pipelines for sponsorship. The dismissal of palliative care as "medically uninteresting" observed by Sudnow in 1967 (p. 91) continues today. Still, the SUPPORT study and the research dollars that followed it have not been in vain. Clinician interest and participation continue to rise, and palliative care models have burgeoned, even as the generous philanthropic and government funding has moved elsewhere.[6]

But this growth has not come without great struggle. Palliative care programs are new arrivals in hospitals, needing visibility, legitimacy, and a foothold in what is still a hostile environment. Their reliability depends on factors that may be beyond their control: hospital buy-in, adequate staff, and economic viability. The state of palliative care in the two sites of my research indicates the difficulties of storming the fortress of rescue. The Catholic community hospital has clear hospital endorsement for the concept of palliative care, but the implementation is fragmented and ineffective. The teaching hospital has a model program with competent and committed trailblazers, but financial footing is tenuous and staffing marginal. How well can palliative care in these institutions exhibit fidelity and inspire trust?

Palliative Care in the Two Hospitals

Catholic Community Hospital: The Mission and the Missionary

The Catholic community hospital's mission statement explicitly endorses the care of the dying patient. Its "Care of the Dying Quality Plan," six single-spaced pages dated September 2001, supposedly incorporates such care into the health system's strategic plan. Further, the hospital bestows an annual award to three clinicians, recognizing them for excellence in end of life care. All of these gestures of support indicate administrative interest, but they amount to window dressing. They do not translate into proactive attention to dying patients. Once unrescuable patients are transferred to the appropriate "less important" bed for watching and waiting, waiting can occur. Dying is certainly not rushed, but the watching portion is less available, as the nurse-to-patient ratio is less favorable on floor units compared to the ICUs. Sometimes patients are found dead, or a family member reports the death.

Nurses referred to a "palliative care pathway" in my interviews, and I asked to see the document. The "Clinical Pathway for Palliative Care" is two foldout pages with holes at the top so that it can be incorporated into the patient record. The inside carries palliative care protocols that constrain physician orders (e.g., "Lab tests: Has to be a reason; no standing orders for routine lab tests"). The outer pages contain six columns relating to eight categories of assessment, totaling forty-eight boxes of very small print. The columns account for "Phases I–V" (no names or labels for the phases) with space to add a date. The sixth column is for "Outcome Indicators," with specific definitions, such as "Spiritual Distress: [Outcome desired:] Patient describes satisfaction with meaning and purpose of illness, suffering, and impending death." This form, designed to be a place to chart about a dying situation, is very complex.

In referring to the palliative care pathway, Mr. Wallace's nurse may have mistaken the six columns for successive days. This is understandable in that the form does not define how the phases should be differentiated. She gave short shrift to the pathway's careful elaboration, even as she voiced her approval of it: "We have a palliative care pathway. The docs know about it. It's a six-day pathway. No vital signs, meds for comfort only, nothing invasive. It's death with dignity, the way I see it. For a patient you know is terminal. Nothing but morphine and turning the patient."

Another nurse spoke of bypassing the pathway for the designation "comfort care," which allowed more flexibility in the design of the patient's care plan:

> RN: The palliative care pathway is different from comfort care. The pathway is very specific. We use comfort care [more often]. If the patient wants to eat, even if they're aspirating everything you put in their mouths [under comfort care we let them].

> HC: For comfort care, then, you have to get the docs to specify everything [separate orders for each comfort measure]?

RN: Yes. If they discontinue everything [stop normal treatment orders], we call them and ask, "Did you want palliative care then?"

Even though I was hoping my question would elicit the differences between comfort care and the palliative care pathway more specifically, her last statement blurred the two once again. Clinicians have clear preferences and are using the tools as they see fit. Another day I asked a nurse if the pathway had been used with her patient who had died. She said: "No pathway. [You get] the name on the pathway and the ink is not dry, and they die. It's not worthwhile."

It is unclear whether the "name on the pathway" is the physician's or the patient's. In either case, the pathway seems to be a lot of trouble to invoke for such a simple plan as "nothing but morphine and turning the patient." It is as if palliative care has no substance to it, especially when compared to the basic importance of having an open code bed (see Chapter 6).

Another nurse indicated a further limitation of the pathway's structure, demonstrating the clinical instinct to work around the system when it became an obstacle: "Many of our physicians won't order the palliative care pathway. But most of them, we can get the same orders out of 'em. They've also come to trust us. When we call and say, 'This patient's dying,' they take us at our word."

Relying on trust in the messenger is more effective than invoking a prescribed format. The form is difficult to read or to use for tracking events in the patient's course. With little room in the boxes to record information, the document's purpose is unclear. Is it meant more as a prompt to preferred practice than a documentation tool? Can one presume that Dying was "good" if all the blocks moving left to right were addressed? Clearly the form and the pathway itself represent careful thought by their designers about the orderliness that a dying situation should assume. It carried a hospital copyright dated seven years before, but at the time of this study, four years had elapsed without a revision. This elaborate gesture toward "good dying" is less of a practice tool than a particular vision cemented into a document that clinicians do not find particularly useful or relevant.

Nor has this pathway enabled the hospital to travel to an effective palliative care program. Despite a remarkable history of activity in this direction, no solidified program is accessible to clinicians or patients. Eight years before my research began, the Catholic community hospital and the teaching hospital had planned a joint venture in palliative care to benefit both their hospitals. Four years of negotiation brought the two parties to the point of contract signing. Just before the deal was finalized, disputes over the care of indigent patients and the ownership of donations caused a falling out. Each hospital went its own way.

When my research began four years later, the palliative clinicians at the teaching hospital had mounted a consultation service and procured a palliative care unit of their own. In the meantime, even though the Catholic hospital had paid an outside consultant to advise them on the best approach, hired a dedicated administrator and physician, and sent them out of state to an education program sponsored by the Center to Advance Palliative Care (see below), no formal palliative care initiative was taking shape. The hospital patients in the four "hospice" beds on three East (with the "pretty beds" and the "nice nurses") do not actually receive hospice care, as no mechanism exists to admit them into the hospital's home hospice program. During the time of my research, talks continued among administrators regarding the imminent implementation of a palliative care program, but it never materialized. My field notes dated September 29 provided a progress report.

> I asked the chaplain for an update on palliative care. She says the effort is now divided up into committees. Educational modules are being prepared. There will probably be a hospital wide educational effort. Her module is on spirituality, and it's two pages. Her committee has the VP for Nursing on it. There is to be a meeting every month, but no meeting so far in September. So it seems that there is some movement, but it's very slow. She confirms there is nothing on the ground yet.

When I left the area at the end of 2004, clinicians were no closer to palliative care expertise than they had ever been before. But they are not without a resource. Nurses and chaplains call on Dr. M, the palliative care physician on staff, a pathologist, and a member of a Catholic order. As such, this physician carries a measure of authority in this Catholic environment at once unrelated to clinical experience and also unavailable to other physicians. This sets up an unusual dynamic. Bedside clinicians see this person as a champion, someone who comes to their rescue when they encounter a physician reluctant to write orders for symptom control. It is hoped that when Dr. M enters the situation, the patient's doctor will bow to Dr. M's dual authority as religious and as "expert" in palliative care. Such an expectation that patient management would automatically be handed over to the palliative physician was odd to me. In my hospice experience, private physicians were encouraged to follow their home-bound or nursing home-bound patients while they were in the program. When I mentioned this practice to the administrator for yet-to-be-realized palliative care, she responded, "But why *not* [give them up] if they don't know how to manage the patient?" It seemed obvious to her that in the face of obvious "wrong," lack of specific hospice expertise, the "right" should prevail.

It is not surprising, then, that Dr. M clashes with physician colleagues. The following comments illustrate the significance of Dr. M to some clinicians and the conflicts that arose.

> RN: We turned to [Dr. M] because we wanted to do more for [the patient]. [Her doctor] wasn't being aggressive enough with her. I don't understand why he wouldn't want to make her as comfortable as possible. We use Dr. M when we feel our backs are up against the wall. Usually they [the docs] don't mind.

> Another RN: We love to have Dr. M who's so good with the meds [drugs and dosages].

> Chaplain: I used a diagram that Dr. M showed us. It's very helpful with DNR discussions. I've used it often. Dr. M's our prizefighter, our second opinion we rely on.

With Dr. M as the sole incarnation of palliative care, a "prizefighter" deployed against unenlightened medical and surgical authority, palliative care as a concept is not likely to win new physician converts at the Catholic community hospital. The impact on patient care was evident at the time: not only were nurses frustrated in their attempts to obtain good palliative care for their patients, but clinicians themselves were sometimes unable to recognize and address palliative care emergencies when they occurred.

It is ironic that in the Catholic community hospital, administrative endorsement of palliative care is quite clear, but real palliative care expertise in the trenches of bedside care (Dr. M notwithstanding) is virtually unavailable to patients or clinicians. It cannot be a trustworthy alternative offered to patients and families. Despite the good intentions of the administration, Dr. M as palliative care's white knight, and the palliative care pathway, palliative care in the Catholic community hospital is unreliable. The double standard of endorsement without a program generates discontent among some clinicians, and trust in palliative care lacks foundation.

Teaching Hospital: The Besieged Base Camp

Unlike the Catholic community hospital's high-level buy-in to palliative care, initiatives at many hospitals are grass-roots in origin, generated by highly motivated individuals anxious for change. Such clinicians at the teaching hospital continued to pursue a way to open a dedicated palliative care unit after their collaboration with the Catholic hospital fell apart. Not long afterward, an unexpected donation and hard negotiation for bed space allowed the unit to become a reality. As long as it pays for itself in real time, the hospital agrees to keep it open. Such a physical underpinning (along with the expertise and dedication of its clinicians) offers palliative care a tangible, visible reality. Such materiality imbues palliative care with an unquestionable force and presence. Its carpeted floors, bright kitchen, family lounge space, curtained windows, and consoling wall coverings assure struggling clinicians, families, and patients that refuge and time to regroup from technology's onslaught might be available to them.

The founders sought an operational unit not only to ground their palliative care consult service, but also because the unit's specialized staff could learn and practice palliative care on a high-volume basis, thus improving their expertise and lowering cost. The unit constitutes a base camp from which its staff fan out and attempt to ingratiate palliative care into the technological overstructure. Its consult service visits the units regularly, answering questions, looking for problems, hoping for referrals, and generally maintaining awareness of the existence of palliative care. One nurse commented, "The consultant from palliative care is very kind. She is reminding us of palliative care. Helping with the bed crunch."

This nurse informant clearly understood palliative care's dual role, to free up beds in the ICU while offering a kinder, gentler alternative. When the palliative care consultant left her job in May, two nurses from the Neuro ICU expressed their dismay at the news, saying that they would miss her expertise and "her ability to talk with authority to those who need it," echoing the shortage of palliative care's clout that the nurses in the Catholic community hospital expressed in their endorsement of Dr. M.

The palliative care unit as base camp is itself in a constant state of barely controlled chaos because of the number of activities forced into its tiny "backstage" common space: in-services and education for staff, lunches, charting, discharge arrangements, and care coordination among different medical and surgical services. The much larger lounge and kitchen across the hall is for family use. Two nurses care for five or six patients each. They cannot leave each other alone on the unit for meals or to run for equipment or medications. The unit cannot afford a higher staffing level and still break even. One nurse on the unit complained to me, "It's way too much work for two people. They say we can only do what we can do. If I could just figure that out! If I could know what I could eliminate that wouldn't be on my evaluation. But I have a good attitude, don't I?"

Beds without palliative care patients often receive "boarders": nonpalliative patients followed by some other service. These are a major problem for the nurses because of the low staffing level. They must scramble to find the correct service and team caring for the patients when they need orders from physicians. I recorded circumstances in the unit during an interview with one of the nurses: "While talking to me she was eating lunch (at 3:15!). We were interrupted many times: to talk to the lab, to respond to patient indigestion (requiring clarification re: which doc to page); interrupted by the doc's callback; interrupted by another nurse offering to teach her how to correct something in the computer system."

Admissions the staff prefers to get are not only dying patients needing palliative care, but also patients on trials of pain medication being infused into the epidural space of the spine, hematology-oncology patients, patients with medication pumps implanted under the skin, and patients with sickle cell anemia. Of course, dying can still occur among nonpalliative patients over days of watching and waiting. One nurse described its nonrescue focus, unique in the hospital: "We don't fix vital signs here. If the blood pressure is low, we don't fix it." The business of palliative care, then, is completely different than what goes on in the rescue environment that houses it.

The attention paid to each dying situation may not occur in measurable chunks, piecework, or interventions that payers understand, but patient stays must still be justified under acute-care standards, never as subacute or custodial care. Discharge planners work constantly to justify lengths of stay to insurance payers and/or to find another home for patients whose need for acute care in the unit can no longer be substantiated. Possible alternative placement sites are hospice home care programs, regular home care, nursing homes, or rehab facilities. The nurse expert in pain management noted that 60 percent of their patients are discharged, sometimes well before death. He explained the unit's predicament.

RN: We get to a place where insurance just stops paying. If they hear that a patient is nursing home material and awaiting placement, they can just stop paying. [To them] the patient doesn't need to be in a hospital. So it makes me need to lie. I won't lie if I'm asked directly, but I don't go out of my way. And nursing homes don't want to take our patients. We didn't know this before we started. The medication requirements [for some of our patients] are too complex, and they don't want a patient who is going to be dead in a week. It hurts their statistics. They don't want patients that have lost 25 percent of their body weight. If they can get a patient [they can classify as] subacute rehab, they're happy. Even if the rehab doesn't work, they've done a good thing and they have a longer term patient. So if we can't find placement, payers say "That's your problem."

All entities—the hospital, the palliative care unit, and the nursing homes—must dance to the payers' tunes. If they fail to mind the steps, reimbursement will falter.

My field notes recorded random palliative care issues in the unit:

> There is a problem for tomorrow. There is a patient who needs to get a one-time dose of chemo, lasting thirty minutes. But not all the nurses who work here can give chemo, so they looked at the schedule to see if patient would need to be transferred to another floor to get that dose, in case the nurses can't do it here.

> The pain specialist, two fellows and two med students are working on dosages of methadone and short acting morphine for "ten out of ten" pain. Very complex. By mouth? IV? Plus the conversions if the medication infused by IV versus a pump controlled by the patient. Equivalencies are difficult, plus they're working on pain not yet controlled.

This concentrated hubbub and the focused attention to both symptom management and patient flow could not form a sharper contrast to the idea of palliative care understood by Mr. Wallace's nurse (above) as "nothing but morphine and turning the patient." Here symptoms command attention, but unlike the Catholic community hospital, excessive waiting cannot occur. Interventions are active, benefiting the patient whether or not death is imminent. Yet to perform these services for patients, it is necessary for the unit staff to fight constantly for their turf, a demonstration of their marginal status in the world of rescue. They struggle to keep the hospital from filling their space with boarders and to justify their patients' lengths of stay with payers. These battles consume huge amounts of the staff's energy.

The problem of legitimacy extends into relationships with other physicians in the teaching hospital. In the Catholic community hospital, Dr. M may offend colleagues by intruding into cases when invited by nurses rather than by attending physicians. Here in the teaching hospital, the palliative care fellows feel they are on the receiving end of disrespect from physicians who do extend invitations for palliative expertise. The palliative care unit held an open house one day for the hospital to enhance its visibility, but the physician showing was poor. The fellow voiced her opinion and her disappointment at the low turnout:

> MD Fellow: I just want docs not to send patients down [to the unit] without consulting us. That's what gets me upset. They're not allowed to—they don't treat us like a real medicine service. That's what I don't get. It's like they say, "We've done all this stuff and now there's nothing else, and you can have her." So there's no idea of teamwork. Like they've exhausted the "real" work. It's a hot potato [the dying patient], get rid of it. They're afraid of dying. Or it's not legitimate. We're so much more than just hospice. If any of them had come [to the open house]—we'd show a great case, complex patient needs, lots of pain issues. How the goals [of care] are difficult to sort out.

Here the fellow defended palliative care as being legitimate and "real work" because of the complexity of symptom control and the murkiness of the goals of care, while she distanced it from being "just hospice." She objected to the fact that palliation is seen as unnecessary and/or premature as long as the project of salvation is in full swing.

Her criticism echoed a common misperception among advocates for palliative care who do not appreciate the significance of the transformation that the ritual of intensification brings about. A pair of graphs illustrates this problem. Palliative care promoters often use similar ones to depict their vision of how palliative care should fit into patient care, called "trajectory" rather than "transition,"[7] shown in Figure 8.1.

The transition graph depicts the ritual of intensification and its tipping point as we know it, the "what is." The trajectory graph is an idealization of what could be, and what many in palliative care believe should characterize the course of serious illness. It shows palliative care's role increasing in a comforting, orderly progression added in as the options for successful curative treatment diminish. Advocates such as the fellow in the teaching hospital's palliative care unit would like to see symptom control assume an important role alongside aggressive medical care, rather than after its exhaustion.

Although the alternative configuration has intuitive appeal, it often encounters puzzling resistance as palliative care advocates work to move "upstream" to improve patients' quality of life before the tipping point. Surely a critical barrier to wider implementation is the fact that in the trajectory model, the discrete, vertical tipping point is missing. Instead, the rising diagonal line implies that minor adjustments to both sides of the care plan

Transition:

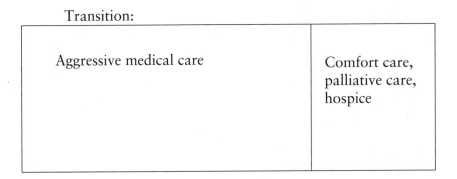

Time → Death

Trajectory:

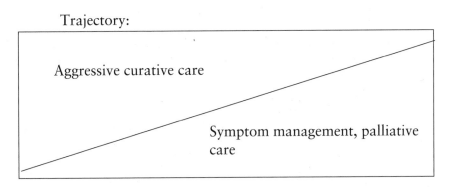

Figure 8.1. Transition and Trajectory Graphs.

could occur over time. Such mixing of the classes of care would necessitate a negotiation of each segment of the treatment plan for each patient to be sure it met the present, fluctuating goal. Clinicians (especially nurses) who are delivering acute care in an environment of rescue and emergency, cannot tolerate fuzzy goals. We saw the confusion that results in the case of Mr. Wallace in the previous chapter. The floor nurse described the situation:

> He was critically ill, very critically ill. When we got out of report, the night nurse said he wasn't breathing, so we went in together. He'd had an elevated temp, he was tachy, he was on a lot of oxygen. The night nurse asked, "If he's comfort care, why am I giving meds every hour?" If there is no order for palliative care, we do every treatment that is ordered.

The ordered treatments congruent with a care plan of rescue made no sense to the night nurse if the patient had been moved out of the rescue environment to comfort care. But because she lacked an explicit plan for comfort from the physician, she was obligated to disturb her dying patient (and herself) regularly and needlessly.

To question the default mode, the archetype of rescue and stabilization, is to destabilize it. It operates through clear algorithms of cascading priorities. If it loses its place as the primary model, *all its accompanying treatments and elaborations become unhinged.* Within an environment designed to stamp out instability, such lack of clarity is untenable. Let us look further into what this means.

In practice, following the trajectory model would distract ritual practitioners from the main job of monitoring every physiologic fluctuation, with the latitude to thwart any that threaten hemodynamic equilibrium. It would require them to delineate instead just how much rescue should be applied to this particular patient today. The resulting confusion, miscommunication, and disorder would bring bedside routines, the application of technology, and patient flow to a crawl. Further, aggressive biomedicine requires an unswerving loyalty to its mandated disturbances from both the patient and the clinicians in the "fight" to save lives. Oncologists may even complain that palliative care seems to be "on the side of the tumor" in the battle against cancer, in the same draconian understanding that specifies that those who are not "for us" must be "against us."

Beyond these considerations are the tipping point and the family hurdle themselves. They play critical roles as a clear demarcation of status. The two designate the completion of a social transformation enacted by clinicians through the ritual of intensification that requires the drawing of a vertical line. No alternative exists as a substitute for indicating this completed work of differentiation (Drought and Koenig 2002). The moral ground for designating the patient to a second-class level of care is the application, display, and (finally) the failure of all-out rescue. Without the ritual and its tipping point, social consensus in the hospital around dying itself cannot occur. Its absence would confound the heroic, egalitarian obligation in U.S. ideology to fight and overcome, to endure (or inflict) whatever is required to maintain anyone's life (before the tipping point). It would also remove the subsequent redemption available to clinicians who can finally make it their business to relieve suffering.

Recently, a tearful wife visited one of my patients for the first time shortly after his cardiac arrest and successful resuscitation. He was unconscious, seriously ill, and barely stable. Clearly, his appearance upset her. At the end of her brief visit, she looked me in the eye and said, "Nurse, will you promise that you'll do everything in your power to save his life?" I felt awkward, put on the spot. But I assured her that I would, that we all would, because I knew the system was designed to do just that. At that moment, despite the technology surrounding her husband, she needed reassurance about the fidelity of our rescue, not about how free of pain we would keep him.

If trust requires consistency and reliability, the paradigm of rescue is more trustworthy than palliative care in these two hospitals, supported as it is by the cultural and economic infrastructure. In the Catholic community hospital, palliative care cannot be reliable or consistent, and its main practitioner lacks the expertise and professionalism that would attract additional powerful allies to the cause. In the teaching hospital, palliative care is on a firmer footing, but it is still struggling, needing to prove itself continuously to its payers and to the institution. How can palliative care gain stature and reimbursement in a framework that sees its efforts as a mop-up operation after the "real" work? In the next section, we examine the palliative care movement on a national level, wondering if its sophisticated strategies will encourage trust from patients and families at the crucial time of the family hurdle. Its approaches offer a foil to the rescue paradigm in hospitals, working around its edges, and finding important ways into the system that reveal the predilections of both.

National Palliative Care Movement: Working with What Is

An important successor to the post-SUPPORT study grants is the Center to Advance Palliative Care (CAPC), a national organization dedicated to the growth of palliative care, now sponsored by five foundations. It is the "go-to" place for start-up programs and a locus for the movement. Through its partnership with the National Palliative Care Research Center, it displays its connection with research, the critical feature of hard science legitimacy.

Local obstacles to palliative care growth in hospitals, such as those encountered by my fieldwork sites, are grist for CAPC's mill. Instead of bemoaning the difficulty of physicians' unwillingness to incorporate palliative care early in the patient's course, or delaying the realization of a palliative care program until the administrative stars of the hospital are in alignment, CAPC encourages palliative care professionals to work with what is, and it gives them practical advice for how to do this. Unfortunately, its sophisticated strategies include a premise that hospitals may embrace at their peril: finding economies by expanding their definition of patients who qualify for palliative care.

One strategy to "grow" palliative care at the time of my research was provided through CAPC's Palliative Care Leadership Conferences, which offered strategies to clinicians with fledgling palliative care programs so that they could overcome obstacles such as those encountered by the teaching hospital and the Catholic community hospital. I attended one of these two-day conferences along with representatives from four hospital sites scattered around the country. Their different programs ranged from consultation services to distinct hospital units, as well as a combination of these models. One of the groups was adamant that their new palliative care unit *not* be known around their hospital as "the death and dying unit."

CAPC literature commonly refers to the patients who would benefit from palliative care as "seriously ill" rather than "dying." All the groups knew they were fighting for a piece of ideological, financial, and physical turf in their hospitals. CAPC's message to them was sophisticated, astute, and multifaceted: they must not attempt to reform administrators and physicians using the "rightness" of their mission on behalf of patients. Rather, they must mobilize palliative care to work within the hospital's unique existing conditions of local hierarchy, payer relationships, and reimbursement. To that end, their programs must distance themselves very deliberately from the "myths" of hospice (specifically that "hospice" means "dying," therefore "not acute care," therefore not reimbursable),[8] so that the models of care they propose are not be perceived as "soft," meaning uncomplicated, not evidence based, not entitled to reimbursement, or solely nurse-driven. The directors of the conference insisted that a physician and/or a hospital financial officer be present in each group, and programs had to submit a comprehensive profile of their hospital's financial standing as a prerequisite for attendance. The CAPC strategy bypasses nurses, families, and patients to concentrate on the power players in three key hospital domains: physicians, finance, and administration.

Physicians

CAPC recommends that palliative care physicians should win over their colleagues by building relationships and by "talking the talk." They should adopt the role of consultant and problem solver, beginning their campaign with the "low-hanging fruit" of sympathetic specialties like hospitalists and oncologists, the primary sources for referrals. Higher "fruit" would be physicians in such specialties as transplant surgery. Every candidate for whole-organ transplant is terminally ill, but their physicians are usually quite closed to palliative care. Palliative care physicians should model their behavior after pharmaceutical company detailers by: (1) using physician-friendly tools; (2) developing talking points of no more than ten minutes; (3) being easy to reach; and (4) demonstrating reliability by giving feedback about each referral. Generally, they should hold themselves accountable to their colleagues rather than appear to them as missionaries seeking converts. Their message must communicate credibility in terms of concrete, dependable interventions supported by research, and emphasize the complexity of patient management. Palliative care's professional standing improved when it became an official subspecialty in medicine, and its advocates must self-consciously incorporate "outcomes data," research grants, publications, and training fellowships to gain the confidence of their peers leading to patient referrals.

Finance

The Palliative Care Leadership Conference instructors emphasized the critical importance of overcoming palliative care's financial handicaps, specifically its virtual absence in the hospital reimbursement structure and its shortage of favors to offer in trade with medical industry. Presenters counseled physicians to mine the ICD-9-CM codebook to find "neglected" codes for patient symptoms and physician time spent rather than the more commonly used codes for diagnosis and interventional procedures. Because of the structure of oncology reimbursement via chemotherapy, palliative interventions are available to oncologists (Cassel, Ludden, and Moon 2000: 66). As part of its start-up, each program should seek out local representatives of insurance companies and educate them regarding the differences between excellent and less than optimal palliative care (which also conveys the "we are not the same as hospice" subtext) to head off denials of reimbursement before they happen. In addition, palliative care advocates received advice to act on these unfriendly reimbursement structures by working with lobbyists in state government regarding budget amendments.

Administration

The CAPC message urges palliative care leaders to use political savvy when dealing with their hospital administrations. They must not only align themselves with the hospital's mission but also point out how their work enables the hospital to comply with quality standards handed down from oversight structures such as The Joint Commission for Accrediting Healthcare Organizations. They must ask themselves who in the organization will be threatened by the success of their program. Hospital accounting officers need to understand that even when families and patients are accepting death, expensive diagnostic and treatment interventions may still occur if palliative care is not a specific part of the care plan (Smith et al. 2003). Key to the conversations is for palliative care to show administrators how this alternative plan for excellent care can offload the ICUs and the ED.

Finally, the Palliative Care Leadership Program demonstrated how to gather the necessary objective data they would need to persuade professionals as to the impact and effectiveness of palliative care in their institutions. They distributed tools and strategies for documenting each patient and each consultation. They advised the groups not to engage in time-consuming chart review to glean outcomes. Instead, they suggested the insertion of a simple tracking code, from which trends and durations could be derived and compared to hospital statistics as a control group. The attendees learned how to use these codes to produce a quick look at usage trends, the practice of dashboarding. The financial data that the groups had produced as a part of the price of admission to the CAPC training laid groundwork for this hands-on exercise, enabling them to produce the data from their programs that would give credibility to their cause.

The message of this set of tactics and CAPC's overall strategy is remarkable in several ways. Cloaking itself in power from the outset, it wastes no time in self-affirmation or "preaching to the choir." Further, its emphasis on the business and politics of hospitals takes account of palliative care's roots in the romance of "good dying" (born from hospice and the revival of death movement), because it assumes that bedside professionals who are on a mission to the improve care for the dying may not have a clear understanding of the nature of the start-up obstacles they face. Tailoring the message for the audience's learning needs is not the sole object for CAPC's emphasis on economic practicalities, however. Palliative care *is* less expensive than rescue care.[9] CAPC advocates the use of economic arguments in financially strapped hospitals to secure its place at the health-care table, and to "institutionalize palliative care," as CAPC puts it: "Experience working on or with a palliative care service will not only effectively educate health professionals across the country, but will also contribute to the social and *culture-change movement* needed to fundamentally improve our health care system (CAPC 2009, emphasis added).

CAPC as an organization and proponents of palliative care as offshoots of the revival of death movement clearly feel the need to make their case to hospitals through cost savings, working to help them survive in the current economic realities of U.S. health-care. CAPC also promotes palliative care as a method to "bridge the quality chasm" for "our most seriously ill and vulnerable" hospitalized patients overall, a signal of reaching out to include patients before they are designated as Dying (CAPC 2008b: 7).

Partnership between hospitals and palliative care, even for less than optimal reasons, promises more success than a link between hospice and hospitals. Not only does its name give it a more medical flavor than hospice (which connotes death and "last resort"), but more importantly, its reimbursement patterns correspond to that of acute care, making it a better fit as the infrastructures now stand. Because it must work within the hospital, it must understand and conform to its culture rather than attempt to reform it. It is the most promising development for attending to the dying situation as an end in itself, rather than a means to an end (Chapple 1999). It restores a sense of personhood to the patient and seeks to preserve the uniqueness of her life until death occurs. One example occurred in the pilot study, when a palliative care nurse described the last hour of Mr. Kiernan's life.

> This man came from MICU with end-stage non-Hodgkins lymphoma. We knew about him at 3:30. He didn't get over to us till five. When he got here he was on [morphine] and an [oxygen mask]. His respiratory rate was 36 and his heart rate was 120. I'd heard it had been much higher. He'd had acute abdominal pain, I was told, but he was unresponsive here. I [adjusted his pain medication per the attending's order]. I proceeded to comfort the patient, to bridge a relationship with the family to gain their trust very quickly. I took the [oxygen mask] off. He didn't need it. The family was relieved when I told them that—he had hated it. They told me that he hated to be seen unshaven, so I used an electric razor and shaved him. His respiratory rate was still high at twenty-eight, so I called the intern for an order to titrate to comfort. I gave him a bolus of eight and kept the [hourly] rate at five. The respiratory rate was distressing to the family. Forty-five minutes later the family came and got me. He had just quit. I was amazed at the speed, and happy that it was peaceful. I sat with them, waiting for others to come.

Even with such a short time in which to know and care for Mr. Kiernan, who was unresponsive and actively dying when he arrived in the palliative care unit, the nurse attended to his physical symptoms (high respiratory rate) and to his unique subjectivity by following the family's characterizations of him: hating the oxygen mask and wanting to be clean-shaven. If he had not worked so deliberately to "gain their trust," they would have been lost in the new surroundings, just as Mr. Kiernan was becoming lost to them. This multifaceted attention was a sharp contrast to the intentional distancing that nonpalliative care nurses often described to me as their habit when they knew a patient was near death.

If the ritual of intensification acts on the patient to "make" her "into a DNR," palliative care can restore a measure of her subjectivity, even if the illness has removed agency, as Mr. Kiernan's case illustrates. The importance of this attention as a cultural exercise cannot be overemphasized, as will become clear in the next chapter. But to anchor the means of obtaining this attention in cost savings places hospitals in the untenable position of promoting second-class citizenship for the marginally rescuable (the aged, the neurologically devastated, the chronically ill) to conserve their scarce resources for the clearly rescuable (young, previously healthy, neurologically intact). Palliative care advocates may not recognize that hospitals' role in rescuing persons who have collapsed may be the only manifestation of universal access to healthcare the United States offers. Although the implementation of rescue may threaten the hospital's bottom line, the capability and willingness to rescue is the bottom line of trust in the health-care system. For palliative care to set itself up as a short circuit to the rescue process for the hospital's benefit could tempt administrations to capitalize on this opportunity, and jeopardize their position as holders of the community's trust (Naik 2004). Economic realities for cash-strapped hospitals may prevent attention to such subtleties, according to a 2005 study of palliative care growth in hospitals: "Our data suggest that although growth in palliative care programs has occurred throughout the nation's hospitals, larger hospitals, academic medical centers, not-for-profit hospitals, and VA hospitals are significantly more likely to develop a program compared to other hospitals" (Morrison et al. 2005: 1127). It is ironic that palliative care's high quality and lower cost works to its disadvantage if Americans associate it only with dying rather than with broader, more customized care that could benefit almost any patient.[10]

Because the economics of health-care finance are so inscrutable in the United States, it may not become widely known that hospitals benefit financially by spending less money on patients who go to palliative care. A more profound danger exists, however. Display and showiness are part and parcel of rescue, demonstrating the social and economic value of persons to whom it is applied. To advocate for balancing the hospital's budget on the backs of unrescuable patients confirms their lack of value. It admits that dying has no need of public attention in the form of hospital prioritizing, because, according to CAPC, first-class care for these patients can be done by scavenging for unused billing codes. Believing that they are part of the "culture-change movement," the advocates for palliative care nevertheless work within prevailing norms that maintain the U.S. "otherness" of dying.

Palliative Care and Pizzazz

Palliative care is critically important in countering the dominance of rescue in cultural and hospital contexts. But for individual patients and families facing the family hurdle, it may not go far enough. In comparison to the intensity and energy expended in stabilization, palliative care efforts struggle to measure up, as we have seen. Even if the gift of palliative care is beautiful, sincere, and benefits the patient greatly, it is not usually offered to those finishing in what is *popularly* considered as first place. Families sense this and may reject the indignity that such an option implies.

An alternative would be to recast the dying situation as social elevation rather than diminishment. Suffering through the ritual of intensification could be a rite of passage that enhances the patient's status visibly and tangibly. It could include significations of honor and acclaim, in the same way that Mrs. Lee in the Catholic community hospital (Chapter 6) was dressed in layers of respect for her personage, her position at the brink of death, and the journey to come. If, in the family hurdle, loved ones must choose whether or not to extend the ritual of intensification on the patient's behalf, palliative care could be seen as ritual display in its own right, carrying even greater public expenditure than the ritual they are being asked to give up. Palliative care might be housed in the hospital's VIP suites, lavishly decorated and staffed. Closing the ritual of intensification and its aftermath could be seen not as disordered rescue gone bad, and therefore disposable and distasteful, but as graduation into a higher order of honor and acclaim.

As we fantasize about an extravagance in palliative care that balances the public "gift" of rescue, it is important also to question the legitimacy of the latter, not only because it compromises the care of dying patients, but also because its domination of health-care is so inefficient and costly. At this writing, the call for health-care reform in the United States is more audible, but it voices no challenge to the sacrosanct position of rescue. It would be disturbing in the extreme to do so, but it is necessary. How is it that rescue, the fighting, is the most legitimate game to play in health-care? Because this approach taps into the combined power of a national self-image of innovation, a self-reliant ideology and a robust economic engine and rallies them all to the struggle. The enemy is universally to be feared, is it not (Bourdieu 1998: 6)? As Kaufman states, "No one wants to choose death if they think there is hope for life" (2005: 187).

The appeal to rescue and stabilization in the face of one individual's oppressive illness resonates powerfully with U.S. national ideals of liberty and freedom, not to mention with salvation from death. Further, the stakeholders in the present system will not hesitate to imply that access to basic health-care for all will require the sacrifice of research and development in technology. By contrast, to express solidarity in shared humanity with fellow Americans through universal access to health-care in search of a healthier nation is a far less compelling set of ideas. The realities of living, aging, and dying do not ring with triumph as Joanne Lynn describes them:

> We hope to live as well as possible, even with serious illness. It matters to ease symptoms, enhance autonomy, avoid bankruptcy, alleviate depression, and otherwise relieve what suffering can be relieved, even in the "valley of the shadow of death." But we can't tackle these urgent issues unless we learn to reach beyond the folly of focusing only on prevention and cure. (2004: 28)

The problem is that neither the dazzle of rescue nor the reparation of palliative care can be completely trustworthy in their present forms because their premises are unstable. Highly elaborated technological care can indeed support vital signs and hold back death under certain circumstances. But it also promotes the illusion that death can be infinitely postponed, and its advocates must capitalize on this fantasy to compete in the marketplace, compromising their credibility. Palliative care is certainly a necessary refuge from the excesses of intense rescue, but it maintains the fallacy that dying itself is not important enough to make material demands on the living. Individual practitioners of both rescue and palliative care may be entirely trustworthy, but the premises under which they operate are unstable because they are both partly true and partly false.

Rescue and palliative care exist in an untrustworthy cultural context that robs each of its chance for reliability. Americans' beliefs dictate that health-care must triage out what appear to be less urgent group needs in favor of the individual now being treated, and they assume that having more time alive in terms of a quantifiable future corresponds with cultural significance. Although rescue from calamity is presumably available to anyone who collapses, any guarantee to basic health-care is unreliable. Even rescue itself is jeopardized for many, especially for those who have been reclassified as Dying after the ritual of intensification. The prospects for a functional future also figure heavily into the status accorded persons in the United States and patients in the health-care system. Those who are deemed less able or immediately subject to finitude may rightly suspect that their conditions could trigger social fears of dependency and dying, opting them out of first-class care.

Americans need to discover the untapped power that rests in the margins, as the palliative care movement is seeking to do in the hospital. It is the need for others, admitting it and drawing on it, that gives humans their strength, not their ability to stand alone and fight off all who would interfere with their projects. What is needed is for U.S. society to embrace and celebrate human frailty as a source of dignity and stature, richness and satisfaction, and as an opportunity to honor humanity, vulnerability, and dependency in common. Even as a counterbalance to the prevailing self-reliance, perhaps this is a pipedream. Nevertheless, with these values, demonstrated in universal access to health-care, for instance, trust in the care of the dying and in the health-care system as a whole might be possible in the United States.

Notes

1. These features recall potlatch, a ritual display used by one group to impress another and encourage reciprocity.
2. Robert Seifert and Mark Rukavina (2006) indicate that medical expenses destabilize the finances of one in six nonelderly Americans, interfering with their access to further care.
3. As Kaufman (2005) and others (Drought and Koenig 2002) have stated, the validity of this "choice" is open to serious question.
4. In the teaching hospital, chaplains were on call for this "real" work when they supported the families of patients arriving with devastating neurological injury. Their role here helped secure consent for organ donation.
5. Unfortunately, these comments can be speculation only, because the study design did not allow for interviews on units the patient occupied prior to the unit where she died. Mr. Nguyen's case in Chapter 6 was an exception to this rule because the circumstances of his death upset both units.
6. CAPC (2008b) figures indicate that palliative care programs in hospitals increased from 500 programs in 2000 to approximately 1,300 in 2007 (Center to Advance Palliative Care & National Palliative Care Research Center 2008b).
7. See Lynn and Adamson (2003: 7). These models differ slightly from both Lynn and Anderson and from Sean Morrison (2005: S-81). Morrison's model adds a block for time in hospice before death. For a more complex graphic of the interaction of palliative care and acute care, see Connor and Fine (2009).
8. The Medicare hospice benefit reimburses through a daily rate rather than through coding for diseases or specific interventions.
9. See Morrison et al. (2008). These savings accrued in the rescue interventions that were *not* done, such as pharmacy and laboratory costs, not because of decreased length of stay, and they applied to patients discharged alive as well as those who died in the hospital.
10. The fear of "death panels" abroad in 2009 reflected these anxieties. For the reaction from palliative care advocates, see Meier et al. (2010).

CHAPTER 9

Making a Place for Dying in the Hospital

Someone was punching me, but I was reluctant to take my eyes from the people below us, and from the image of Atticus's lonely walk down the aisle.

"Miss Jean Louise?"

I looked around. They were standing. All around us and in the balcony on the opposite wall, the Negroes were getting to their feet. Reverend Sykes's voice was distant as Judge Taylor's:

"Miss Jean Louise, stand up. Your father's passin'."

—Lee (1961: 241)

Having learned how to bring some people back from death in some circumstances has caused Americans (and other peoples as well) to reconstruct death. U.S. society, steeped in individualism, egalitarianism, and abhorrence of the powerlessness embodied by dying and death, carries out an urgent social obligation to provide this boon of attempted rescue to everyone. Having little else on the menu of health-care that can be offered to all comers, the culture and the society are in the position of having to grant explicit permission for dying and death in many cases. At the same time, society's complacent confidence that its agents' ability to perform life-saving miracles distracts the group from the inevitability of the death of its members. Meanwhile, the responsibility to grant or deny this permission is a great burden to carry and to carry out, especially when its torturous machinations occur in the very midst of rescue itself. Of course it would be preferable to push it off somewhere else—to the patient's body as having an irreversible condition;

to the patient's wishes, however they might be expressed; or to the family in the family hurdle. Having discharged this difficult responsibility, society (through its hospital representatives) distances itself from the dying situation, often taking refuge in the easier-to-justify beneficence of universal rescue.

The hospital is a meeting place for major forces such as drama, altruism, heroic display, egalitarianism, and individual rights. How a given hospital negotiates its own tensions between maintaining both an operating margin and an altruistic mission (Pearson, Sabin, and Emanuel 2003) influences the ways in which dying will be minimized within it, as we have seen. The ritual of intensification serves as a mechanism to discharge public responsibility to persons in crisis because it fulfills expectations to explore every contingency before death is allowed. It suspends time to resolve uncertainty.

Each hospital is a conduit holding an untold number of supply chains and constituencies together, including the obvious ones of equipment, staff, patients, and documentation. The hospital also contains financial opportunities, profit centers, professionalism, heroicism, hopes, dreams, love, attention, compassion, and overcoming. Because the intense national energy of acute care is concentrated on the identified lives within its walls, the amorphous health-care needs on the outside pale into insignificance. The contrast between "opening a jar when your arthritis acts up" (Lynn 2004) and resuscitating a fibrillating heart is so dazzling that the amazing ability to do the latter whenever it is required seems to mitigate the social need to address the former.

Seeing the diverse needs of dying patients in the hospital through the lens of status and equity enables a clearer view of acute care and dying in the U.S. hospital and their uneasy coexistence. Dying is minimized in many ways as the hospital serves as a broker among major forces, many of them buttressed by dollars. Hospital cultures themselves mandate various ways to make dying disappear without completely abandoning the patient and sometimes without rescuing him from anything, either death or troubling symptoms. In their zeal to relieve suffering in general, whether physical, spiritual, emotional, existential, or that of simple impatience, clinicians may sedate persons who are dying more than necessary, such as Ms. Snyder (Chapter 8). The failure to hold difficult conversations at inconvenient times (Mr. Gomez, Chapter 1) can be excused by the more pressing and more legitimized demands of rescuable patients. It is acceptable for cross-cover physicians to do only what is needed in the moment to get them all through until the primary team returns, without an expectation of a more comprehensive plan from them or from the primary physician, as happened for

Mr. Diangelo. Practicing with outcomes and goals in mind, unspoken cultural permission and lack of review allows clinicians to expedite patient deaths, as happened for Mrs. Harper. The goal when life support is withdrawn may not be supporting the dying situation or simply being rid of unwanted treatments, but getting to the death itself, as it became in Ms. Hunter's case when methods were accelerated.[1] Basically, the situations of dying patients can be easily manipulated to suit whatever need in the system asserts its priority in the moment. Or aggressive treatment may continue outright to maintain fidelity in the patient-physician relationship, so that the dying situation is not officially acknowledged. As sincerely as hospitals and clinicians intend to operate in good conscience on the patient's behalf, they are subject to forces beyond their understanding or control.

Persons who are dying in the hospital are minimized to the point of disappearance. How would it be possible to make a place for them in the hospital? This chapter is a thought experiment to answer this question. We begin by considering the idea of empowerment. Power and control mesh well with rescue and stabilization, and it is logical to believe that enhancing these attributes among dying patients, or broadening the knowledge base of clinicians, or both, would reify the status of persons who are dying in the hospital. We will see that as tempting as these strategies are, empowerment leads us down the wrong road. If reasserting personhood is so difficult to do, why should the effort even be made? We consider the arguments for and against bringing dying out of the closet and the private reaches of the hospital into a more recognizable space. At the end, we arrive at a different approach for returning the dying patient to the social realm. It may be more appropriate to relinquish power in favor of recognition and witness so that dying can find its own place among the living.

The Fallacy of Empowering the Dying Patient

Last year, a former nurse with recurrent cancer gave a presentation about using art therapy during her journey through terminal illness. In the discussion that followed her formal remarks, she mentioned that she had been hospitalized recently with pneumonia. She was being treated with IV antibiotics, and her physicians recommended that she have a bronchoscopy[2] to pin down the source of the infection. She found the suggestion superfluous as the antibiotics were showing signs of success. She refused the procedure saying, "I'm a dying patient. I don't need a bronch." In telling this story, she indicated nothing remarkable in having so identified herself. But I found it startling. Here was someone who embraced a culturally stigmatized status.

To claim dying as a part of her identity enabled her to rank and dictate her own treatment priorities, and the bronchoscopy was not among them. Her posture expanded even the agency in dying that hospice and palliative care promote: that patients use their autonomy to leave the rescue camp and expand their horizons in what time remains, even as the disease continues its advance.

The ability to determine and state one's autonomous choices is not a feature that characterizes every part of the dying situation, however, and for patients actively dying in the hospital it is rarely available. Certainly someone as alert and interactive as this nurse would not have been considered by her hospital clinicians to be a dying patient, simply because of her high level of function. To hear her inform them of her mortality and how it should define her treatment plan would have surprised them. As we saw in the discussion of clinical features that lengthen or shorten the ritual of intensification (Chapter 7), it is very difficult for clinicians in acute-care settings to perceive conscious patients as dying. By the same token, many clinicians are hard pressed to consider permanently unconscious patients as viable.

Although it is salutary, this nurse's experience cannot give us a model for dying patients in the hospital. It is unrealistic and perhaps even unkind to expect someone who is seriously ill or dying to assume the responsibilities of a (well) moral agent, a fact recognized and accommodated in many cultures (Blackhall et al. 2001). And empowering the actively dying patient as discourses in bioethics suggest can be a fruitless exercise. Lionizing such an individual in terms of autonomy and choice does not enable them (or their advocates) to challenge the cultural forces swirling around them in the hospital bent on "moving things along," as Sharon Kaufman succinctly puts it (2005).

I offer a situation that occurred in my unit as illustration of the difficulty in empowering patients who are dying. Mrs. Russell was elderly and intubated. Her lung problems were unfixable, and she could not be weaned from the ventilator. She had been somnolent for days, and no one knew why. Late one afternoon with family in to visit, she perked up somewhat. Her nurse had Mrs. Russell sitting up in a chair, and she seemed to be unusually attentive to her surroundings. This auspicious change motivated the nurse's desire that the physicians and the family seize the moment to find out what Mrs. Russell's treatment preferences were.

The resident started the conversation, and the daughter quickly took over. Mrs. Russell was hard of hearing, and the daughter had to shout to be heard. She yelled, "Do you want to go to Jesus?" Mrs. Russell mouthed that she wanted to go home, according to the nurse's report. She did not answer the Jesus question. Undaunted, her daughter continued to press for guidance from Mrs. Russell: "Do you know that this machine is keeping you alive? Do you know that? If we take it out and let you go home, you will die. Do you want to die? This machine is keeping you alive."

The resident wished to understand Mrs. Russell's mental state to evaluate her capacity to make any decision. He asked, "Do you have a son Jack?" She didn't, but she nodded yes. "Are you in school?" She nodded yes. Her erroneous responses indicated that even though she was responsive and interactive for the first time in days, Mrs. Russell was not the autonomous decision-maker that they hoped she could be. Nor did this fact really matter, because Mrs. Russell would not have survived a trip home. Her choices were truly nonexistent. Even so, she had certainly expressed her preference, to go home, one that no one could grant to her.

Appealing to preferences about life-sustaining measures does not allude to the existential struggle and search for meaning that comes with facing mortality, and to focus on the technology-driven choices enables one to sidestep the need to do so. Empowering personal choice in those who are actively dying in the hospital is not the path to take to ensure that they are not minimized, and simply reaffirming individualism in this way may amount to a distraction. On the other hand, seeking to understand the personal style of the one who is dying, such as Mrs. Lee in Chapter 6, is an important alternative to explore.

If empowering the dying patient is not the most effective way to ensure a place for dying in the hospital, then patient advocates could surely be of more service to the patient's cause if they had greater familiarity with the territory of dying. In the next section, we explore this territory and consider whether the knowledge of it brings us closer to making a place for dying in the hospital.

In Search of Hospital Dying: Knowledge to Empower Advocates of the Dying

It is in the U.S. hospital that the cultural forces standing against death are most highly developed. Rescue and stabilization are the stars around which the hospital navigates, even though these beacons fail to dispel the shadows of death itself. Between the close of the ritual of intensification on one side and the death of the patient on the other is an interval of time bracketed by these two events. This interval is defined by what has come before and the unknown of what lies ahead, and the details it contains are different for every dying person. What does this interval entail? Acknowledging that hindsight's representation of order is illusory, a retrospective look at that interval can still yield some useful information.

Myriad forms of dying occur in the hospital. By focusing on dying situations in two of them, we have seen that seriously ill and dying patients are managed through norms that are specific to the sites and the clinicians within them. The Catholic community hospital, with fewer resources to explore all the contingencies of rescue and fluttering attempts at palliative care, can still be relaxed about the duration of the dying interval. The teaching hospital's higher intensity and more patterned practice allows less room for modification while displaying higher elaborations of rescue and palliative care. These are variations on the aspiration they have in common: to accommodate but also to minimize dying while maximizing rescue.

From the clinicians' perspective, the dying situations may be linear and orderly, such as what happens in the withdrawal of life support (Chapter 4), or chaotic and very troubling, such as having to call a code for a patient who could have benefited from a DNR order or palliative care (Chapter 7). Every dying situation is unique, of course. Perhaps it dishonors the persons who have died to use any vantage point that sorts or categorizes them, but if we found it difficult to learn from them as death loomed large for them and for us, perhaps we can be forgiven for seeking the insights their experiences can offer retrospectively. An attempt to group them can provide tools for thinking.

The dying situations themselves can shed light from their interaction with rescue. Death cannot be allowed in the United States without specific exemption from rescue. Its mandate requires that every dying situation interact with it in some way, making this a feature they hold in common. Using the closing down of the ritual of intensification and the death of the patient as bookends for the dying situation, it is possible to sort the 211 study cases of death in the hospitals (two research sites plus the pilot) accordingly, helping to bring hospital dying into a better view. Defined on either end by the brackets of the ritual of intensification and death, seventeen separate trajectories/scenarios of dying situations present themselves (see Figure 9.1 and the list defining these categories that follows it and see Table 9.1).[3]

In Chapter 4, we attempted to separate this wide variety of dying situations into those that clinicians see as orderly or disorderly. The situations of orderly dying (withdrawal of life support and patients with do not resuscitate orders who received at least some palliative measures) accounted for almost half of the sample (98 of 211, or 46 percent). (Of course, these situations themselves contained more disorder than the categories would imply.) Beyond these instances of orderly dying, two patterns

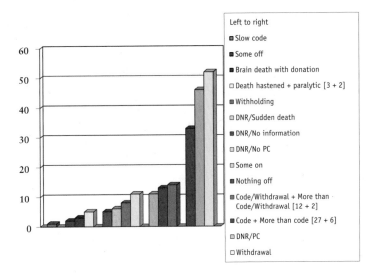

Figure 9.1. Hospital Dying Situations.

in the domain of disorderly dying deserve comment because of the particular ambiguities they reveal, "starting then stopping" and "the many manifestations of DNR."

Starting then Stopping

When a patient showed signs of deterioration, clinicians might intervene quickly first and then change their minds: starting then stopping. The most aggressive examples of starting then stopping occurred when an attempt at resuscitation was transformed into a withdrawal of life support, if a discussion with the family occurred while it was in progress. In these situations, the tipping point, the family hurdle, and the closing of the ritual of intensification occurred all at once. The insertion of family consultation at this crucial moment gave the dying situation a different cast than resuscitation attempts that were halted by physician edict. Such on-again-off-again efforts happened in other instances as well. Despite strenuous efforts to establish the certainty of dying through the ritual of intensification, a surprising amount of ambivalence and desire to rescue often persisted after its close. Patient deterioration prompted a response to restart rescue efforts at different levels and for different motivations before those efforts were abandoned, as happened in the case of Mr. Diangelo. But at a less aggressive level, even when patients had been "made a DNR," clinicians might

Table 9.1. Categories of Dying Situations.

1. Code: Persons may have had one or more, but for the purposes of this retrospective study, it was the last code that counted. Resuscitative efforts continued until the physician called the code off. Total: 27

2. More than Full Code: An unstable patient received more aggressive measures than CPR, such as open chest massage, ECMO (extracorporeal membrane oxygenation), or surgical exploration. Total: 6

3. Code/Withdrawal: Code was called with chest compressions; discussion with family resulted in resuscitation being called off, and life support was withdrawn. Total: 11

4. More than Code/Withdrawal: Discussion with family resulted in an end to aggressive stabilization measures, or surgeons realized irreversibility and returned the patient to the ICU for death. Total: 2

5. DNR Sudden Death: Patient was DNR but died suddenly; was not considered a dying patient prior. No code was called, no interventions were attempted. Total: 6

6. Withholding, or Code/Withholding: Rescue treatment was deliberately withheld by the physician before or after patient received some resuscitative efforts. Different from Code/Withdrawal because it was the physician's decision and family may have protested. Total: 5

7. Some Interventions Added On: A patient with a DNR order began to die actively. Limited interventions were started to stabilize the patient and later discontinued. May or may have not received palliative care. Total: 11

8. Some Interventions Taken Off: DNR was written when the patient destabilized, and some interventions were discontinued at that time. Total: 2

9. Nothing Off: DNR written for ICU patient, but no changes to life supportive measures (adding or subtracting) were made. Patient dwindled and died. Total: 13

10. Brain Death with Organ Donation: Brain death was declared and patient went to OR several hours later when workup for organ procurement completed. Total: 3

11. Withdrawal: Life supportive measures were withdrawn after discussion with the family. Total: 53

12. Withdrawal with Paralytic Infusion: Life support was withdrawn, but paralytic was not discontinued, either deliberately or through an oversight. Death was not "natural" but imposed, since no breathing was possible. Total: 2

13. Death Hastened: After an agreement to withdraw life support was reached, clinicians took action to hasten the death, such as removing the trach and covering the hole; starting drips deliberately to hasten death rather than to treat pain. (Does not include opioids given during withdrawal of life support. Does not include trach removal alone.) Total: 3

14. DNR with Palliative Care: Patient expected to die and some effort to provide palliation was reported. Does not indicate that patient was in a palliative care unit or that palliative care consult service was involved, but those patients are included in this category. Total: 46

(Continued)

Table 9.1.   Continued

---

15. DNR, No Palliative Care: Patients did not receive palliative care while actively dying. Total: 13
16. DNR, No Information About Palliative Care: DNR order in place; patient may or may not have received palliation. Total: 8
17. "Slow Code:" Clinicians deliberately delayed calling for or implementing resuscitative measures for a patient with no DNR order. Total: 1

---

still institute some interventions to stabilize the patient, such as increasing Mr. Diangelo's respiratory support or starting fluids to hold a blood pressure, before surrendering these efforts.

The Many Manifestations of DNR

At the point of the family hurdle, some families elected to forgo resuscitation for a patient receiving life-supportive interventions, so that the patient "became a DNR." After chest compressions had been taken out of the equation, family members at times wished to continue every intervention already in place without addition or subtraction. In these cases, the patient eventually dwindled and died. Besides such a stipulation of "turning nothing off," a patient exempt from cardiopulmonary resuscitation could have other particularities attached to the care plan after the DNR was established, such as "some off" (discontinue some interventions such as dialysis, but leave others, such as the ventilator, in place); "some on" (e.g., in case of deterioration, start IV blood pressure medication and call the family). At times, clinicians made these decisions on their own to start interventions in the moment—starting then stopping. Palliative measures might or might not have been instituted for these patients at the time the DNR decisions were made, and in some instances no determination about palliative care could be discerned from the information at hand. The territory of DNR by itself did not necessarily signal imminent death or the need for palliative care. Some patients with DNR orders died very suddenly, which was upsetting to clinicians who had not pictured death to be at all imminent. Mr. Gomez's vascular surgery team thought he was fine the day before he died. It is not uncommon for DNR patients to stabilize and to be discharged from the hospital, but methodology of this research did not include these patients (see Appendix).

The key to understanding both of these examples of disorder in a dying situation is to realize that the territory of dying continues to frustrate human efforts to control it. Any dying situation, therefore, may not unfold in a clear or linear way just because the ritual of intensification has settled the patient's rescue status. Ongoing ambivalence, starting and stopping, unpredictability, uncertainty, surprises, and chaos sometimes characterized this interval between the ritual of intensification and death. From this information, one gleans that despite clinicians' best efforts, unknowns may persist through every point of the Dying situation. The ritual of intensification may, therefore, designate patients as Dying to staff, for instance, but not to family. Patients with DNR orders may die without having been considered as dying patients. Palliative measures are underused outside of palliative care, and many patients will never have the opportunity to find refuge there. Deaths and the dying that precede them are both tamed and untamed, under control, or beyond human management (Aries 1974). Attempts to manipulate the patient's physiology and maintain one's composure are imperfect. In the morass that is dying, these findings are not unexpected. The wide-ranging variability of dying situations occurring in the U.S. hospital makes finding a way to incorporate dying patients into the mainstream appear even farther out of reach.

Using the ritual of intensification to define, describe, and categorize the territory of dying is a good exercise to undertake. Even as it offers perspective on the wide variation of hospital dying, imposing such a superstructure does not provide a way into the dying situations themselves, however. Empowering oneself with empirical knowledge about the territory of dying does not bring one closer to finding a way to legitimize it. Before speculating on what else might work, it is important to take stock of the reasons for seeking a remedy at all.

Why Not Continue to Minimize Dying in the Hospital?

Certainly the territory of dying involves helplessness, fear, waiting, unpredictability, and awareness of personal vulnerability. These features offer experiences and feelings avoided by most Americans with a choice in the matter, and the social and collective wisdom for taking a different tack is not evident. To minimize dying may, then, seem to be a completely appropriate response. On its face, it may seem more profitable on many levels to maintain the present strategy: attempting to capitalize and grow humanity's way out of dying by investing in rescue and stabilization efforts so that the ritual of intensification has even more contingencies to explore before admitting defeat and closing down.

And perhaps this is as it should be. Surely social norms serve important purposes. Why not allow what has evolved to prevail? I have heard several clinicians express the wish to me that their own dying be so brief and uneventful when the time comes as to go virtually unnoticed. If such is their own preference, many a clinician would argue, why isn't extending that courtesy to others a form of compassion?

Despite the strong tendency to minimize the awareness of dying, which is a broadly felt desire well honed in the U.S. hospital, significant reasons exist to challenge its dominance. Allowing the fear of death unconsciously to collude with economic forces in the hospital is frighteningly convenient. Arguments that oppose these forces by championing the individual have been unsuccessful in stemming this tide. Although family and clinicians continue to strive for what they believe is best for each seriously ill patient, "moving things along" exerts irresistible pressure to minimize exposure to the experience of dying in the two hospital study sites.

Making hospitals safe for dying patients and improving quality of their lives are not the only reasons to question the status quo. Allowing the ritual of intensification to pronounce the last word on who is legitimate to receive the gold standard of health-care allows power and profitability to be mixed with the demand that vulnerability always be overcome, an unrealistic and alienating premise. By the time the tipping point and the family hurdle arrive and the ritual has resolved the uncertainty, often it has made the patient's severance from legitimate society permanent and unchangeable.

Once the dying of this patient has been exorcised from collective concern, society presumably has been made safe from death once again. At least it is safe from this death, as it has been carefully confined to this patient's body alone. Seeing dying and death as happening to one individual at a time makes it possible to see any particular dying situation as exceptional, applying to that person only, rather than as common or shared. This act of singling out the dying patient from those who are (still) rescuable is one of the functions of the ritual of intensification.

The still-living patient has been placed in a dangerous place. One may be subject to banishment or to being hastened into the beyond presumably for one's own or for society's protection. Can persons who die in the hospital regain legitimacy? With the exception of hospital chaplains, no one outside the boundaries of palliative care claims them. They have no voice. It seems that almost no one is held accountable on their behalf. An entire ritual has grown up to do the work of naming them and justifying disengagement with them. Society's felt need to protect itself from the dangers of dying patients is not to be sneezed at.

The ritual of intensification is remarkable for its efficacy in protecting society. But it is also limited. Unlike many rituals celebrating the transitions of life, it demotes and isolates rather than honors the patient. It does not provide transcendence or adequate room for lamentation at a time when both are needed (Myers 2003). It has no way of accomplishing a triumphal reentry of the person back into the social world, as its purpose is to close off this possibility. What is needed is to see the ritual of intensification for what it truly is—something that has redefined both dying and death, but as only part of what could be a larger and more successful effort of a culture to come to terms with its mortality.

When hospitalized dying patients are minimized, each member of the society is shortchanged. Allowing such a tendency to prevail decreases one's awareness of personal limitations, the fact of human interdependency, the need for solidarity, the positive aspects of vulnerability, and the possibility of getting in touch with something bigger and more transcendent than one's own important projects. Even though they are potentially contaminating, persons who are dying are also teachers and models, going before us and others we love, representing what may be in store for us more assuredly than perhaps other groups of underserved persons. Doing one's best by all dying persons acknowledges their value and serves the larger society.

Strategies for Making a Place for Dying

We have already seen that neither direct empowerment of dying patients nor of their advocates can reverse the prevailing cultural tendencies toward death with as little dying as possible (although according them more authority is not ill advised on its own merits). Ascribing dignity, autonomy, and choice to patients themselves who may be dying does not protect them when social and cultural agendas purporting to serve their best interests play out in the hospital. Arming the supporters of dying patients with greater understanding will not serve as the antidote to the ill effects of the ritual of intensification. The answer has to lie with the society itself, through self-exploration and through imagining alternative cultural agendas. If empowerment is unhelpful, our thought experiment may find another path. Let us move out from the ritual of intensification to look more closely at how rites of passage work in general to ease social transitions.

Dying as a Rite of Passage and the Effects of the Ritual of Intensification

Using Arnold van Gennep's terms (1960), rites of passage that occur during important life transitions include three consecutive phases: rites of separation that move the person apart from society; rites of transition that enact the transformation; and rites of incorporation to bring the person back into society in her new position. The ritual of intensification would satisfy the middle portion, the rite of transition, but it has turned the rite of passage itself on its head. Instead of being followed by a rite of incorporation, the ritual of intensification works backward to isolate the person who is dying from society at large.

In general, a rite of passage develops to reduce the harmful effects of changes in life conditions to persons and to the society. But in this case, the omission of the opportunity to reconnect increases the harm. The enforced isolation results in alienation and greater disturbance. It is emblematic of modernity, "marked by a superstitious worship of oppressive force and by a concomitant reliance on oblivion. Such forgetfulness is willful and isolating: it drives wedges between the individual and the collective fate to which he or she is forced to submit."[4] The "oppressive force" in this case is the ritual of intensification. The "reliance on oblivion" is the isolation of the dying and the interest in keeping dying and death from intruding on the cultural consciousness. The "individual" refers not only to the dying person but also to the living persons around her. It is the [very] collectivity of the "fate to which he is forced to submit" that becomes lost. A rite of incorporation would work to remove these wedges of isolation.

In the ritual of intensification, the society deploys ideological and economic power to stand against death, offering a boon to the society. But when the patient must be surrendered to the inevitability of finitude, the society turns its back on both death and the patient. This odd denouement for a ritual fosters social estrangement, signifies the strength of the felt need for self-protection, and reinforces both. Any larger understanding of this time of life that strives to include a rite of incorporation will need to take account of both the need to include the dying and the fear of doing so.

Imagining a Rite of Incorporation

One may prescribe or create a rite; it costs little to use imagination. It is something else again (and perhaps quite implausible) to expect that any social entity would take up such ideas. Nonetheless, let us imagine a few elements that such a rite could contain. Considering the gulf that sometimes separates the dying from society after the ritual of intensification, it is unlikely that wholesale embrace of the dying can be expected. And any incorporation would require enough flexibility to account for wide variation in the duration and circumstances of hospital dying described earlier.

To undergird the feasibility of a rite of incorporation, two cultural shifts would be beneficial. The first is to eliminate the extraneous honorifics now associated with rescue, stabilization, and the ritual of intensification. These activities acquire inflated status when they must function as the major proofs of equal opportunity in health-care delivery. The connection between rescue and egalitarianism puts an unrealistic burden on efforts to salvage and stabilize patients. Clinicians, patients, and families cleave to them not only because they promise more time alive, but also because they confer validity and social worth on the patient. If new economic configurations and methods of delivering health-care could display comprehensive equity, then rescue and stabilization could take their places simply as forms of treatment rather than as demonstrations of democracy in the realm of health-care. Universal access to affordable health-care for all comers would be an obvious choice. The honor that rescue bestows on the individual would be appropriated and redistributed by the health-care delivery system as a whole. Who can say what it would mean to individuals in the United States to understand that their health is important to the society as a whole for the duration of their existence as human beings on U.S. soil? What if this dignifying value could be demonstrated by providing ready access to preventative and maintenance health measures as well as to rescue?

The second cultural shift would be to endow palliative care efforts with so much social and economic capital that they become at least equal in the cultural imagination to the legitimacy now conferred by the ritual of intensification. One can imagine palliative care service as a source of good will for the hospital, a magnet for investment, philanthropic, and research dollars, touted as a model of innovation with the same pride used to describe the Women's Center or Cardiac Care. If palliative care enjoyed this much stature and economic investment in the hospital and in the culture at large, the options posed at the point of the family hurdle would be more evenly balanced.[5]

Failing these developments, how can a rite of incorporation for dying persons in the hospital decrease the alienation left by the ritual of intensification? What would it encompass? Imagining answers to these questions is difficult because dying persons really *are* on the margins. It is no wonder that they may be shunted away from public concern when hospice and palliative care give them quarter. How can this obstacle of stigmatization be overcome? How does the hospital staff, acculturated to rescue, care for the living persons in their midst whose dying seems to define them so utterly? The imagined rite of incorporation must allow not only for bringing dying persons back into the midst of the living, but also for a measure of self-protection from their contaminating effects.

Recognition

Accordingly we will think small. To begin imagining a rite of incorporation, one must relinquish power in a way that coincides with what the person approaching death faces. Let us start with a deliberate act of recognition only. This recognition could take Glaser and Strauss's (1965) open awareness of dying and add a personal element: identifying the person and the dying situation as entities both familiar and distant. In fact, dying persons have what every person has, but for everyone else, it is *not yet* (rather than not ever). As the dying person in the bed occupies a space in the margins between life and death (and gives evidence that life there is still possible), those standing near the bed can recognize and claim their own space alongside. Such a perspective may affirm all of life while acknowledging that finitude can be close by or far off for any given person. It admits that a different order of being is possible for all of us. It can encourage a fellow feeling while retaining some level of detachment.

This recognition might be coupled with appreciation for the position that the dying person occupies. He has come a long way already, farther than anyone else there. The rite of incorporation would accord stature to the person who is dying, as a pilgrim, an older soul. His profound vulnerability and proximity to death contain the power to bring humanity more fully to those around him. Much of the path ahead (for him and for the rest of us) is murky. Now is not our time to die, but it is the time to extend ourselves for one who might be. What might slowing down and attending to the situation before us bring to our awareness?

A bedbound person approaching death is vulnerable and must rely on her companions. Because some of her path ahead can be anticipated, such as symptoms and likely course, it is the responsibility of the relatively healthy to look ahead and navigate on her behalf. Even though Mr. Diangelo may not have appeared to be a dying patient at the time that the DNR order was written for him, twin realizations informed the rationale behind that order: the expectation of respiratory difficulty prior to death and the understanding that a full rescue and stabilization measures in his case would only delay the inevitable. The primary physician might have recognized a prelude to active dying in these realizations. He might have looked ahead with Mr. Diangelo and his family at that point, hoping for the best, but prudently preparing for the worst. Together they might have formulated a plan of care reflecting this possibility, one that would have persisted whether or not the physician was on service. Deliberately embracing the dichotomy of hoping for the best while admitting that death could happen allows for a more open discussion.[6] Alternatively, one can imagine that a robust culture of incorporating the dying, if it existed, might override the tendency for off-shift personnel to avoid substantive decisions regarding the care of patients such as Mr. Diangelo. Recognizing his DNR order and the probability that he was now dying, the weekend staff would seek to create a plan of care with the family that accommodated this change.

Along with recognition of the dying situation, a rite of incorporation would seek to overcome isolation and exclusion. That is, its application could not be confined to the palliative care unit or just to situations of withdrawal of life support. A positive initiative to mark the significance of the event (notifying the family, the nearby staff, and the chaplain) could be seen as appropriate for persons known to be dying anywhere in the institution at any point in their situation, even if the event itself is tragic. It would sweep in anyone nearby who could be aware of the dying situation. The rite would have to be flexible enough to allow dying to unfold in any possible way because of the differing amounts of warning, preparation, and/or control afforded by the wide-ranging territory of dying in the hospital.

The demands on even a simple rite of incorporation would thus be formidable. Its enactment would need to be very deliberate to counteract the isolating power of the ritual of intensification. It would display an expansive attitude, the opposite of minimizing. It would bring the dying situation into the light, not exactly as welcoming the death to come, but acknowledging it as real. The rite would counter alienation by exploring ways of making meaning. It would allow for lamentation, for admitting one's anxiety, for finding hope in relationships and in outcomes other than prolonged time alive, for opportunities to "connect personal occasions of suffering with larger universalizing contexts of meaning," (Myers 2003: 382) and for transcendence.[7] If a rite of incorporation had been culturally available, Mrs. Russell's caregivers and her family might have continued the conversation with her by saying, "Mom, you might die before we get you home. You've been very sick; we've been worried about you. We love you."

Recognition and the Role of Witness

In the previous section, we imagined the act of recognition as a foundational assumption, a first step needed for a rite of incorporation. How would recognition take shape in the clinical encounter with the dying situation? How would it play out for individuals, the institution, and society as a whole? I propose that the idea of witness solidifies this concept of recognition in a helpful way and moves us toward a rite of incorporation.

In the film *Taking Chance*, a Marine officer finds himself accompanying a soldier's body home to its final resting place. At each transfer point while the casket is in sight, he salutes it, prompting others to show signs of respect as well. Toward the end of his journey, he expresses his doubts as to the significance of his having taken up this duty. A veteran enlightens him by saying: "You're his witness. Without a witness, they just disappear" (Katz 2009). Many social and cultural agendas in the United States conspire to make persons who are dying in the hospital disappear as well.

To be a witness is a bivalent term meaning to observe and also to testify or authenticate. To be aware to any degree of dying occurring nearby suggests the role of witness when rescue is not an option. To consciously take on the role of witness *in addition to whatever roles one has already* would be a decision of agency in the face of the unknown, as it was for the puzzled officer in the film. To be a witness allows one to recognize the dying situation for what it is, and to enter into it with empathy, even if one must stand apart. It is to choose in some way to occupy that marginal space along with the person who is dying. It rescues the human and social connection to the dying patient from the exile imposed after the ritual of intensification.

To take the opportunity to be a witness is a role that stands in opposition to simply feeling helpless or assuming there is nothing to do. To be a witness is to acknowledge the gravity of someone else's journey, not in an intrusive or voyeuristic way, but with a view toward being of service to the situation, or even just to maintain vigilance from a distance. Envisioning such a role opens up possibilities, depending on the situation and the amount of control one is able or privileged to use. Witnesses confirm one another's life and vitality during rituals that they share (Myerhoff 1996). As a witness, one must deploy time, energy, and focus to be sensitive to changing opportunities for leading, following, or simply watching for cues.

How would adopting the role of witness influence one's approach to the dying situation? The witness could step into and out of the situation as needed, being fully present without being overwhelmed. The witness would assist with opportunities to seek and make meaning, with inclusion and expansion in mind rather than minimizing. Conversely, the role of witness offers meaning and participation to the bystander even if she has little control, which is common in situations of dying. Mr. Gomez's nurse was at least a witness and could attend to the course of his death, even though she could not change the events that preceded the code. It is the role of the witness to seek out the family to be present during resuscitation attempts, if they desire to do so, so that they also can be witnesses (Baumhover and Hughes 2009; Mohammed and Peter 2009). After the withdrawal of life support, the witness would allow the dying person's unique physiology to dictate the style and manner and duration of the journey (as long as overt suffering is not an issue). One would allow time to pass, inviting interaction among family members to recall important life events (Chapple 1999). The witness recognizes that unpredictability is part of the territory of dying, and there is stature in this act of waiting (Vanstone 2004). It is the role of witness to call for a moment of silence after the unsuccessful attempt at resuscitation is called off, marking and incorporating the dying situation into the life of the living. Hospital workers who transport the body in draped gurneys to the morgue complain that they are shunned by hospital staff who see them pass by. To be a witness might change this behavior, suggesting instead that one stop one's work, perhaps nod, and wait until the body passes. The role of witness honors the particular life of the patient who is dying. It points also to the significance that the concluding moments in any life may hold for persons in the vicinity.

Recognition and Witness on an Institutional Level

Hospitals could also adopt the role of witness. Recognizing dying situations at a system level would incorporate the delivery of care to patients prior to their death into normal quality measures. But achieving such a goal is more difficult than it might appear, because it involves not only noticing and including but evaluating as well. At this writing, the goals and standards that would ground mechanisms of quality measurement for dying situations in the hospital are in their infancy.[8] Postdischarge quality assurance surveys carefully bypass the family members of persons who died in the hospital.[9] Retrospective chart audit is a difficult, time-consuming, and unreimbursable exercise requiring a high level of motivation. And because dying situations vary so widely, goals of care with broad applicability are difficult to establish. What does "patient safety" mean after life support has been withdrawn? At a minimum, it should provide guidelines for symptom control that do not hasten the patient's death.

Standards of care for patients in situations when death is expected are now legion as such programs as End of Life Nursing Education Consortium (ELNEC), Education on Palliative and End of Life Care (EPEC), and other palliative care initiatives have gained in popularity. Measuring how well these standards are met is routine in the domain of hospice and palliative care, as opposed to the hospital as a whole. Pain management has been designated a key quality indicator for hospitals by The Joint Commission, applying to all hospitalized patients (Quill 2002). But measuring the quality of care delivered to patients who are dying outside palliative care, when death may or may not be expected, is far rarer.

Staff members seeking to foster a hospital culture that bears witness to the dying situations in its midst may not be welcomed. Where will they find allies? Supporters might be sought among the less-empowered segments of the hospital, including chaplaincy. Connecting recognition of the dying and the importance of witness explicitly to the mission of the institution will be a necessary step.

Recognition and Witness on a National Level

A rite of incorporation on a national level would require grappling more openly with the dependency and vulnerability that is part of the human condition. As long as unfettered self-realization remains an icon of U.S. ideology, it will be difficult to buy into the freedom that comes from letting go of that idea. When one is accustomed to operating from the more powerful position of giver, to be compelled to receive care from others is an unwelcome surprise. It is not part of the national conversation that such a change in position is both inevitable and extremely difficult for most Americans to accept, schooled as they are in the virtues of self-reliance. Nor is it widely understood that a state of dependence is completely unrelated to one's personal dignity, Christopher Reeve being a case in point. The avenues to transcendence as a means for coping with the limitation of the human condition are not thought to be needed often in the United States, so they are very poorly marked.

Recognizing persons who are dying as full members of the societal family is a leap for a society so engaged in overcoming its mortality as to have brought forth the ritual of intensification. The "aspiration to reach a higher or more intense humanity" is clearly not for everyone (August 1981: 94). All the same, cultivating one's awareness of those who are in vulnerable situations in quotidian life would be a start. The next step in being a witness would be to consider such vulnerability not always as an adversity to be overcome, but as an untapped reservoir of possibilities.

Reintegrating persons who are dying may seem only to remind us of our limitations. But in fact they alert the worried well that mysteries and the unknowable still abound, and it is possible by drawing near to the veil to recognize and be reassured by the connection. Those willing and able to accord honor to the dying give honor to themselves. By excluding dying persons from society at large, the public at large denies itself the opportunity to benefit from their pilgrimage.

Notes

1. Death as objective is acknowledged in David Asch's research. See Chapter 6.
2. Bronchoscopy involves inserting a flexible tube into the lungs with a camera and suction capabilities. Without proper anesthetic it can cause gagging.

3. Two other dying situations resisted categorization and were left on their own.
4. Carolyn Forche (1993: 32) is characterizing the arguments of philosophers Walter Benjamin and Theodor Adorno's arguments here.
5. A test case for these two cultural shifts could be the Veterans Administration hospitals where access to health care for veterans is unquestioned and palliative care has been more widely embraced (Quill 2002).
6. Back et al. (2009), Casarett and Quill (2007), and West et al. (2005) give guidelines about these discussions with patients and families. The problem is that opportunities to express preferences have already passed for many hospitalized dying patients.
7. Myers (2003) contains a nice discussion of possibilities for implementing these ideas. See Howe (2008) for further suggestions.
8. Significant work has been done in the area of introducing palliative care into the ICU and measuring its impact, but the distribution and uptake of this work is uncertain. See Mularski (2006), Levy et al. (2005), Fowler et al. (1999), and Glavan et al. (2008) for discussions of techniques and challenges.
9. Quality of Death and Dying instruments include interviews with bereaved family members.

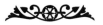

Appendix

Standing on shifting ground makes it clear that every view is a view from somewhere and every act of speaking a speaking from somewhere.

—Abu-Lughod (1991: 468)

This text purports to represent meaning made from ethnographic fieldwork. Although my methodology in studying dying was retrospective rather than prospective, the meaning making took place in multiple, ongoing, unfolding *prospective* contexts of data gathering over fifteen months. I spent weekdays in two hospital cultures and weekends working in a third. I attempted to get interviews within days of a patient's death in the two research sites while clinician memories of the events were still fresh and to follow up on deaths of all ages throughout each "house." Retrospective methodology reflects meaning backward, reorders events, and puts more order on them than existed in the moment. Eye-witness accounts of events in the past are notoriously unreliable. Ethnography requires that the fieldworker be in continuous dialog with daily experiences, data from informants, reflections, and analysis of findings to date. But meaning making and ethnographic texts that present this meaning are all retrospective in the end, even if they are eye-witness accounts by the ethnographer. The present is already past, and truths are always incomplete.

By way of illustration, I could look back on the day I stalked Margaret Mead and say "There. That's the day when it all started." This was back in the 1970s. Stalking may or may not be an overstatement. I was a Washington, DC stockbroker going out to get an allergy shot, not very interested in anthropology, but a fan of Margaret Mead. I recognized her walking ahead of me on the sidewalk with that wooden staff she always used, a dead giveaway. What did it matter that she had two people with her? I knew that she lived in New York, so she had to be in town for a reason. Such a thing didn't happen every day. So I followed her, all of them, to the parking garage that turned out to be their destination. I could say that because she told me she was giving a talk in Georgetown that night, because I hung around after the talk long enough to realize that her ride wasn't coming for her, and because she accepted my offer to drive her back to her hotel, giving me the unparalleled opportunity to have a private conversation with the common man's icon of anthropology, wherein we happened to discuss my dead-end career, that my life was changed forever. I could say all that, and give it that meaning. And maybe on some level it would be true. But it took a *very* long time to show—decades, in fact.

The less-than-tidy unfolding of life that followed that event is typical of ethnography, anthropology's signature method of research. It reflects life's messiness as it is lived and meaning as it is made, on the fly and reinterpreted in the light of reflection and subsequent events. As "outcomes" and "evidence based" have become watchwords in the hard sciences and now in health-care, the process that is working its way toward these ends itself often seems superfluous. The critical ethnographic tension continuously negotiated over time between the close-in perspective and a systems viewpoint seems not to fit and not to matter. It seems a paradox that exploring individual contexts deeply would bring one closer to the answers to moral questions, as Kleinman describes below, but it does. How does one go about studying "a culture"? How does one make sense of one's findings and present them? Anthropologists have worked to analyze, define, and explain ethnographic methods for the last half century as the discipline has struggled to overcome its culpability in colonization, where ethnography was used as a tool in domination.[1] One's position and stance are critical in evaluating three domains of ethnography: location of the fieldwork, both in terms of physical location and the researcher's relationship to that location; ethnographic methods; and text production.

Spending time in the field, preferably quite a long time, is central to ethnography. The field is the place where "culture" as a supposedly definable entity of Otherness is encountered (Abu-Lughod 1991). Field locations need no longer be remote and exotic, but the field must still be defined as somehow distinct from "home" (Gupta and Ferguson 1997). Or does it? Arthur Kleinman suggests that because local moral worlds "are *particular, intersubjective, and constitutive* of the lived flow of experience" (1995: 123, and see Gupta and Ferguson 1997), the encounter with culture might be achieved simply by defining a local moral world. Certainly any hospital location would qualify. Kleinman emphasizes the "moral processes" of these particular contexts because they are the glue, the critical connection between the human and the wider world. They anchor body experience with its surroundings of relationships, history, and identity through what is most at stake for both. Examining this shifting world of life experience by focusing on its moral processes as they are contested over time offers a unique way of knowing that is invisible to more reductionist methods of inquiry.

And how does the examination proceed? Through participant observation, by putting one's body in position so that it is a part of the field itself, and taking notes about one's observations and experiences while there. Of course, "the observer becomes a party to what is being observed" (Dewalt, Dewalt, and Wayland 1998: 261), so some enmeshment, with its opportunities for bias and subjectivity must be acknowledged as a part of the territory of participant observation. The use of physical presence makes the knowledge personal.

Along with the immediacy of field experience is the need to withdraw from it periodically to type up and flesh out the notes, reflect on what one has been seeing, explore the scene's periphery, and draw out new hypotheses regarding the threads of meaning one is perceiving. This withdrawal is a luxury not often or easily accomplished in some field sites. The shift in focus from near to far to close in again makes ethnography both iterative and a process, "both delimited and open ended" and "not straightforward," as Sharon Kaufman points out (2005: 327).

In exploring "local moral worlds," ethnography is uniquely suited for the moral work of "tallying body counts," critical to the meaning making in this book's body of research. Along with the characteristics of inherently messy, lengthy, personal fieldwork with iterative mechanisms, understanding those local worlds requires a weaving together of history and political economy. Without considering these issues, "we risk seeing only the residue of meaning. We see puddles, perhaps, but not the rainstorms and certainly not the gathering thunderclouds" (Farmer 2004: 308–309). The ethnographer's awareness must be constantly moving from noticing the puddles in the path and analyzing the wind direction to considering the path itself. What made those depressions that allowed the water to collect? What do they imply? Close-in knowledge of life activities woven together with reflections and explorations becomes personal, subsidiary, and tacit knowledge (Kleinman 1995: 76). A tension exists between the personal investment and the detached observation. How to participate without "going native," to maintain both detachment and the susceptibility to being wounded (Dewalt, Dewalt, and Wayland 1998: 263).

Ethnographic work most often speaks its findings (including its interpretations, its meaning making) through text, and here also the position of the ethnographer is key. "Finding somewhere to stand in a text that is supposed to be at one and the same time an intimate view and a cool assessment is almost as much of a challenge as gaining the view and making the assessment in the first place."[2] And how does one turn active or observed practice into words? Regardless of the position they choose, ethnographers are caught up in the invention rather than the representation of culture, because everyone, the researchers and the voices informing the research, speaks from a certain position. Every participant conveys a partial narrative, an incomplete truth (Clifford 1986). Participant observation and its reporting involves choices in every step—the recording of data, the reflections, the producing of the text that conveys it. Further, the informants make choices as to how to filter what they know, what to convey to the anthropologist. The ethnographer is positioned between systems of meaning (Clifford 1986: 2–3), with a personal lens refracting what she receives and what she describes. Her position and the lens she uses are unique. Neither the position nor the lens can be exactly duplicated.

Hence, the positioning of the ethnographer and the lens are keys to understanding and evaluating the work that flows from both. How "close" is the ethnographer in space and time to the culture under study? Certainly my double enmeshment in both the United States and in acute care affects my "lens," and disclosure cannot fully mitigate this. Rather than speculating about whether "going native" is getting too close, and whether placing boundaries around culture makes "the natives" too distant, too Other,[3] it is preferable to notice Elisa Sobo's observation that "people may belong to many cultures and most cultures are partial; that is most cultures (e.g., organizational cultures, professional cultures) do not cover all life's questions" (2009: 116). The question of insider/outsider status is likewise partial and difficult to define. In the interests of transparency, I offer this (fuller, but admittedly partial) description of my position and stance.

On my introduction into the discipline of anthropology, I realized that I had been in the field since I entered nursing school and then began work thirteen years before. If nurses with some level of experience usually enjoy the phenomenon of suddenly feeling absorbed in the routine, a sense of belonging in the nursing world, as Daniel Chambliss found,[4] then my nursing experience has been aberrant. I have always been on the outside looking in, wondering "what is up with this?" Perhaps I came to the profession too late in life to be resocialized. This is not to say that I did not develop confidence and comfort as a nurse. I affirm also that many if not most clinicians are also fraught with moral questions and misgivings about their practices much of the time. It is to say that I never found the work to be easy, nor that it was ever routine. I marveled at the nurses around me who, with the ease of those born with a "feel for the game" (Bourdieu 1990: 67), seemed to be able to deliver fine patient care and mentor a new graduate without missing a beat, for instance. For me, patient care took every ounce of my concentration. How is it determined that one does or does not belong in a social field? If it seemed that most clinicians made the transition into the mother tongue of routinization in the hospital, grammar and syntax kept tripping me up. I could sometimes achieve fluency, but my accent never disappeared.

Anthropology and ethnography gave me the tools to grind my own axe, so to speak. I came to the discipline with my question already formulated, filtered, and honed through experience in various acute-care venues, cancer research nursing, a clinical ethics masters program and still unanswered: why don't more people find hospice before they die? Now I had found the method of inquiry that would help me examine my assumptions and notice at least some of my biases, while providing me with the tools to sharpen observations, notice patterns, probe variations. Here I came to see that hospice/palliative care was simply one of many cultural formations along with being the best approach to the management of dying persons that the world had ever seen.

I continued to do clinical work while I studied anthropology. I began this research with an IRB-approved pilot study conducted in the hospital where I worked over two months in the summer of 2001. Of the fifty-six cases in the pilot, ten were from my own unit, and three were patients I had cared for myself. This initial foray was a kind of autoethnography, and I interviewed every clinician I could find regarding deaths occurring anywhere in the hospital. The content analysis of the data in the pilot revealed that clinicians spoke often about the failings of the system, a finding that the subsequent research elsewhere did not duplicate. I attribute this important discrepancy to informants seeing me as one of them, expecting that a researcher who was a fellow employee might be able to change the system. In any case, it was clear to me that further research would have to be conducted in a selection of acute-care settings strange to me. Eventually, I received funding from the National Science Foundation that made such a project possible.

A new question arose with fresh IRBs looking at the project. Who are the actual research subjects, the patients who died or the clinicians being interviewed about their deaths? If my research subjects were no longer living, then presumably they would not need human subject protection. Such requirements for neat categorization stymie ethnographers perhaps more than researchers who are conducting randomized clinical trials. The issue of power in the relationships formed between the anthropologist and members of the culture being studied is understood quite differently in anthropology than it is by IRBs. On the one hand, anthropological discourse about ethnography wonders how informants may be treated as partners in the research rather than subjects, equalizing the balance of power. At the same time, Charles Bosk points out, "Ethnographers do not inform subjects that the world from their point of view is the starting point for our interpretive activities," making some level of deception and betrayal inevitable (2001: 213). In my study, some of the subjects were beyond the purview of the IRB. They included the persons who died, many of the clinicians (although interviewees signed consent forms), and the hospitals in the foreground, with the economics of health-care and the ideology of the nation as coactors. If I had looked for a connection between patient death and IRB operations, perhaps these bodies might have needed human subject protection.

From the pilot I learned that structured questions did not always elicit the full story of the patient's dying situation from my informants. So in the formal study that followed I abandoned this approach in favor of an open-ended interview. The in-person patient hand-off or shift report that clinicians use with each other to talk about patients often takes a narrative shape using a chronological sequence, and the fluent narrative that poured out of most informants often took this form. Sometimes I needed a beginning prompt, such as "How did he present?" or "Was the death expected or unexpected?" In the majority of cases, clinicians told the patient's story with great intensity and little or no encouragement. If they faltered, I fell into the nurse mode, asking questions that would have been important to me in assessing the patient. My agenda was to get the story, and when fluency was not forthcoming, or if I wanted particular information, I pushed. I wanted the narrative to open up the dying situation when the informant might be inclined to dismiss it. Being a practicing ICU nurse enabled me to elicit a level of detail that a nonclinician could not have obtained. It also means that the information is filtered through that lens, introducing its own bias. Because I often thought I knew what was meant by a statement, I failed to ask a question for clarification or confirmation. I did not "play dumb" often enough (Bosk 2001: 218).

Using a retrospective methodology certainly brings in another form of bias, that of working backward from the known outcome. A prominent ICU physician where I worked complained about this stance during the pilot, disallowing the research itself because of this premise. His objection was similar to one leveled at narrative in general—that hindsight brings about an illusion of order missing in real time when the future is unknown and still unpredictable.[5] To answer this objection, I planned to use the groundwork laid during the retrospective portion in terms of site knowledge and relationships to launch a prospective "arm" of the study. Here, I would narrow the focus to particular units in the two hospitals and follow a few patients prospectively. Unfortunately, constraints imposed by the IRB and the additional time it required prevented implementation of that phase. This objection is thus unanswered.

The methodology required me to follow up with clinicians who cared for patients in the places where the patients actually died. But if these clinicians received the patient in transfer very shortly before the patient died, they might not know the patient's history well. If the ritual of intensification was completed at a distance in time and place from the location of the death, I could not learn the details that precipitated the transfer. In this aspect, the opportunity for hindsight did not impart order, and a prospective look would have been preferable.

Besides the detective work to find the units and the clinicians I needed within days of a death and the interviews that were its end product, I supplemented my interview time in the two hospitals with ancillary conversations and interviews wherever I could get them: with hospitalists on and off duty, EMTs, drug and device reps, volunteers in both hospitals, nurse educators, dietary staff. I interviewed staff during their day or night shifts regarding deaths of all ages, including newborns and children (although the examples in this text are confined to the dying situations of adults). I interviewed managerial staff at both field sites. I attended meetings (staff, care plan, ethics, bereavement, management) and in-service sessions at the field sites along with seminars about health-care in the city itself. I scoured the local media for news and advertisements originating from any local hospitals to understand the public face they wanted to present and the national media to track the portrayal of acute care in the culture at large. I overheard conversations in hallways and nearby bus stops that enlarged my perspective of each hospital's culture. I visited hospitals in two other cities when the opportunity arose, gathering further perspective.

My travels within the hospitals' hallways (carpeted or linoleum?); lobbies, with the seasonal changes made to their public displays; cafeterias (name-brand fast food, shipped in, or "home-cooked"?), gift shops (boutique or convenience orientation?), unit break rooms (separate for physicians and nurses, or shared?), chapels (obvious or hidden?) and services within them; stairwells, elevators, administrative office areas, all helped me understand the hospitals' inside and outside faces and their multiple, layered corporate personalities. Access to the NICU's patient care area in the teaching hospital required approved entry through five separate doors, for instance. The shiny areas displaying recent renovation in each hospital and the shabbier areas waiting for attention spoke of administrative priorities.[6]

Meanwhile, the iterative operations of fieldwork proceeded apace. The two field sites, the work site, and these myriad experiences triggered more reading and reflection, sending me in new directions seeking new conversations and answers as I began to trace the connections between business, medicine, power, economics, and ideology that became apparent. In this way, ethnography is both summative and generative (Sobo 2009: 160).

Because I depended on on-site interviews, it was not possible for me to gain regular access to some areas and personnel that I needed, and this obstacle could not be overcome. Some nurse managers did not approve of my presence, and I could not reach the nurses who were involved with deaths in those areas for interviews. With few exceptions, the residents in the teaching hospital were too overwhelmed to talk, and except for palliative care, attending physicians were not visible outside of morning rounds. Most private-practice physicians visited their patients in the Catholic community hospital when I was not present. My access to physicians in general was much less as an outsider during the study than it was in the pilot, when I was an insider. The ED at the teaching hospital was chaotic, without possibility for me to navigate with this methodology. In the Catholic community hospital I never found an expedient way to learn about the deaths that occurred in the ED. I was able to mitigate these difficulties when I encountered some ED clinicians and physicians in staff meetings and in venues outside of patient care.

On weekends I worked in a hospital nearby, where I could supplement my field data with perspective gained through informal conversations with residents and physicians who saw me as a colleague rather than as a researcher. Physicians here explained the differences between working in private practice or in research facilities. Residents shared their perspectives about serving as the critical labor force in teaching institutions while advancing their education and the career opportunities and recruitment strategies used to attract them to postresidency positions. Seeing their future possibilities as they saw them opened worlds to me that would never have concerned me simply as a bedside nurse.

Even with two levels of removal or distance from the hospitals and clinicians under study (the ongoing lack of fit with nursing and the strangeness of the field sites themselves), some amount of enmeshment over time was unavoidable. I attended staff and unit retreats, happy to be included. I was invited to serve on a multidisciplinary committee in the teaching hospital that was trying to create a protocol for the withdrawal of life support that all critical-care units would use. After a chaplain in the Catholic community hospital discovered that I had copied the cartoons they had displayed on their office bulletin board, she said, "You're studying us, too!" The relationships that formed in the two systems gave me entrée into meetings that were critical to my understanding and interpretation, and for this "enmeshment" I am very grateful.

Regarding confidentiality: it was impossible to obtain consent from patients and families because I was blinded to all identifying information. Patient information spilled out from clinician narratives in dazzling particularity, but I have omitted or disguised identifying details (e.g., permutations of illness and treatment, gender, nationality, ethnicity) to make patients less recognizable in this text. I assigned pseudonyms to patients, while clinicians remain unnamed. Certainly the need to cloak identifying nuance implies a level of generalizability that cannot be justified on its face. Because its usual purpose is to bring particular cultures to life through specific details of very specific sites, ethnography itself is not overtly expandable. In fact, the pendulum has often swung in the other direction. Anthropological scholars have argued that ethnography and the study of culture sets the Other even more apart, (even as it "makes strange" what is familiar) (Abu-Lughod 1991; Fabian 1983). This problem can be compounded by use of the past tense. Although the past tense increases the distance between the reader and the subject of ethnography, it also allows the text to imply that "that was there and then, this is here and now," and because cultures are not static or frozen, the past tense indicates that some things have undoubtedly changed since the ethnographer made her observations.

At the same time, one might remember that intimate exposure to and knowledge of any culture is self-reflexive. One studies the Other to explore congruencies and divergences relating to the Self, a phenomenon making ethnography and its findings inherently not restricted only to the sites of research. I make these points because I have chosen to use a combination of tenses: the past tense when referring to a specific observation taken from the fieldwork and the present tense almost everywhere else. This widespread use of the present tense is not meant to mislead. I recognize that conditions in both hospitals have changed since the fieldwork was completed. I further recognize that all health-care is local and that the conditions in no U.S. hospital will precisely match those of the two described in this study. However, it is my view that the ideology that forms the economic and ideological backdrop of acute care in general and hospital dying in particular is broadly applicable to hospitals beyond these two. These conditions and their consequences for dying patients are widespread enough and immediate enough to allow, even to justify, the use of the present tense.

A word about diversity. Although I documented the race and ethnicity of patients and informants, clinician narratives rarely included the kind of information that would have allowed me to trace any specific correlations between a given dying situation and the patient or the clinician's race or ethnicity. Mrs. Lee (Chapter 6) stands out as a clear exception.

What meaning is being made after a life-changing event such as a death depends on its context and the one who is making the meaning. Mary Frances O'Connor differentiates between responses that seek to make meaning and those that seek to "return to baseline" after a traumatic event, pointing out that one looks back and one looks forward (Drought and Koenig 2002: 159; O'Connor 2002). Certainly my chance encounter with Margaret Mead was not traumatic. And the meaning I took from it was much less than life-changing. But I never forgot the incident, or our conversation, even though at the time I dismissed its implications out of hand (that I could go back to school and consider anthropology). I gave myself credit for interrupting my routine to seize a sudden opportunity and milk it for all it could give me; somewhere in the mix of impressions from that incident some small seed may have been planted, and the fruit that appeared later might be related to it (along with other seeds) in some way.

Notes

1. Clifford and Marcus (1986), Behar and Gordon (1995), Abu-Lughod (1991), Geertz (1973, 1988), and Gupta and Ferguson 1997) are suggested readings.
2. See Geertz (1988:10).
3. See Narayan (1993), Abu-Lughod (1991), and Weston (1997) for excellent discussions of these issues.
4. Reported by Daniel Chambliss (1996: 39, 55–57).
5. This problem has been cited elsewhere when retrospective research purports to estimate the costs of end of life care, because the survivors are excluded from the data (Abelson 2009).
6. Although such details would be critical to a pre-HIPAA ethnography, they must be omitted here.

References

Abella, B. S., Alvarado, J. P., Myklebust, H., Edelson, D. P., Barry, A., O'Hearn, N. et al. (2005). Quality of cardiopulmonary resuscitation during in-hospital cardiac arrest. *Journal of the American Medical Association, 293*(3), 305–310.

Abelson, R. (2009). Months to live: Weighing the medical costs of end-of-life care. *New York Times*, 22 December, p. A1.

Abu-Lughod, L. (1991). Writing against culture. In R. G. Fox (Ed.), *Recapturing anthropology: Working in the present* (pp. 137–154). Santa Fe, NM: School of American Research Press.

Adam, B. (1995). *Timewatch: The social analysis of time*. Cambridge: Polity Press.

Adloff, F., & Mau, S. (2006). Giving social ties, reciprocity in modern society. *European Journal of Sociology, 47*(1), 93–123.

Agency for Healthcare Research and Quality (AHRQ). (2005). *Total number of people accounting for expenditures by site of service: United States, 2003*. Washington, DC: Agency for Healthcare Research and Quality.

Agency for Healthcare Research and Quality (AHRQ). (2008). In U.S. Department of Health and Human Services (Ed.), *National healthcare disparities report* (p. 7). Rockville, MD: Agency for Healthcare Research and Quality.

Aiken, L. H., Clarke, S. P., Sloane, D. M., Sochalski, J., & Silber, J. (2002). Hospital nurse staffing and patient mortality, nurse burnout, and job dissatisfaction. *Journal of the American Medical Association, 288*(16), 1987–1993.

American Hospital Association. (2008). *AHA central office: About us.* Retrieved December 27, 2009, from http://www.ahacentraloffice.org/ ahacentraloffice/html/aboutus_index.html

American Medical Association (AMA). (2009). *CPT process—how a code becomes a code.* Retrieved May 12, 2009, from http://www.ama-assn. org/ama/no-index/physician-resources/3882.shtml

Angell, M. (2000). The pharmaceutical industry—to whom is it accountable? *The New England Journal of Medicine, 342*(25), 1902–1094.

Angell, M. (2009). Drug companies & doctors: A story of corruption. *The New York Review of Books,* January 15, p. 56.

Angus, L. D. G., Cottam, D. R., Gorecki, P. J., Mourello, R., Ortega, R. E., & Adamski, J. (2003). DRG, costs and reimbursement following roux-en-Y gastric bypass: An economic appraisal. *Obesity Surgery, 13*(3), 591–595.

Apolone, G. (2000). The state of research on multipurpose severity of illness scoring systems: Are we on target? *Intensive Care Medicine, 26,* 1727–1729.

Aries, P. (1974). *Western attitudes toward death from the Middle Ages to the present* (P. M. Ranum, Trans.). Baltimore: Johns Hopkins University Press.

Aries, P. (1981). *The hour of our death.* New York: Oxford University Press.

Asch, D. A. (1996). The role of critical care nurses in euthanasia and assisted suicide. *New England Journal of Medicine, 334*(21), 1347–1379.

August, E. R. (1981). The only happy ending: Divine comedy in Western literature. *The Bulletin of the Midwest Modern Language Association, 14*(1), 85–99.

Bach, P. B., Schrag, D., & Begg, C. B. (2004). Resurrecting treatment histories of dead patients: A study design that should be laid to rest. *Journal of American Medical Association, 292*(22), 2765–2770.

Back, A. L., Young, J. P., McCown, E., Engelberg, R. A., Vig, E. K., Reinke, L. F., Wenrich, M. D. et al. (2009). Abandonment at the end of life from patient, caregiver, nurse, and physician perspectives. *Archives of Internal Medicine, 169*(5), 474–479.

Baer, H. A. (2001). *Biomedicine and alternative healing systems in America: Issues of class, race, ethnicity, and gender.* Madison: University of Wisconsin Press.

Baker, R. J. (1978). Emergency medical services categorization and regionalization. *Archives of Surgery, 113,* 1133–1134.

Barger-Lux, M. J., & Heaney, R. P. (1986). For better and worse: The technological imperative in health care. *Social Science and Medicine, 22*(12), 1313–1320.

Batt, S. (2007). Limits on autonomy: Political meta-narratives and health stories in the media. *American Journal of Bioethics, 7*(3), 23–25.

Baudrillard, J. (1976). *Symbolic exchange and death.* London: Sage.

Baudrillard, J. (1993). Symbolic exchange and death [L'échange symbolique et la mort] (I. H. Grant, Trans.). London: Sage.

Bauman, Z. (1992). *Mortality, immortality, and other life strategies.* Cambridge: Polity Press.

Baumhover, N., & Hughes, L. (2009). Spirituality and support for family presence during invasive procedures and resuscitations in adults. *American Journal of Critical Care, 18*(4), 357–366.

Baynton, D. C. (2001). Disability and the justification of inequality in American history. In P. K. Longmore & L. Umansky (Eds.), *The new disability history: American perspectives* (pp. 33–57). New York: New York University Press.

Beachley, M. (2002). Evolution of the trauma cycle. In K. A. McQuillan, K. Truter Von Rueden, R. L. Hartsock, M. B. Flynn, & E. Whalen (Ed.), *Trauma nursing: From resuscitation through rehabilitation,* (3rd ed., pp. 2–18). Philadelphia: Saunders.

Beardsley, E. H. (1987). Desegregating southern medicine, 1945–1970. *A history of neglect: Health care for Blacks and mill workers in the twentieth-century South.* Knoxville: The University of Tennessee Press.

Becker, E. (1973). *The denial of death.* New York: The Free Press.

Becker, G. (2004). Deadly inequality in the health care "safety net": Uninsured ethnic minorities struggle to live with life-threatening illnesses. *Medical Anthropology Quarterly, 18*(2), 258–275.

Behar, R., & Gordon, D. A. (Eds.). (1995). *Women writing culture.* Berkeley: University of California Press.

Bell, C. (1992). *Ritual theory, ritual practice.* New York: Oxford University Press.

Berliner, H. S. (1985). *A system of scientific medicine: Philanthropic foundations in the Flexner era.* New York: Tavistock.

Bernato, A. E., Lucase, F. L., Staiger, D., Wennberg, D. E., & Chandra, A. (2005). Hospital-level racial disparities in acute myocardial infarction treatment and outcomes. *Medical Care, 43*(4), 308–319.

Blackhall, L. J. (2006). Why physicians avoid straight talk about CPR. *Virtual Mentor, American Medical Association Journal of Ethics, 8*(9), 602–608.

Blackhall, L. J., Frank, G., Murphy, S., & Michel, V. (2001). Bioethics in a different tongue: The case of truth-telling. *Journal of Urban Health, 78*(1), 59–71.

Bodenheimer, T. (2005). High and rising health care costs. Part 2: Technologic innovation. *Annals of Internal Medicine, 142*(11), 932–937.

Bodenheimer, T. (2005). High and rising health care costs. Part 3: The role of health care providers. *Annals of Internal Medicine, 142*(12), 996–1002.

Bosk, C. L. (2001). Irony, ethnography, and informed consent. In B. Hoffmaster (Ed.), *Bioethics and social context* (pp. 199–220). Philadelphia: Temple University Press.

Bourdieu, P. (1990). *The logic of practice* (R. Nice, Trans.). Stanford, CA: Stanford University Press.

Bourdieu, P. (1998). *Practical reason: On the theory of action.* Stanford, CA: Stanford University Press.

Bowker, G. C., & Star, S. L. (2000). *Sorting things out: Classification and its consequences.* Cambridge, MA: The MIT Press.

Brewster, L. R., & Felland, L. E. (2004). *Emergency department diversions: Hospital and community strategies alleviate the crisis.* Retrieved December 30, 2009, from http://hschange.org/CONTENT/651/651.pdf

Brieger, G. H. (1992). From conservative to radical surgery in late nineteenth-century America. In W. F. Bynum & R. Porter (Eds.), *Medical theory, surgical practice: Studies in the history of surgery* (pp. 219–221). London: Routledge.

Brody, H. (1992). *The healer's power.* New Haven, CT: Yale University Press.

Buchman, T. G., Cassell, J., Ray, S. E., & Wax, M. L. (2002). Who should manage the dying patient? Rescue, shame, and the surgical ICU dilemma. *Journal of the American College of Surgeons, 194*(5), 665–673.

Buntin, M. B., & Huskamp, H. (2002). What is known about the economics of end-of-life care for Medicare beneficiaries? *The Gerontologist, 42*(3), 40–48.

Burns, J. P., Mitchell, C., Outwater, K. M., Geller, M., Griffith, J. L., Todres, D. et al. (2000). End-of-life care in the pediatric intensive care unit after the forgoing of life-sustaining treatment. *Critical Care Medicine, 28*(8), 3060–3065.

Burt, R. A. (2009). Invitation to the dance: Lessons from Susan Sontag's death. *Hastings Center Report, 39*(2), 38–45.

Byrd, W. M., & Clayton, L. A. (2000). Black health in the Republican era. *An American health dilemma, Volume One: A medical history of African Americans and the problem of race: Beginnings to 1900* (pp. 205–250). New York: Routledge.

California HealthCare Foundation. (2006). *Snapshot: Health care costs* 101., 2006, from http://www.chcf.org/documents/insurance/HealthCareCosts06.pdf

California Newsreel (Producer), & Adelman, L. (Director). (2008). *Unnatural causes: Is inequality making us sick?* [Video/DVD]. National Minority Consortia of Public Television; Joint Center for Political and Economic Studies Health Policy Institute. Retrieved December 27, 2009, from http://www.unnaturalcauses.org

Callahan, D. (1993). *The troubled dream of life: In search of a peaceful death.* New York: Simon and Schuster.

Callahan, D. (1995). Frustrated mastery: The cultural context of death in America. *Western Journal of Medicine, 163*(3), 226–231.

Callahan, D. (2000). Death and the research imperative. *The New England Journal of Medicine, 342*(9), 654–656.

Callahan, D. (2003). *What price better health? Hazards of the research imperative.* Berkeley: University of California Press.

Casarett, D. J., & Quill, T. E. (2007). "I'm not ready for hospice": Strategies for timely and effective hospice discussions. *Annals of Internal Medicine, 146,* 443–449.

Casarett, D. J., Stocking, C. B., & Siegler, M. (1999). Would physicians override a do-not-resuscitate order when a cardiac arrest is iatrogenic? *Journal of General Internal Medicine, 14,* 35–38.

Cassel, C. K., Ludden, J. M., & Moon, G. M. (2000). Perceptions of barriers to high-quality palliative care in hospitals. *Health Affairs, 19*(5), 166–172.

Cassell, E. J. (1974). Dying in a technological society. In P. Steinfels & R. M. Veatch (Eds.), *Death inside out* (pp. 43–48). New York: Harper and Row.

Cassell, E. J. (1991). *The nature of suffering and the goals of medicine.* New York: Oxford University Press.

Cassell, J., Buchman, T. G., Streat, S., & Stewart, R. M. (2003). Surgeons, intensivists, and the covenant of care: Administrative models and values affecting care at the end of life. *Critical Care Medicine, 31*(4), 1263–1270.

Center to Advance Palliative Care. (2008a). *Letter to The Joint Commission.* Retrieved July 22, 2009, from http://www.capc.org/tjc-letter.doc

Center to Advance Palliative Care & National Palliative Care Research Center (CAPC). (2008b). *America's care of serious illness: A state-by-state report card on access to palliative care in our nation's hospitals.* Retrieved June 23, 2009, from http://www.capc.org/reportcard/state-by-state-report-card.pdf

Center to Advance Palliative Care. (2009). *Frequently asked questions: How is CAPC maintaining momentum in the field?* Retrieved December 28, 2009, from http://www.capc.org/about-capc/faqs

Centers for Medicare and Medicaid Services, & Statistics (2005). *ICD-9-CM official guidelines for coding and reporting.* Washington, DC: U.S. Department of Health and Human Services.

Central Intelligence Agency. (2005). *The World FactBook.* Retrieved 3 May, 2006, from https://www.cia.gov/library/publications/the-world-factbook/index.html

Central Intelligence Agency. (2009). *The World FactBook.* Retrieved 25 December, 2009, from https://www.cia.gov/library/publications/the-world-factbook/index.html

Chambliss, D. (1996). *Beyond caring: Hospitals, nurses and the social organization of ethics.* Chicago: University of Chicago Press.

Chan, J. D., Treece, P. D., Engelberg, R. A., Crowley, L., Rubenfeld, G. D., Steinberg, K. P. et al. (2004). Narcotic and benzodiazepine use after withdrawal of life support: Association with time to death? *Chest, 126*(1), 286–293.

Chapple, H. S. (1999). Changing the game in the intensive care unit: Letting nature take its course. *Critical Care Nurse, 19*(3), 25–34.

Christakis, N. A. (1999). *Death foretold: Prophecy and prognosis in medical care.* Chicago: University of Chicago Press.

Clifford, J. (1986). Introduction: Partial truths. In J. Clifford & G. E. Marcus (Eds.), *Writing culture: The poetics and politics of ethnography* (pp. 1–26). Berkeley: University of California Press.

Clifford, J., & Marcus, G. E. (Eds.). (1986). *Writing culture: The poetics and politics of ethnography.* Berkeley: University of California Press.

Comaroff, J. (1984). Medicine, time and the perception of death. *Listening, 19*, 155–169.

Commission on Social Determinants of Health. (2008). *Closing the gap in a generation: Health equity through action on the social determinants of health.* Retrieved December 30, 2009, from http://whqlibdoc.who.int/publications/2008/9789241563703_eng.pdf

Committee on the Future of Emergency Care in the United States Health System, Board on Health Care Services, & Institute of Medicine. (2006). *Hospital-based emergency care: At the breaking point.* Washington, DC: National Academies Press.

Committee on Trauma Research, National Research Council, & Institute of Medicine. (1985). *Injury in America: A continuing public health problem.* Washington, DC: National Academies Press.

Connor, S. R., & Fine, P. G. (2009). Lessons learned from hospice in the United States of America. In G. Hanks, N. I. Cherny, N. A. Christakis, M. Fallon, S, Kaasa, & R. K. Portenoy (Eds.), *Oxford textbook of palliative medicine* (4th ed., pp. 17–22). New York: Oxford University Press.

Connor, S. R., Pyenson, B., Fitch, K., Spence, C., & Iwasaki, K. (2007). Comparing hospice and nonhospice patients who die within a three-year window. *Journal of Pain and Symptom Management, 33*(3), 238–246.

Connor, S. R., Tecca, M., LundPerson, J., & Teno, J. (2004). Measuring hospice care: The national hospice and palliative care organization national hospice data set. *Journal of Pain and Symptom Management, 28*(4), 316–328.

Coppens, C. (1897). *Moral principles and medical practice: The basis of medical jurisprudence* (2nd ed.). New York: Benziger Brothers.

Corr, C. A., Nabe, C. M., & Corr, D. M. (1994). *Death and dying, life and living.* Belmont, CA: Brooks/Cole.

Crawley, L. M. (2005). Racial, cultural, and ethnic factors influencing end-of-life care. *Journal of Palliative Medicine, 8*(Supplement 1), S58–S69.

Daniels, N. (1986). Why saying no to patients in the United States is so hard. *New England Journal of Medicine, 314*(21), 1380–1383.

Dartmouth Atlas Project, Center for Evaluative Clinical Sciences. (1998). The American experience of death. In A. H. Association (Ed.), *The Dartmouth Atlas of Health Care 1998* (pp. 81–106). Chicago: American Hospital Publishing.

Davies, C. (1996). Dirt, death, decay and dissolution: American denial and British avoidance. In G. Howarth & P. C. Jupp (Eds.), *Contemporary issues in the sociology of death, dying and disposal* (pp. 60–71). New York: St. Martin's Press.

Davies, K. (1994). The tensions between process time and clock time in care-work: The example of day nurseries. *Time and Society, 3*(3), 277–303.

Day, L. (2005). Life-support technology, enframing, and disclosing. *American Journal of Critical Care, 14*(6), 551–554.

Dewalt, K. M., Dewalt, B. R., & Wayland, C. B. (1998). Participant observation. In H. R. Bernard (Ed.), *Handbook of methods in cultural anthropology* (pp. 259–299). Walnut Creek, CA: AltaMira.

Diem, S. J., Lantos, J. D., & Tulsky, J. A. (1996). Cardiopulmonary resuscitation on television—miracles and misinformation. *The New England Journal of Medicine, 334*(24), 1578–1582.

Douglas, M. (1966). *Purity and danger: An analysis of the concepts of pollution and taboo.* London: Routledge & Kegan.

Drought, T. S., & Koenig, B. A. (2002). "Choice" in end-of-life decision making: Researching fact or fiction? *The Gerontologist, 42*(Special Issue 3), 114–128.

Dula, A. (1994). Bioethics: The need for a dialogue with African Americans. In A. Dula & S. Goering (Eds.), "*It just ain't fair*": *The ethics of health care for African Americans* (pp. 11–23). Westport, CT: Praeger.

Dula, A., & Williams, S. (2005). When race matters. *Clinics in Geriatric Medicine, 21*, 239–253.

Eisenberg, L. (1996). Medicine and the idea of progress. In L. Eisenberg (Ed.), *Progress: Fact or illusion?* (pp. 45–64). Ann Arbor: University of Michigan Press.

Eisenberg, M. (1997). *Life in the balance: Emergency medicine and the quest to reverse sudden death.* New York: Oxford University Press.

Engelhard, C. L. (2005). *Why does the U.S. spend more than other countries?* Unpublished manuscript.

Fabian, J. (1983). *Time and the other: How anthropology makes its object.* New York: Columbia University Press.

Fadiman, A. (1997). *The spirit catches you and you fall down: A Hmong child, her American doctors, and the collision of two cultures.* New York: Farrar, Straus & Giroux.

Fagerlin, A., & Schneider, C. E. (2004). Enough. The failure of the living will. *Hastings Center Report*, March–April, 30–42.

Farmer, P. (2004). An anthropology of structural violence. *Current Anthropology, 45*(3), 305–325.

Farmer, P. (2005). *Pathologies of power: Health, human rights and the new war on the poor.* Berkeley: University of California Press.

Fins, J. J. (2009). Lessons from the injured brain: A bioethicist in the vineyards of neuroscience. *Cambridge Quarterly of Healthcare Ethics, 18*, 7–13.

Flannery, K. V., & Marcus, J. (1993). What is cognitive archaeology? *Cambridge Archaeological Journal, 3*(2), 260–270.

Flexner, A. (1960 [1910]). *Medical education in the United States and Canada: A report to the Carnegie Foundation for the Advancement of Teaching.* Washington, DC: Science and Health Publications.

Flory, J., Young-Xu, Y., Gurol, I., Levinsky, N., Ash, A., & Emanuel, E. (2004). Place of death: U.S. trends since 1980. *Health Affairs, 23*(3), 194–200.

Forche, C. (1993). Introduction. In C. Forche (Ed.), *Against forgetting: Twentieth-century poetry of witness* (pp. 29–47). New York: W. W. Norton.

Foucault, M. (1977). *Discipline and punish: The birth of the prison* (A. Sheridan, Trans.). New York: Vintage Books.

Foucault, M. (1994). *The birth of the clinic: An archaeology of medical perception* (A. M. S. Smith, Trans.). New York: Vintage Books.

Fowler, F. J., Jr., Coppola, K. M., & Teno, J. M. (1999). Methodological challenges for measuring quality of care at the end of life. *Journal of Pain and Symptom Management, 17*(2), 114–119.

Fox, D. M. (1993). *Power and illness: The failure and future of American health policy.* Berkeley: University of California Press.

Fox, E., Landrum-McNiff, K., Zhong, Z., Dawson, N. V., Wu, A. W., & Lynn, J. (1999). Evaluation of prognostic criteria for determining hospice eligibility in patients with advanced lung, heart, or liver disease. *Journal of the American Medical Association, 282*(17), 1638–1645.

Freymann, J. G. (1977). *The American health care system: Its genesis and trajectory.* Huntington, NY: Robert E. Krieger Publishing.

Fuchs, V. R. (2005). Health care expenditures revisited. *Annals of Internal Medicine, 143*(1), 473–475.

Gabriel, R. A., & Metz, K. S. (1992). *A history of military medicine from the Renaissance through modern times.* New York: Greenwood Press.

Garza, A. G., Gratton, M. C., Salomone, J. A., Lindholm, D., McElroy, J., & Archer, R. (2009). Improved patient survival using a modified resuscitation protocol for out-of-hospital cardiac arrest. *Circulation, 119*(19), 2597–2605.

Gawande, A. (2005). Piecework. *The New Yorker,* April 4, pp. 44–53.

Gawande, A., Caplan, A., Truog, R. & Annas, G. (2008). *Perspective roundtable: Organ donation after cardiac death.* Retrieved October 17, 2008, from http://content.nejm.org/cgi/content/full/359/7/669/DC1

Geertz, C. (1973). Ideology as a cultural system. *The interpretation of cultures.* New York: Basic Books.

Geertz, C. (1988). *Works and lives: The anthropologist as author.* Stanford, CA: Stanford University Press.

Gerardi, D. (2007). The emerging culture of health care: Improving end-of-life care through collaboration and conflict engagement among health care professionals. *Ohio State Journal on Dispute Resolution Symposium Issue, 23,* 105–142.

Geyman, J. P. (2003). The corporate transformation of medicine and its impact on costs and access to care. *Journal of the American Board of Family Medicine, 16*(5), 443–454.

Gilligan, T., & Raffin, T. A. (1996). Withdrawing life support: Extubation and prolonged terminal weans are inappropriate. *Critical Care Medicine, 24*(2), 352–353.

Gilman, S. (1988). Depicting disease: A theory of representing illness. *Disease and representation: Images of illness from madness to AIDS* (pp. 1–17). Ithaca, NY: Cornell University Press.

Glaser, B. G., & Strauss, A. L. (1965). *Awareness of dying.* Chicago: Aldine.

Glaser, B. G., & Strauss, A. L. (1968). *Time for dying.* Chicago: Aldine.

Glavan, B. J., Engelber, R. A., Downey, L., & Curtis, J. R. C. (2008). Using the medical record to evaluate the quality of end-of-life care in the intensive care unit. *Critical Care Medicine, 36*(4), 1138–1146.

Goffman, E. (1959). *The presentation of self in everyday life.* Garden City, NY: Doubleday.

Good, B. J. (1994). *Medicine, rationality, and experience: An anthropological perspective.* Cambridge: Cambridge University Press.

Gordon, D. (1988). Tenacious assumptions in Western medicine. In M. Lock & D. Gordon (Eds.), *Biomedicine examined* (pp. 19–56). Dordrecht, The Netherlands: Kluwer Academic Publishers.

Gordon, D. (1990). Embodying illness, embodying cancer. *Culture, Medicine, and Psychiatry, 14*(2), 275–297.

Grumbach, K., & Bodenheimer, T. (1995). The organization of health care. *Journal of the American Medical Association, 273*(2), 160–167.

Guillemin, J. (1998). Bioethics and the coming of the corporation to medicine. In R. DeVries & J. Subedi (Eds.), *Bioethics and society: Constructing the ethical enterprise* (pp. 60–77). Upper Saddle River, NJ: Prentice-Hall.

Gupta, A., & Ferguson, J. (Eds.). (1997). *Anthropological locations.* Berkeley: University of California Press.

Hahn, R. A., & Kleinman, A. (1983). Biomedical practice and anthropological theory: Frameworks and directions. *American Review of Anthropology, 12,* 305–333.

Hamric, A. B. (2002). Moral distress in everyday ethics. *Nursing Outlook, 48*(5), 199–201.

Hansen, L., Goodell, T. T., DeHaven, J., & Smith, M. (2009). Nurses' perceptions of end-of-life care after multiple interventions for improvement. *American Journal of Critical Care, 18*(3), 263–271.

Harmon, L. (1998). *Fragments on the deathwatch.* Boston: Beacon.

Hartzband, P., & Groopman, J. (2009). Money and the changing culture of medicine. *The New England Journal of Medicine, 360*(2), 101–103.

Hauerwas, S. (1986). *Suffering presence: Theological reflections on medicine, the mentally handicapped, and the church.* Notre Dame, IN: University of Notre Dame Press.

Hazinski, M. F., Nadkarni, V. M., Hickey, R. W., O'Connor, R., Becker, L. B., & Zaritsky, A. (2005). Major changes in the 2005 AHA guidelines for CPR and ECC: Reaching the tipping point for change. *Circulation, 112,* IV206–IV211.

Hilfiker, D. (2005). *Medicine as if justice mattered.* Retrieved October 23, 2009, from http://www.davidhilfiker.com/docs/Justice/Medicine%20As%20if%20Justice%20Mattered.htm

Howe, E. G. (2008). Red towels: Maximizing the care of patients who are dying. *Journal of Clinical Ethics, 19*(2), 99–109.

Hsu, F. L. K. (1972). American core value and national character. In F. L. K. Hsu (Ed.), *Psychological anthropology* (pp. 241–262). Cambridge, MA: Schenkman Publishing.

Huskamp, H., Buntin, M. B., Wang, V., & Newhouse, J. P. (2001). Providing care at the end of life: Do Medicare rules impede good care? *Health Affairs, 20*(3), 204–211.

Illich, I. (1995a). Death undefeated: From medicine to medicalisation to systematisation. *British Medical Journal, 311*(7021), 1652–1653.

Illich, I. (1995b [1976]). *Medical nemesis: The expropriation of health.* London: Marion Boyars.

Institute for Healthcare Improvement. (2003a). *Move your dot: Measuring, evaluating, and reducing hospital mortality rates.* Cambridge, MA: Institute for Healthcare Improvement.

Institute for Healthcare Improvement. (2003b). *Optimizing patient flow: Moving patients smoothly through acute care settings.* Cambridge, MA: Institute for Healthcare Improvement.

Institute of Medicine. (2003). *Unequal treatment: Confronting racial and ethnic disparities in health care.* Washington, DC: National Academies Press.

Jacobs, J. (2003). *Body trauma TV: The new hospital dramas.* London: British Film Institute.

Jameton, A. (1984). *Nursing practice: The ethical issues.* Englewood Cliffs, NJ: Prentice-Hall.

Johnson, N., Cook, D., Giacomini, M., & Willms, D. (2000). Towards a "good" death: End-of-life narratives constructed in an intensive care unit. *Culture, Medicine, and Psychiatry, 24,* 275–295.

Joint Commission, The. (2008). *The Joint Commission introduces draft palliative care standards available for comment.* Retrieved March 17, 2008, from http://www.jointcommission.org/NewsRoom/NewsReleases/nr_03_11_08_2.htm

Joint Commission, The. (2009). *The Joint Commission: Accreditation program: Hospitals; chapter: National patient safety goals, prepublication version.* Retrieved 24 December, 2009, from http://www.jointcommission.org/NR/rdonlyres/31666E86-E7F4-423E-9BE8-F05BD1CB0AA8/0/HAP_NPSG.pdf

Jones, G. K., Brewer, K. L., & Garrison, H. G. (2000). Public expectations of survival following cariopulmonary resuscitation. *Academic Emergency Medicine, 7*(1), 48–53.

Jost, T. S. (2004). Why can't we do what they do? National health reform abroad. *National Health Reform and America's Uninsured, American Society of Law, Medicine & Ethics,* (Fall 2004), 433–441.

Kastenbaum, R. (1978). In control. In C. A. Garfield (Ed.), *Psychosocial aspects of the dying patient* (pp. 227–244). New York: McGraw-Hill.

Katz, R. (Director). (2009). *Taking chance* [Motion Picture]. HBO. Retrieved February 25, 2009, from http://www.imdb.com/video/imdb/vi113247001/.

Kaufman, S. R. (2000). In the shadow of "death with dignity": Medicine and cultural quandaries of the vegetative state. *American Anthropologist, 102*(1), 69–83.

Kaufman, S. R. (2005). *… And a time to die: How American hospitals shape the end of life.* New York: Scribner.

Keenan, S. P., Busche, K. D., Chen, L. M., Esmail, R., Inman, K. J., & Sibbald, W. J. (1998). Withdrawal and withholding of life support in the intensive care unit: A comparison of teaching and community hospitals. *Critical Care Medicine, 26*(2), 245–251.

Kellum, M. J., Kennedy, K. W., & Ewy, G. A. (2006). Cardiocerebral resuscitation improves survival of patients with out-of-hospital cardiac arrest. *American Journal of Medicine, 119*(4), 335–340.

Kirchhoff, K. T., Walker, L., Hutton, A., Spuhler, V., Cole, B. V., & Clemmer, T. (2002). The vortex: Families' experiences with death in the intensive care unit. *American Journal of Critical Care, 11*(3), 200–209.

Kirchhoff, K. T., Anumandla, P. R., Foth, K. T., Lues, S. N., & Gilbertson-White, S. H. (2004). Documentation on withdrawal of life support in adult patients in the intensive care unit. *American Journal of Critical Care, 13*(4), 328–334.

Kleinman, A. (1995). *Writing at the margin: Discourse between anthropology and medicine.* Berkeley: University of California Press.

Koenig, B. (1988). The technological imperative in medical practice: The social creation of a "routine" treatment. In M. Lock, & D. Gordon (Eds.), *Biomedicine examined* (pp. 465–495). Dordrecht, The Netherlands: Kluwer Academic Press.

Kübler-Ross, E. (1976). *Death: The final stage of growth*. Englewood Cliffs, NJ: Prentice Hall.

Kuhn, T. S. (1996). *The structure of scientific revolutions*. Chicago: University of Chicago Press.

Lagnado, L. (2004). Medical markup: California hospitals open books, showing huge price differences. *The Wall Street Journal*, December 27, p. A1.

Lang, M. P. (2004). DRG assurance. *Clinical byte: Economic challenges of healthcare*. Richmond, VA, conference proceedings.

Last Acts. (2002). *Means to a better end: A report on dying in America today*. Washington, DC: National Program Office, Partnership for Caring, Inc.

Latour, B., & Woolgar, S. (1986). The construction of a fact: The case of TRF(H). *Laboratory life: The construction of scientific facts* (2nd ed., pp. 105–150). Princeton, NJ: Princeton University Press.

Laubach, W., Brown, C. E. M., & Lenard, J. (1996). Nurses and physicians evaluate their intensive care experiences. *Heart & Lung, 25*(6), 475–482.

Lawler, P. A. (2004). *Caregiving and the American individual*. Retrieved October 7, 2005, from http://www.bioethics.gov/background/lawler_paper.html

Lawrence, C. (1992). Democratic, divine and heroic: The history and historiography of surgery. In C. Lawrence (Ed.), *Medical theory, surgical practice: Studies in the history of surgery* (pp. 1–47). London: Routledge.

Lawton, J. (2000). *The dying process: Patients' experiences of palliative care*. New York: Routledge.

Leach, W. (1993). *Land of desire: Merchants, power, and the rise of a new American culture*. New York: Vintage Books.

LeBlanc, T. (2006). CPR—Is it always an appropriate option? *Virtual Mentor, American Medical Association Journal of Ethics, 8*(9), 586–589.

Lee, H. (1961). *To kill a mockingbird*. New York: Harper Perennial.

Levine, A. (2004). *The American ideology: A critique*. New York: Routledge.

Levy, C. R., Ely, E. W., Payne, K., Engelberg, R. A., Patrick, D. L., & Curtis, J. R. (2005). Quality of dying and death in two medical ICUs. *Chest, 127*, 1775–1783.

Lipset, S. M. (1991). American exceptionalism reaffirmed. In B. E. Shafer (Ed.), *Is America different? A new look at American exceptionalism* (pp. 21–45). Oxford: Clarendon Press.

Lock, M. (2002). *Twice dead: Organ transplants and the reinvention of death*. Berkeley: University of California Press.

Lombardo, P. (2008). *Three generations, no imbeciles: Eugenics, the Supreme Court, and Buck v. Bell*. Baltimore: Johns Hopkins University Press.

Lynn, J. (2004). *Sick to death and not going to take it anymore! Reforming health care for the last years of life*. Berkeley: University of California Press.

Lynn, J. (2005). Living long in fragile health: The new demographics shape end of life care. *Hastings Center Report, 35*(6), S1–S5.

Lynn, J., & Adamson, D. M. (2003). *Living well at the end of life: Adapting health care to serious chronic illness in old age*. Retrieved October 9, 2006, from http://www.rc.rand.org/pubs/white_papers/2005/WP137.pdf

Matsuyama, R., Reddy, S., & Smith, T. J. (2006). Why do patients choose chemotherapy near the end of life? A review of the perspective of those facing death from cancer. *Journal of Clinical Oncology, 24*(21), 3490–3496.

McConnell, K. J., Richards, C. F., Daya, M., Weathers, C. C., & Lowe, R. A. (2005). The economic impact of ambulance diversions. *Academic Emergency Medicine, 12*(5, Suppl 1), 8–9.

Meier, D. E., Casarett, D. J., von Gunten, C. F., Smith, W. J., & Storey, C. P. (2010). Palliative medicine: Politics and policy. *Journal of Palliative Medicines,*13(2), 1–6.

Mello, M., & Jenkinson, C. (1998). Comparison of medical and nursing attitudes to resuscitation and patient autonomy between a British and an American teaching hospital. *Social Science and Medicine, 46*(3), 415–434.

Mellor, P. A., & Shilling, C. (1993). Modernity, self-identity and the sequestration of death. *Sociology, 27*(3), 411–432.

Metcalf, P. (1982). *A Borneo journey into death: Berawan eschatology from its rituals*. Philadelphia: University of Pennsylvania Press.

Metcalf, P., & Huntington, R. (1991). *Celebrations of death: The anthropology of mortuary ritual* (2nd ed.). Cambridge: Cambridge University Press.

Middleton, B. (2004). Deriving value from IT: Designing for quality and patient safety. *Embracing the Future: Fourth Annual VIPC&S Conference on Patient Safety*, Richmond, VA.

Moerman, D. E., & Jones, W. B. (2002). Deconstructing the placebo effect and finding the meaning response. *Annals of Internal Medicine, 136*(6), 471–476.

Mohammed, S., & Peter, E. (2009). Rituals, death and the moral practice of medical futility. *Nursing Ethics, 16*(3), 292–301.

Moore, S. F., & Myerhoff, B. G. (1977). Secular ritual: Forms and meanings. In S. F. Moore & B. G. Myerhoff (Eds.), *Secular ritual* (pp. 3–24). Amsterdam: Van Gorcum.

Morrison, S. R. (2005). Health care system factors affecting end-of-life care. *Journal of Palliative Medicine, 8*(Supplement 1), S-79–S-87.

Morrison, S. R., Maroney-Galin, C., Kralovec, P. D., & Meier, D. E. (2005). The growth of palliative care programs in United States hospitals. *Journal of Palliative Medicine, 8*(6), 1127–1134.

Morrison, S. R., Penrod, J. D., Cassel, J. B., Caust-Ellenbogen, M., Litke, A., Spragens, L., and Meier, D. E. (2008). Cost savings associated with US hospital palliative care consultation programs. *Archives of Internal Medicine, 168*(16), 1783–1790.

Moyers, B. (2000). *On our own terms*. Boston: WNET.

Mularski, R. A. (2006). Defining and measuring quality palliative and end-of-life care in the intensive care unit. *Critical Care Medicine, 34*(11 [Suppl.]), S309–S316.

Muller, J. H., & Koenig, B. (1988). On the boundary of life and death: The definition of dying by medical residents. In M. Lock & D. Gordon (Eds.), *Biomedicine examined* (pp. 351–376). Dordrecht, The Netherlands: Kluwer Academic Publishers.

Munn, N. D. (1970). The effectiveness of symbols in Murngin rite and myth. In R. F. Spencer (Ed.), *Forms of symbolic action: Proceedings of the 1969 annual spring meeting of the American Ethnological Society* (pp. 178–207). Seattle: University of Washington Press.

Myerhoff, B. G. (1996). Death in due time: Construction of self and culture in ritual drama. In R. L. Grimes (Ed.), *Readings in ritual studies* (pp. 393–412). Upper Saddle River, NJ: Prentice-Hall.

Myers, G. E. (2003). Restoration or transformation? Choosing ritual strategies for end-of-life care. *Mortality, 8*(4), 372–387.

Nader, L. (1996). The three-cornered constellation. In L. Nader (Ed.), *Naked science: Anthropological inquiry into boundaries, power, and knowledge* (pp. 259–275). New York: Routledge.

Naik, G. (2004). Final days: Unlikely way to cut hospital costs: Comfort the dying. *The Wall Street Journal* (Eastern Edition), March 10, p. A1.

Narayan, K. (1993). How native is a "native" anthropologist? *American Anthropologist, 95*(3), 671–686.

Nathaniel, A. K. (2006). Moral reckoning in nursing. *Western Journal of Nursing Research, 28*(4), 419–438.

National Center for Health Statistics. (2007). *Death by place of death, age, race and sex, United States.* Retrieved July 23, 2009, from cdc.gov/nchs/datawh/statab/unpubd/mortabs/gmwk309_10.htm

National Institutes of Health. (2007). *Legislative chronology—National Institutes of Health.* Retrieved December 25, 2009, from http://www.nih.gov.cuhsl.creighton.edu/about/almanac/historical/legislative_chronology.htm

Navarro, V. (1976). *Medicine under capitalism.* New York: Prodist.

Norton, S. A., & Bowers, B. J. (2001). Working toward consensus: Providers' strategies to shift patients from curative to palliative treatment choices. *Research in Nursing and Health, 24,* 258–269.

Nurok, M. (2001). The death of a princess and the formulation of medical competence. *Social Science and Medicine, 53,* 1427–1438.

Nye, D. E. (2001). Technology and cultural difference. In D. Carter (Ed.), *American exceptionalism revisited* (pp. 94–111). Amsterdam: Aarthus University Press.

Oberle, K., & Hughes, D. (2001). Doctors' and nurses' perceptions of ethical problems in end-of-life decisions. *Journal of Advanced Nursing, 33*(6), 707–715.

O'Connor, M. F. (2002). Making meaning of life events: Theory, evidence, and research directions for an alternative model. *Omega—Journal of Death and Dying, 46*(1), 51–75.

O'Malley, A. S., Gerland, A. M., Pham, H. H., & Berenson, R. A. (2005). Rising pressure: Hospital emergency departments as barometers of the health care system. *Center for Studying Health System Change: Issue Brief, 101,* November 20.

Osherson, S. D., & Amara-Singham, L. R. (1981). The machine metaphor in medicine. In E. G. Mishler, L. R. AmaraSingham, S. D. Osherson, S. T. Hauser, N. E. Waxler, & R. Liem (Eds.), *Social contexts of health, illness and patient care* (pp. 218–249). Cambridge: Cambridge University Press.

Paz, O. (1969, 1974). *Conjunctions and disjunctions* (H. R. Lane, Trans.). New York: The Viking Press.

Pearson, S. D., Sabin, J. E., & Emanuel, E. J. (2003). *No margin, no mission: Health-care organizations and the quest for ethical excellence.* New York: Oxford University Press.

Pew Research Center. (1999). *Introduction and summary: Technology triumphs, morality falters.* Retrieved November 3, 2005, from http://people-press.org/report/57/technology-triumphs-morality-falters.

Prendergast, T. J., Claessens, M. T., & Luce, J. M. (1998). National survey of end-of-life care for critically ill patients. *American Journal of Respiratory Critical Care Medicine, 158,* 1163–1167.

Prendergast, T. J., & Luce, J. M. (1997). Increasing incidence of withholding and withdrawal of life support from the critically ill. *American Journal of Respiratory Critical Care Medicine, 155,* 15–20.

Prendergast, T. J., & Puntillo, K. A. (2002). Withdrawal of life support: Intensive caring at the end of life. *Journal of the American Medical Association, 288*(21), 2732–2740.

President's Council on Bioethics, The. (2009). *Controversies in the determination of death.* Washington, DC: The President's Council on Bioethics.

Puntillo, K. A., Benner, P., Drought, T., Drew, B., Stotts, N., Stannard, D. et al. (2001). End-of-life issues in intensive care units: A national random survey of nurses' knowledge and beliefs. *American Journal of Critical Care, 10*(4), 216–229.

Putsch, R. W., & Pololi, L. (2004). Distributive justice in American healthcare: Institutions, power, and the equitable care of patients. *The American Journal of Managed Care, 10*(Special Issue), SP45–SP53.

Quill, T. E. (2002). In-hospital end-of-life services: Is the cup 2/3 empty or 1/3 full? *Medical Care, 40*(1), 4–6.

Ramsey, P. (1970). *The patient as person: Explorations in medical ethics.* New Haven, CT: Yale University Press.

Rappaport, R. A. (1971). Ritual sanctity and cybernetics. *American Anthropologist, 73*(1), 59–76.

Reinhardt, U. E. (2006). The pricing of U.S. hospital services: Chaos behind a veil of secrecy. *Health Affairs, 25*(1), 57–69.

Reinhardt, U. E., Hussey, P. S., & Anderson, G. F. (2004). U. S. health care spending in an international context: Why is U.S. spending so high, and can we afford it? *Health Affairs, 23*(3), 10–24.

Rhea, T. D., Eisenberg, M. S., Sinibaldi, G., & White, R. D. (2004). Incidence of EMS-treated out-of-hospital cardiac arrest in the United States. *Resuscitation, 63*(1), 17–24.

Riddick, F. A. (1989). *Hsiao report receives limited blessing—William Hsiao, report on resource-based relative value scales.* Tampa, FL: Physician Executive.

Roberts, D., Hirschman, D., & Scheltema, K. (2000). Adult and pediatric CPR: Attitudes and expectations of health professionals and laypersons. *American Journal of Emergency Medicine, 18*(4), 465–468.

Rosenberg, C. E. (1987). *The care of strangers: The rise of America's hospital system.* New York: Basic Books.

Rosenberg, C. E. (1992). Introduction: Framing disease: Illness, society, and history. In C. E. Rosenberg, & J. Golden (Eds.), *Framing disease: Studies in cultural history* (pp. xiii–xxvi). New Brunswick, NJ: Rutgers University Press.

Rosenberg, C. E. (2006). Anticipated consequences: Historians, history, and health policy. In R. A. Stevens, Charles E. Rosenberg, & L. R. Burns (Eds.), *History and health policy in the United States: Putting the past back in* (pp. 13–31). New Brunswick, NJ: Rutgers University Press.

Rothman, D. J. (1991). *Strangers at the bedside: A history of how law and bioethics transformed medical decision-making.* New York: Basic Books.

Rothman, S. M., & Rothman, D. J. (2003). *The pursuit of perfection: The promise and perils of medical enhancement.* New York: Vintage Books.

Sandelowski, M. (1991). Compelled to try: The never-enough quality of conceptive technology. *Medical Anthropology Quarterly, 5*(1), 29–47.

Savitt, T. L. (1982). The use of Blacks for medical experimentation and demonstration in the old South. *The Journal of Southern History, 48*(3), 331–348.

Scarry, E. (1985). *The body in pain: The making and unmaking of the world.* New York: Oxford University Press.

Schulman, K. A., Berlin, J. A., Harless, W., Kerner, J. F., Sistrunk, S., Gersh, B. J. et al. (1999). The effect of race and sex on physicians' recommendations for cardiac catheterization. *The New England Journal of Medicine, 340*(8), 618–626.

Scott, S. S., & Elliott, S. (2009). Implementation of a rapid response team: A success story. *Critical Care Nurse, 29*(3), 66–74.

Seale, C. (1998). *Constructing death: The sociology of dying and bereavement.* Cambridge: Cambridge University Press.

Seifert, R. W., & Rukavina, M. (2006). Bankruptcy is the tip of a medical-debt iceberg. *Health Affairs, 25*, w89–w92.

Seymour, J. E. (2000). Negotiating natural death in intensive care. *Social Science and Medicine, 51*(8), 1241–1252.

Shield, R. R., Wetle, T., Teno, J., Miller, S. C., & Welch, L. (2005). Physicians "missing in action": Family perspectives on physician and staffing problems in end of life care in the nursing home. *Journal of the American Geriatrics Society, 53*(10), 1651–1657.

Singer, M. (1989). The coming of age of critical medical anthropology. *Social Science and Medicine, 28*(11), 1193–1203.

Smith, D. B. (2005a). Racial and ethnic health disparities and the unfinished civil rights agenda. *Health Affairs, 24*(2), 317–324.

Smith, D. B. (2005b). The politics of racial disparities: Desegregating the hospitals in Jackson, MI. *The Milbank Quarterly, 83*(2), 247–269.

Smith, T. J., Coyne, P., Cassel, B., Penberthy, L., Hopson, A., & Hager, M. A. (2003). A high-volume specialist palliative care unit and team may reduce in-hospital end-of-life care costs. *Journal of Palliative Medicine, 6*(5), 699–705.

Sobo, E. J. (2009). *Culture & meaning in health services research: A practical field guide.* Walnut Creek, CA: Left Coast Press.

Society for Critical Care Medicine Ethics Committee, American College of Critical Care Medicine. (2001). Recommendations for nonheartbeating organ donation. *Critical Care Medicine, 29*(9), 1826–1831.

Sprung, C. L., Geber, D., Eidelman, L. A., Baras, M., Pizov, R., Nimrod, A. et al. (1999). Evaluation of triage decisions for intensive care admission. *Critical Care Medicine, 27*(6), 1072–1079.

Stace-Naughton, D. (1999). *Coding and reimbursement: The complete picture within health care.* Chicago: American Hospital Association Press.

Starr, P. (1982). *The social transformation of American medicine.* New York: Basic Books.

Stein, H. F. (1990). *American medicine as culture.* Boulder, CO: Westview.

Stevens, R. (1999). *In sickness and in wealth: American hospitals in the 20th century.* Baltimore: Johns Hopkins University Press.

Strathern, M. (1992). Greenhouse effect. *After nature: English kinship in the late twentieth century.* Cambridge: Cambridge University Press.

Sudnow, D. (1967). *Passing on: The social organization of dying.* Englewood Cliffs, NJ: Prentice Hall.

Sulmasy, D. P. (1995). Killing and allowing to die. Doctor of Philosophy, Georgetown University, pp. 1–506.

Sulmasy, D. P., & Pellegrino, E. D. (1999). The rule of double effect: Clearing up the double talk. *Archives of Internal Medicine, 139*(6), 545–549.

SUPPORT Principal Investigators. (1995). A controlled trial to improve care for seriously ill hospitalized patients. *Journal of the American Medical Association, 274*(20), 1591–1598.

Swigart, V., Lidz, C., Butterworth, V., & Arnold, R. (1996). Letting go: Family willingness to forgo life support. *Heart & Lung, 25*(6), 483–494.

Taheri, P. A. (2004). The cost of trauma center readiness. *The American Journal of Surgery, 187*(1), 7–13.

Taheri, P. A., Butz, D. A., Dechert, R., & Greenfield, L. J. (2001). How DRGs hurt academic health systems. *Journal of the American College of Surgeons, 193*(1), 1–8.

Tambiah, S. J. (1990). *Magic, science, religion, and the scope of rationality.* Cambridge: Cambridge University Press.

Task Force of the International Liaison Committee on Resuscitation. (2004). Cardiac arrest and cardiopulmonary resuscitation outcome reports: Update and simplification of the Utstein templates for resuscitation registries. *Circulation, 110*(21), 3385–3397.

Taussig, M. T. (1980). Reification and the consciousness of the patient. *Social Science and Medicine, 148*(1), 3–13.

Taylor, R., & Rieger, A. (1985). Medicine as a social science: Rudolf Virchow on the typhus epidemic in Upper Silesia. *International Journal of Health Services, 15*(4), 547–557.

Teno, J. (2004). Measuring outcomes retrospectively. *National Institutes of Health State-of-the-Science Conference on Improving End-of-Life Care.* Bethesda, MD, companion book to conference proceedings, pp. 35–37.

Timmermans, S. (1999). *Sudden death and myth of CPR.* Philadelphia: Temple University Press.

Timmermans, S., & Berg, M. (2003). *The gold standard: The challenge of evidence-based medicine and standardization in health care.* Philadelphia: Temple University Press.

Titmuss, R. M. (1997 [1970]). *The gift relationship: From human blood to social policy.* New York: The New Press.

Toner, E., Waldhorn, R., Maldin, B., Borio, L., Jennifer B. Nuzzo, Clarence Lam et al. (2006). Meeting report: Hospital preparedness for pandemic influenza. *Biosecurity and Bioterrorism: Biodefense Strategy, Practice and Science, 4*(2), 1–11.

Truog, R. D., Cist, A. F. M., Brackett, S. E., Burns, J. P., Curley, M. A. Q., Danis, M. et al. (2001). Recommendations for end-of-life care in the intensive care unit: The ethics committee of the society of critical care medicine. *Critical Care Medicine, 29*(12), 2332–2348.

Turner, T. (1977). Chapter IV: Transformation, hierarchy and transcendence: A reformulation of Van Gennep's model of the structure of rites de passage. In S. F. Moore & B. G. Myerhoff (Eds.), *Secular ritual* (pp. 53–73). Amsterdam: Van Gorcum.

Turner, V. (1967). *The forest of symbols: Aspects of Ndembu ritual*. Cornell, NY: Cornell University Press.

Ulrich, L. T. (1990). December 1793 "birth 50. birth 51." *A midwife's tale: The life of Martha Ballard, based on her diary, 1785–1812* (pp. 162–203). New York: Vintage Books.

United States Department of Health and Human Services. (2005). *HHS— fact sheet: Your rights under the community service assurance provision of the Hill-Burton act.* Retrieved December 25, 2009, from http://www.hhs.gov/ocr/civilrights/resources/factsheets/hillburton.pdf

U.S. Department of Health and Human Services Public Health Service. (1994). *For a healthy nation: Returns on investment in public health.* Washington, DC: U.S. Government Printing Office.

van der Geest, S., & Finkler, K. (2004). Hospital ethnography: Introduction. *Social Science and Medicine, 59*, 1995–2001.

van Gennep, A. (1960). *The rites of passage* (M. B. Vizedom & G. L. Caffe, Trans.). Chicago: University of Chicago Press.

Vanstone, W. H. (2004). *The stature of waiting*. Norwich, Norfolk England: Page Brothers.

Vohs, K. D., Mead, N. L., & Goode, M. R. (2006). The psychological consequences of money. *Science, 314*(5802), 1154–1156.

VonRueden, K. T., & Hartsock, R. L. (2002). Nursing practice through the cycle of trauma. In K. A. McQuillan, K. T. Von Rueden, R. L. Hartsock, M. B. Flynn, & E. Whalen (Eds.), *Trauma nursing: From resuscitation through rehabilitation* (3rd ed., pp. 107–128). Philadelphia: Saunders.

Waitzkin, H. (1983). Technology, health costs, and the structure of private profit. *The second sickness: Contradions of capitalist health care.* New York: The Free Press.

Walter, T. (1994). *The revival of death*. New York: Routledge.

Wangensteen, O. H., & Wangensteen, S. D. (1978). *The rise of surgery: From empiric craft to scientific discipline*. Minneapolis: University of Minnesota Press.

Waters, C. M. (2001). Understanding and supporting African Americans' perspectives of end-of-life care planning and decision making. *Qualitative Health Research, 11*(3), 385–398.

Wennberg, J. E. (2006). *The care of patients with severe chronic illness: A report on the Medicare program by the Dartmouth Atlas Project*. Retrieved 6/5/2006, from http://www.dartmouthatlas.com/atlases/2006_Chronic_Care_Atlas.pdf

West, H. F., Engelberg, R. A., Wenrich, M. D., & Curtis, J. R. (2005). Expressions of nonabandonment during the intensive care unit family conference. *Journal of Palliative Medicine, 8*(4), 797–807.

Weston, K. (1997). The virtual anthropologist. In A. Gupta & J. Ferguson (Eds.), *Anthropological locations: Boundaries and grounds of a field science* (pp. 163–184). London: University of California Press.

Wilson, D. M., Truman, C. D., Thomas, R., Fainsinger, R., Kovacs-Burns, K., Froggatt, K. et al. (2009). The rapidly changing location of death in Canada, 1994–2004. *Social Science and Medicine, 68*(10), 1752–1752.

Wilson, M. J., & Nguyen, K. (2004). *Bursting at the seams: Improving patient flow to help America's emergency departments.* Washington DC: George Washington University.

Wilson, W. C., Smedira, N. G., Fink, C., McDowell, J. A., & Luce, J. M. (1992). Ordering and administration of sedatives and analgesics during the withholding and withdrawal of life support from critically ill patients. *Journal of the American Medical Association, 267*(7), 949–953.

Young, K. (1997). *Presence in the flesh: The body in medicine.* Cambridge, MA: Harvard University Press.

Zawistowski, C. A., & DeVita, M. A. (2004). A descriptive study of children dying in the pediatric intensive care unit after withdrawal of life-sustaining treatment. *Pediatric Critical Care Medicine, 5*(3), 216–223.

Zingmond, D. S., & Wenger, N. S. (2005). Regional and institutional variation in the initiation of early do-not-resuscitate orders. *Archives of Internal Medicine, 165*, 1705–1712.

Zussman, R. (1992). *Intensive care medical ethics and the medical profession.* Chicago: University of Chicago Press.

Index

About the Author

Helen Stanton Chapple, PhD, RN, CCRN, CT, is the Nurse Ethicist at Creighton University's Center for Health Policy and Ethics. Her twenty years of bedside nursing include oncology, research, hospice home care, cardiac and neuroscience critical care. A persistent interest in thanatology and the fate of hospitalized dying patients prompted her to pursue graduate degrees in bioethics and anthropology at the University of Virginia. She is the author of several articles in anthropology and nursing journals.